The Neurobiology of Learning and Memory

THIRD EDITION

.

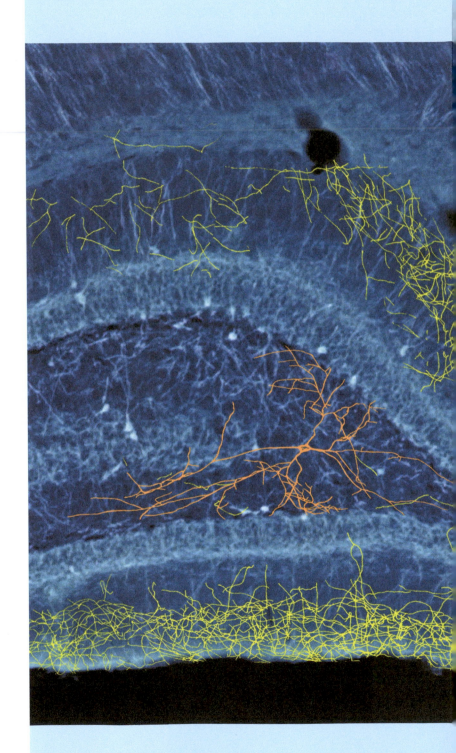

About the cover image

The image shows a single neuron's soma and dendrites (at center, orange) and the dense branches of its axon (yellow) spreading throughout the entire dentate gyrus. The overall structure of the mouse's hippocampus is outlined in the background in blue. Image courtesy of György Buzsáki.

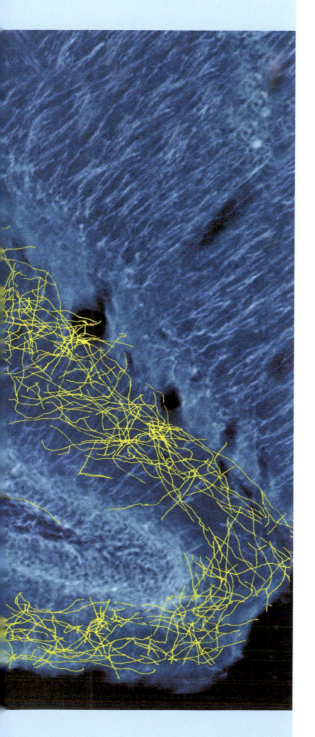

The Neurobiology of Learning and Memory

THIRD EDITION

JERRY W. RUDY

University of
Colorado Boulder

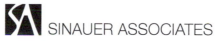 SINAUER ASSOCIATES

NEW YORK   OXFORD

OXFORD UNIVERSITY PRESS

The Neurobiology of Learning and Memory, Third Edition

Oxford University Press is a department of the University of Oxford. It furthers the University's objective of excellence in research, scholarship, and education by publishing worldwide. Oxford is a registered trademark of Oxford University Press in the UK and certain other countries.

Published in the United States of America by Oxford University Press
198 Madison Avenue, New York, NY 10016, United States of America

For titles covered by Section 112 of the US Higher Education Opportunity Act, please visit www.oup.com/us/he for the latest information about pricing and alternate formats.

Address editorial correspondence to:

Sinauer Associates
23 Plumtree Road
Sunderland, MA 01375 U.S.A.

Address orders, sales, license, permissions, and translation inquiries to:

Oxford University Press U.S.A.
2001 Evans Road
Cary, NC 27513 U.S.A.
Orders: 1-800-445-9714

Library of Congress Cataloging-in-Publication Data

Names: Rudy, Jerry W., 1942- author.

Title: The neurobiology of learning and memory / Jerry W. Rudy, University of Colorado, Boulder.

Description: Third edition. | New York : Sinauer Associates : Oxford University Press, [2021] | Includes bibliographical references and index.

Identifiers: LCCN 2020003936 (print) | LCCN 2020003937 (ebook) | ISBN 9781605359342 (hardcover) | ISBN 9781605359359 (epub)

Subjects: LCSH: Memory--Textbooks. | Learning--Textbooks. | Neurobiology--Textbooks.

Classification: LCC QP406 .R83 2021 (print) | LCC QP406 (ebook) | DDC 612.8/23312--dc23

LC record available at https://lccn.loc.gov/2020003936

LC ebook record available at https://lccn.loc.gov/2020003937

5 4 3 2 1

Printed in the United States of America

Preface

As this will be the last edition of *The Neurobiology of Learning and Memory* that I will author, I would like to share a little personal history relevant to this project. I was trained as an experimental psychologist in the animal conditioning and learning tradition. For over 30 years, I taught undergraduate and graduate courses on the subject. However, I abandoned my research interests in traditional issues in this field in the mid-1970s to focus instead on the development of the processes that support learning. At that time, I had no exposure to neuroscience or interest in the field. However, the developmental changes discovered by my students (Laurel Camp, Tom Moye, Rick Hyson, Mark Vogt, Carl Castro, Richard Paylor, and Susan Stadler-Morris) had to relate in some way to changes in the brain. So I started to read some of the behavioral neuroscience literature and interpreted the results in terms of developmental changes in neural systems.

In the mid-1980s I co-opted the psychology department colloquium budget to support a graduate seminar on the neurobiology of learning and memory. This allowed me to invite a number of scientists to participate in the seminar (Dan Schacter, Tom Carew, Jocelyne Bachevalier, the late David Olton, and Rob Sutherland, who was on sabbatical at the University of Colorado Boulder at the time). This seminar was very stimulating and led to Rob and I collaborating on a theoretical paper on the role of the hippocampus in memory. This collaboration and a subsequent one with Randy O'Reilly on the same topic pushed me toward getting serious about my understanding of the neurobiology of memory. My interest in the cellular–molecular aspects of memory was especially motivated by Julietta Frey and Richard Morris's papers on synaptic tagging and an in-class lecture by Jeanne Wehner on Gary Lynch and Michel Baudry's paper on the chemical basis of memory, featuring the uncovering of glutamate receptors (which in my humble opinion is a true classic).

Unfortunately, I rapidly found that I didn't have a clue about how to approach this field. Two of my graduate students, Kevin Bolding and Joe Biedenkapp, spent many hours trying to enlighten me about the molecular aspects of memory. In spite of their efforts I remained largely in the dark; I just didn't have the necessary background. (They must have had some good laughs at my expense after they left my office.) However, these discussions played a major role in the critical decision that ultimately resulted in the first edition of this book. I decided that the only way to understand this field was to teach an undergraduate course on the topic.

My first task was to find a suitable textbook. I thought I had found one but as the moment of truth was getting close I realized that this book required a background in cell and molecular biology, and I had none. So now I was challenged to create a course without a book and to learn some cell–molecular biology so that I could teach the course. In looking back, I somehow arrived at an organization for the course and created a detailed set of PowerPoint lectures, which subsequently proved to be a good starting point for a textbook (and which was fairly close to the first edition of this book). But the thought of writing a textbook on the subject was the last thing on my mind!

I had thoroughly enjoyed creating the course and cornering colleagues to tell them how much I had learned and about the extensive set of lectures I had created for the class. At some point one of them—and I don't remember who (maybe Randy O'Reilly?)—said, "Why don't you turn this material into a textbook?" I was quite taken aback. It seemed absurd that someone with my very limited knowledge of basic cell and molecular biology and neurophysiology could pull off such a project. However, gradually these reservations turned into a challenge. I then remembered that several years previously I had told Peter Farley (who at that time represented Sinauer Associates) that if I ever wrote a book I would like to publish with Sinauer. So I called up Andy Sinauer (whom I had confused with Peter Farley) and reminded him of our conversation a few years before and told him that I might have a book for Sinauer. I could tell that Andy (whom I had never met or talked to) was trying to get his head around this. He rightfully had no recollection of the conversation and must have thought I was nuts. Nevertheless, he agreed to put me in touch with Greg Donini to review my proposal. It was not until a few years later when Peter Farley's name came up in a conversation with Mark Bouton, who also published with Sinauer, that I realized my faux pas.

The most enjoyable part of creating this book was getting a handle on cell and molecular biology and gaining an understanding of the conceptual basis of long-term potentiation that was necessary to appreciate its molecular underpinnings. I can honestly say that I had no clue about any of this when I started. I had many private moments of delight as I began to gain insight into the big picture and could fill in the details in a narrative that I intended to be informative but not overly tedious.

I believe that my approaching this field as a true novice with no experts around to lean on was ultimately a great benefit to students. At the beginning, I was very uncomfortable with the obscure (to me anyway) language of cell and molecular biology. So I tried to eliminate as much of the technical language as possible and to create narratives around the topics that hopefully would convey the essential points without bludgeoning the students (and myself) with tedious details. Had I been a true expert in these domains I am sure that I would have been compelled to unintentionally overwhelm the students with my mastery of the molecular gymnastics of the field. From comments I have received on the previous editions I think this turned out to be the correct approach. So now we roll out the third edition.

The study of learning and memory belongs to scientists trained in a variety of disciplines that include psychology, biochemistry, cellular–molecular biology, electrophysiology, neuroanatomy, and neuropsychology. As I noted in the preface to the second edition: "The work of hundreds of scientists from these diverse fields has produced an explosion of knowledge about the neurobiological basis of learning and memory that almost defies comprehension." In the six years since that edition the explosion has continued, driven in part by the incredible advances in technologies that permit neurobiologists to probe the brain in previously unimaginable ways. The challenge again was to decide what new information should be included in this edition and what old stories could be eliminated. Ironically, in some cases the "new" information comes from research that existed prior to the second edition. This is because it has since become foundational material for new discoveries and ideas. I am sure that not everyone will agree with my choices but there was no way to tell every story and the book is not encyclopedic.

Readers of the second edition will find the basic organization of the third edition and its general goal to be the same—to integrate some of what we have learned from this multidisciplinary field into a framework that can be understood by students who have a rudimentary background in biology, psychology, and neuroscience, as well as by the wider scientific community.

The third edition again consists of three sections and the story is told from the bottom up: it progresses from neurons, synapses, and molecules that provide the synaptic basis of memories to the neural systems that capture the rich content of our experience. Although the organization remains the same, many of the chapters have been extensively revised to accommodate new material and to provide a more coherent presentation of the material. These changes are reflected in the new titles of many of the chapters and the addition of new ones.

Writing this book has been a wonderful experience. My respect and admiration for the talented and brilliant scientists that have created this field have doubled with each edition. I have tried to provide a broad context in which to introduce the key concepts and facts that are central to a particular topic. I have made no attempt to be comprehensive in the material I covered. Instead, I have tried to maintain a level of description and discussion that was sufficient to ensure a basic understanding of the relevant principles and processes, without getting to a level of detail that would be tedious. I hope this approach does justice to the field and provides the reader with a foundation to continue an in-depth exploration of some of the topics and an appreciation of some of the remarkable achievements of many wonderful researchers who have made this field one of the great scientific adventures of our time.

Summary of Changes

Chapter 1 again provides a brief conceptual and historical overview of the field. Part 1, *Synaptic Basis of Memory,* introduces the idea that synapses modified by experience provide the basis for memory storage. It describes the long-term potentiation methodology used to study how synapses are modified and the concepts needed to understand the organization of synapses. The eight chapters in Part 1 are organized around the idea that the synaptic changes that support long-term potentiation evolve in four overlapping stages referred to as generation, stabilization, consolidation, and maintenance. The goal of each chapter is to reveal that each stage depends on unique molecular processes and to describe what they are.

The six chapters in Part 2, *Molecules and Memory,* build on this foundation to illustrate how molecules and cellular processes that have been identified from studies of synaptic plasticity also participate in the making of memories. Chapter 9 discusses some of the basic conceptual issues researchers face in trying to relate memory to synaptic molecules and describes some of the behavioral and biological methods that are used. Chapter 11, on memory consolidation, has been significantly revised to provide a more integrated view of the underlying processes, and Chapter 13, on memory maintenance, has been completely rewritten to recognize advances in the neurobiology of forgetting. (It is now titled *The Yin and Yang of Memory: Forgetting versus Maintenance.*) An entirely new chapter, *Hunting for Engrams* (Chapter 14) describes progress in the development of the methods needed to find the neurons supporting memory and some of the new findings they have yielded.

The five chapters in Part 3, *Neural Systems and Memory,* are organized around the multiple memory systems view—that different neural systems have evolved to store the content contained in our experiences. Three chapters are devoted to the role of the hippocampus in episodic memory and begin with the story of Henry Molaison (H.M.) to establish the historical foundation linking the medial temporal hippocampal system to episodic memory. Although much of the content remains the same, the chapters on the hippocampus have been reorganized and updated to include new findings. The most significant change in Part 3 is an entire chapter (Chapter 18) on what happens when memories age. I made very few changes to the chapter on actions and habits (now Chapter 19) or to the chapter on learning about danger (now Chapter 20).

Acknowledgments

All credit goes to the brilliant scientists who created this field and produced the remarkable achievements described here. I have told some of the important stories and regret that I was unable to include more.

Many thanks go to my Colorado colleagues, Dr. Robert Spencer and Dr. Michael Barrata. Bob often served as a sounding board for the new material and helped to shape my thoughts. Mike did his best to educate me on the new techniques used to find engrams and provided a critical reading on the new chapter of finding engrams. Cristina Alberini generously contributed her thoughts on the new chapter on consolidation. The chapter on the neurobiology of forgetting and memory maintenance benefitted from the comments of Oliver Hardt, Virginia Migues, and Lucas Alvares. Jonathan (Joff) Lee provided helpful advice on the revised chapter on the fate of retrieved memories. I thank Robert Sutherland for his comments and many discussions of the material presented in the new chapter on what happens when memories age.

Until you write one, you have no idea of what is involved in turning your material into a textbook. So it is a pleasure to recognize the staff at Sinauer Associates. Special thanks go to Linnea Duley, Production Editor, who did a fantastic job keeping the ball rolling and ensuring the consistency of the material. I also thank other members of the Sinauer staff for their contributions: Joan Gemme, Production Manager and Art Director; Mark Siddall, Photo Research Editor; Rick Neilsen, Production Specialist and Book Designer; Michele Beckta, Permissions Supervisor; Jess Fiorillo, Executive Acquisitions Editor; Peter Lacey, Digital Resource Development Editor; Jan Troutt, Illustrator; and Grant Hackett, Indexer.

For the third time, my wife, Julia A. Rudy, assumed major editorial duties and was the frontline defense against my attack on the English language. Her editorial skills and commitment to excellence are responsible for the book's organizational clarity and readability. This was a collaborative effort and without Julie's involvement there is no way that I would have started this project, let alone finished it.

In many ways this book is the product of a community of neuroscientists. I especially thank the following colleagues who, through the years, have provided important critique and commentary on prior editions of this book.

Arnold Bakker, *The Johns Hopkins University School of Medicine*
Sondra Bland, *University of Colorado Denver*
Marsha Dopheide, *Monmouth College*
Mike Ferragamo, *Gustavus Adolphus College*
Roberto Galvez, *University of Illinois at Urbana-Champaign*
Laura Harrison, *Tulane University*
Fred Helmstetter, *University of Wisconsin, Milwaukee*

Michael Hylin, *Southern Illinois University*
Rick Hyson, *Florida State University*
William Kennedy, Emeritus, *Michigan Technological University*
Christopher Kliethermes, *Drake University*
Monica Linden, *Brown University*
Christa McIntyre, *University of Texas, Dallas*
Tom Newpher, *Duke University*
Gina O'Neal-Moffit, *Florida State University*
Barbara Oswald, *Miami University*
Kathleen Page, *Bucknell University*
Marise Parent, *Georgia State University*
Vinay Parikh, *Temple University*
Jessie Peissig, *California State University, Fullerton*
Marsha Penner, *University of North Carolina, Chapel Hill*
Zach Reagh, *University of California, Davis*
Peter Serano, *CUNY Hunter College*
Jeffrey S. Taube, *Dartmouth College*
Tuan Tran, *East Carolina University*
Natalie Tronson, *University of Michigan*
Linda Wilbrecht, *University of California, Berkeley*
Brian Wiltgen, *University of California, Davis*

Digital Resources to accompany

The Neurobiology of Learning and Memory THIRD EDITION

Enhanced eBook (ISBN 978-1-60535-935-9)

Ideal for self-study, *The Neurobiology of Learning and Memory* enhanced eBook delivers valuable digital resources in a format that is independent from any courseware or learning management system platform. Features include newly developed learning objectives for each chapter, end-of-section study questions (aligned to learning objectives), and embedded animations that provide a dynamic look at key figures in the text. The enhanced eBook is available through leading higher education eBook vendors.

For the Instructor (Available at oup.com/he/rudy3e)

The digital resources that accompany *The Neurobiology of Learning and Memory* provide instructors with a wealth of content for use in course planning, lecture development, and assessment. Resources include:

TEXTBOOK FIGURES AND TABLES   All the figures and photos from the textbook are provided as JPEGs, optimized for use in presentation software (such as PowerPoint).

POWERPOINT RESOURCES   Two ready-to-use presentations are provided for each chapter:

- A lecture presentation that includes text covering the entire chapter, with selected figures
- A figures presentation that includes all the figures and photos from the chapter, with titles on each slide, and complete captions in the notes field

TEST BANK   The Test Bank consists of a broad range of questions in a variety of formats—such as multiple choice, fill-in-the-blank, and short answer—covering all the key facts and concepts in each chapter. Available in both MS Word format and common cartridge format, for use in all major learning management systems.

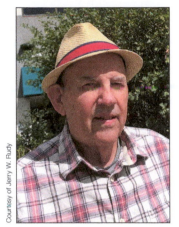

Courtesy of Jerry W. Rudy

Jerry W. Rudy

About the Author

Jerry W. Rudy is College Professor of Distinction in the Department of Psychology and Neuroscience at the University of Colorado Boulder. He received his Ph.D. in psychology from the University of Virginia in 1970, and joined the CU Boulder faculty in 1980. He served as Department Chair for 10 years and was instrumental in creating the undergraduate Neuroscience degree and served as the Director of that program for several years. The author of over 150 peer-reviewed research papers and book chapters, Dr. Rudy has served on the editorial boards of the *Journal of Experimental Psychology: Animal Behavior Processes, Psychobiology, Developmental Psychobiology* (Editor in Chief), *Behavioral Neuroscience, Neuroscience & Biobehavioral Reviews, Learning and Memory*, and *Neurobiology of Learning and Memory* (Associate Editor). He also served on the governing board and as President of the International Society for Developmental Psychobiology. He has received grant support from the National Science Foundation, the National Institute of Mental Health, and the National Institute of Health. Professor Rudy's research interests center on learning and memory processes. His research focused primarily on memory development and understanding the complementary contributions the hippocampus and neocortex make to learning and memory. Professor Rudy retired in June 2019.

Table of Contents

PART 1 ■ Synaptic Basis of Memory   17

PART 2 ■ Molecules and Memory 151

17 The Hippocampus Index and Episodic Memory   317

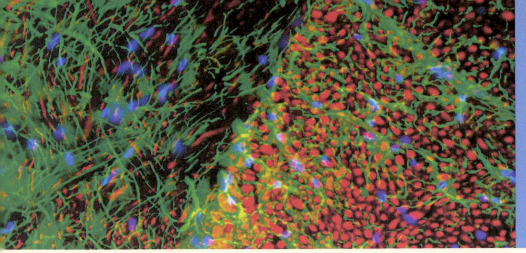

Introduction: Fundamental Concepts and Historical Foundations

Our uniqueness as human beings derives in large part from evolutionary adaptations that permit experience to modify connections linking networks of neurons in the brain. Information conveyed into the brain by our sensory channels can leave a lasting impression on neural circuits. These networks not only can be modified, the information contained in the modifications can be preserved and later retrieved to influence our behavior. Our individual experiences act on these networks to make us who we are. We have the ability to learn a vast array of skills. We can become musicians, athletes, artisans, skilled craftsmen, or cooks. Experience tunes our emotions to our environments. We acquire food preferences and aversions. Incredibly, without intention, we also lay down an autobiographical record of the events, times, and places in which our experiences occur. We are connected with our past and can talk about it. We learn and we remember.

Historically, the study of learning and memory has been the domain of philosophers and psychologists who have defined the relevant phenomena and many of the important variables that influence them. Only recently have brain scientists seriously weighed in on this topic. Armed with sophisticated methods to measure and manipulate brain processes and conceptual frameworks to guide their application, neurobiologists have now made enormous inroads into the mystery of how experience modifies the brain.

Consequently, an important field now exists called the **neurobiology of learning and memory**. Scientists working in this field want to know how the brain stores and retrieves information about our experiences. The goal of this book is to present an account of some of the major accomplishments of this field and to provide a background that will facilitate the understanding of many of the issues and central assumptions that drive research in this field.

Learning and Memory Are Theoretical Concepts

The terms "learning" and "memory" are often used as if they are directly observable entities, but they are not. *Learning and memory are theoretical concepts used to explain the fact that experience influences behavior* (Figure 1.1). A familiar example will suffice to make the point.

You have an exam tomorrow. So over the next few hours you closet yourself with your books and class notes. You take the test and answer the questions to the best of your knowledge. Later you receive your grade, 90%. Assuming that your grade would have been 50% if you had not studied, then a reasonable person (the professor) would assume that you learned and remembered the information needed to pass the test. The key phrase here is "would assume." Learning and memory were never directly observed. The only directly observable events in this example are that (a) you spent time with your notes and books, and (b) you took the test and performed well. That you learned and remembered is inferred from your test performance and the professor's knowledge that you studied.

Larry Squire (1987) has provided a useful definition of the terms learning and memory: "Learning is the process of acquiring new information, while memory refers to the persistence of learning in a state that can be revealed at a later time" (p. 3). Other, more restrictive definitions have been proposed.

Learning and memory are theoretical concepts

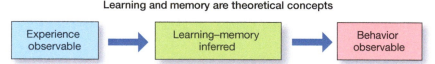

FIGURE 1.1 Learning and memory are unobservable, inferred processes used to explain the fact that our past experience influences our behavior.

They usually also stipulate what learning and memory are not. For example, a restricted definition would appropriately exclude fatigue, maturation, and injury that might result from or be associated with experience.

Although learning and memory are theoretical concepts, neurobiologists are motivated by the belief that they have a physical basis in the brain. A slight modification of Squire's definition provides a useful definition of the field: The goal of neurobiologists working in this field is to understand how the brain acquires, stores, and maintains representations of experience in a state that permits the information contained in the representation to be retrieved and influence behavior.

Psychological and Neurobiological Approaches

The study of learning and memory is the domain of both psychology and neurobiology. It is useful to point out some fundamental differences between the two approaches.

Psychological Approach

The general goal of psychology is to (a) derive a set of empirical principles that describe how variation in experience influences behavior, and (b) provide a theoretical account that can explain the observed facts. The study of memory became a science when Hermann Ebbinghaus developed the first methods for assessing the acquisition and retention of a controlled experience. He recognized that to study "pure memory" required a methodology that could separate what the subject already has learned from what the subject is now being asked to remember (Ebbinghaus, 1913). To do this, he invented what are called **nonsense syllables**. A nonsense syllable consists of a vowel placed between two consonants, such as *nuh*, *vag*, or *boc*. These syllables were designed to be meaningless so they would have to be learned without the benefit of prior knowledge. Thus, for example, *dog*, *cat*, or *cup* would be excluded. Ebbinghaus made up hundreds of nonsense syllables and used them to produce lists that were to be learned and remembered. Among the task variables he manipulated were factors such as the number of times a given list was presented during the memorization phase and the interval between the learning and the test phase.

Ebbinghaus worked alone and was the only subject of his experiments. He found that his test performance increased the more he practiced a given list. He also documented the fact that retention performance was better when he spaced the repetition of a given list than when the list was repeated without inserting a break between the learning trials. He also documented the first "forgetting curve." As is illustrated in Figure 1.2, retention was excellent when the test was given shortly after the learning trial, but it fell off dramatically within the first hour. Remarkably, the curve stabilized thereafter.

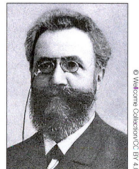

Hermann Ebbinghaus

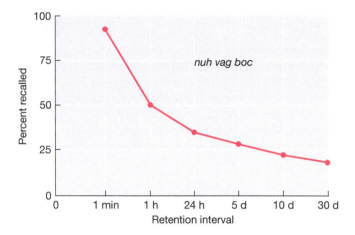

FIGURE 1.2 Ebbinghaus documented the first forgetting curve. Note that substantial forgetting occurs in the first hour after learning, but thereafter recall is fairly stable. (Inspired by H. Ebbinghaus. 1913. *Memory: A Contribution to Experimental Psychology*. Trans. by H. A. Ruger and C. E. Bussenius. New York: Teachers College, Columbia University.)

Empirical principles such as those produced by Ebbinghaus's experiments led to theoretical questions about the underlying structure of the memory (Figure 1.3). Consider Ebbinghaus's forgetting curve. One could imagine that this behavioral function is a direct reflection of the property of a single memory trace—a sustained neural representation of a behavioral experience—the strength of which declines monotonically as a function of the retention interval. In essence, the behavioral function directly represents the decay properties of the memory trace. Another theorist looking at the same data might be struck by the fact that although the rate of forgetting is initially rapid there is very little change after the first hour. This theorist might propose that the forgetting

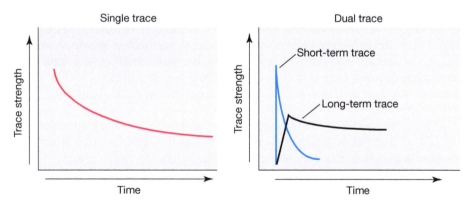

FIGURE 1.3 The single-trace theory explains Ebbinghaus's forgetting curve by assuming that the strength of a single memory trace declines monotonically as a function of time between learning and the retention test. The dual-trace theory explains that the forgetting curve results from two memory traces whose strength decays at different rates.

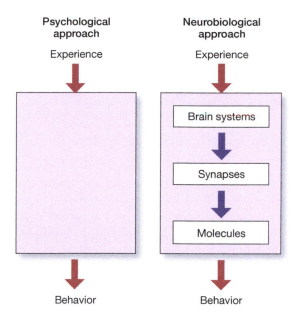

Psychological approach

Experience

Neurobiological approach

Experience

Brain systems

Synapses

Molecules

Behavior

Behavior

FIGURE 1.4   Psychologists study only the relationship between experience and behavior. Neurobiologists study how experience influences memory-dependent behavior by its influences on brain systems, synapses, and molecules.

curve is a product of two memory traces with different decay rates: a short-term memory trace that decays relatively rapidly and a long-term memory trace that has a much slower decay rate. Note in both cases hypotheses are put forth that point to properties—memory strength and memory traces with different decay rates—that defy direct observation.

A fundamental feature of the traditional psychological approach is that a single methodology is used to collect the data and to test theory. Psychologists do not directly manipulate or measure brain function. They vary only the nature of experience and measure only behavior (Figure 1.4). Thus the psychological approach can be described as operating at a single level of analysis. Psychological research has identified critical phenomena and concepts that provide the starting point for neurobiological investigation.

Neurobiological Approach

Psychologists study only the relationship between experience and behavior. Neurobiologists study how experience influences memory-dependent behavior by its influences on brain systems, synapses, and molecules.

The goal of neurobiology is to relate the basic facts of learning and memory to events happening in the brain. If, in the above example, the dual-trace theory was established as valid by psychological experiments, the neurobiologist would want to know what are the properties of the brain that support two different memory traces. This goal requires a multilevel approach. In addition to using the behavioral methods of psychology that reveal how task variables such as trial spacing and repetition influence learning and retention, the neurobiological approach requires methods for:

- determining the regions of the brain that make up the brain system supporting the memory;
- determining how synapses that are potential storage mechanisms are altered by experience; and
- manipulating and measuring molecules in neurons that ultimately support the memory.

Thus the neurobiological approach is an interdisciplinary, multilevel approach. It combines the behavioral methods of psychology with the methods of anatomy, electrophysiology, pharmacology, biochemistry, and genetics. Because the methodologies of each discipline are complex and require specialized training to learn, different scientists often combine their individual skills to attack the problem.

Historical Influences: The Golden Age

The full-scale application of neurobiological methods to the study of learning and memory is a relatively new development. However, many of the important phenomena, concepts, insights, and methods that drive the field emerged over 100 years ago. Forty-four years ago, in his comprehensive review of the psychobiology of memory, Paul Rozin (1976) described the last decade of the nineteenth century as the Golden Age of Memory because many of the basic phenomena and ideas emerged during that period.

Phenomena and Ideas

It was at the beginning of that decade that the French psychologist Théodule Ribot published his classic *Diseases of Memory* (1890). He was motivated by the belief that the study of brain pathology could provide insights into the normal organization of memory. His studies of many clinical cases led him to believe that the dissolution of memory accompanying pathology or injury followed an orderly temporal progression. He proposed that recent memories are the first to be lost, followed by autobiographical or personal memories that also have a temporal gradient (Figure 1.5). He believed that habits and emotional memories were the most resistant to dissolution. Ribot's insight anticipated the modern development—termed the multiple memory systems perspective—that is discussed in Chapter 16. This is because his insight implies that there are different categories of memory and they are supported by different neural systems.

The idea that there is a temporal progression to memory loss—that old memories are more resistant to disruption than new ones—is often referred to as Ribot's Law (see Figure 1.5). This generalization begs the question,

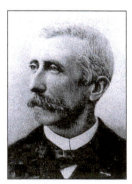

Théodule Ribot

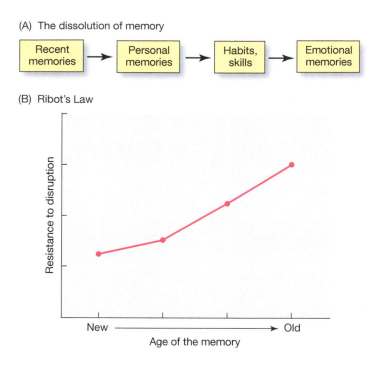

(A) The dissolution of memory

| Recent memories | → | Personal memories | → | Habits, skills | → | Emotional memories |

(B) Ribot's Law

Resistance to disruption

New ——————————→ Old

Age of the memory

FIGURE 1.5   (A) Ribot believed that after a brain pathology or injury the dissolution of memory followed an orderly temporal progression. Recent memories are the first to be lost, followed by autobiographical or personal memories that also have a temporal gradient. He believed that habits and emotional memories were the most resistant to dissolution. (B) Ribot proposed that older memories are more resistant to disruption by traumatic events than newer memories. This hypothesis is called Ribot's Law.

what is it about old memories that makes them resistant to disruption? This question, which remains at the center of contemporary research and is the source of both excitement and controversy, is more fully discussed in Chapter 18.

It was also during this period that Sergei Korsakoff (1897) described the amnesic syndrome that now bears his name. Patients with this syndrome display what would now be called a severe **anterograde amnesia**. They are not able to remember events experienced after the onset of the syndrome. However, early in the disease, memories established before the onset of the syndrome are generally preserved. Thus, they initially display very little **retrograde amnesia**.

Korsakoff believed that the primary defect was an inability to form new memories. His interpretation of the deficit included two ideas. One idea was that the pathology impaired the physiological processes needed to establish and retain the memory. Today one might say that the mechanisms of memory storage or consolidation are impaired. The second idea was that the pathology in some way weakened the associative network that contained the memory or, in modern terms, produced a retrieval deficit, that is, the core memory trace is established but cannot be accessed. Korsakoff believed both factors contributed to the syndrome. Whether memory impairment is the result of a storage or retrieval failure can still be the source of heated debate in the contemporary literature.

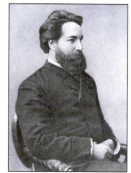

Sergei Korsakoff

FIGURE 1.6 William James proposed that memories emerge in stages. The after image is supported by a short-lasting trace, then replaced by the primary memory trace. Secondary memory is viewed as the reservoir of enduring memory traces.

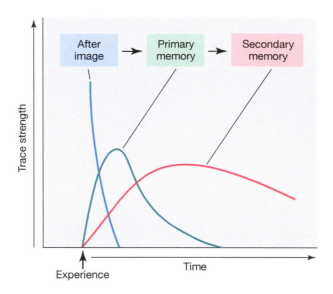

One can only marvel at the insights contained in William James's *Principles of Psychology* (1890). An often noted contribution was his conception of memory as a sequence of processes initiated by an experience that begins with a briefly lasting sensation he called **after images**, then to the stage he called **primary memory**, and to the final stage he called **secondary memory** or **memory proper** (Figure 1.6).

Primary memory was viewed as the persisting representation of the experience that forms part of a stream of consciousness. Secondary memory contained the vast record of experiences that had receded from the stream of consciousness but could be later retrieved or recollected: "It is brought back, fished up, so to speak, from a reservoir in which, with countless other objects, it lay buried and lost from view" (James, 1890, p. 646). An object in primary memory is not brought back: it was never lost. Thus, we have the roots of the modern distinction between short-term memory and long-term memory that remain central to modern investigations of the neurobiological bases of memory.

James devoted an entire chapter to the brain. However, the absence of any relevant information precluded an attempt to directly relate memory phenomena to any specific regions of the brain or mechanisms. Nevertheless, he strongly believed that the retention of experience was not a mysterious mental property but that it was "a purely physical phenomenon, a morphological feature…" (p. 655). He even provided a connectionist model of the memory trace to bolster his belief. In at least two places he used the term **plasticity** to describe the property of the brain that allows it to be modified by experience. For example, in his discussion of memory he wrote, "What happens in the nerve-tissue is but an example of that

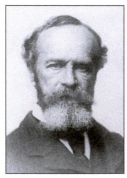

William James

plasticity or of semi-inertness, yielding to change…" (p. 655). Thus, modern developments would come as no surprise to him.

The Neuron Doctrine and Synaptic Plasticity

During this era, the foundation for modern neuroscience—**the neuron doctrine**—emerged (see Shepard, 1991). Camillo Golgi had developed a method (now called the Golgi Stain) that allowed what came to be called neurons to be visualized. However, there was debate about how these elements were organized to support brain function.

A prominent idea that was backed by Golgi was called **reticulum** (network) **theory**. According to this theory the nervous system represented an exception to **cell theory**—the idea that the fundamental element in the structure of living bodies is a cell. Instead, nerve tissue was organized into a continuous network rather than discrete independent units. Golgi believed that the branches from the cell body we now call **dendrites** were in contact with blood vessels and functioned only to provide nutrients to the cell. The business end of the nerve cells was carried out by what are now called **axons**, which he believed were continuous (fused) with each other and formed the reticulum or network (Figure 1.7). A significant problem with this view is that it prohibits the formulation of a principle for how transmission between nerve cells could occur.

Many individuals contributed to the dismissal of reticulum theory (Shepard, 1991); however, the great Spanish neuroanatomist Santiago Ramón y Cajal is generally acknowledged as the most important opponent of reticulum theory and father of the neuron doctrine—the idea that the brain is made up of discrete cells called nerve cells or neurons that are the elemental signal units of the brain (Ramón y Cajal, 1894–1904). (See Box 1.1 for a list of key elements of the neuron doctrine.) He refined Golgi's method to increase its reliability and, based on his anatomical descriptions, forcefully argued that neurons are

(A)

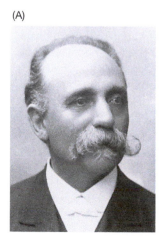

(B)

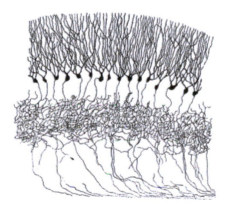

FIGURE 1.7 (A) Camillo Golgi. (B) Golgi developed a method (now called the Golgi Stain) that allowed what are now called neurons to be visualized. Based on his observations, he believed in the reticulum or network theory of the organization of nerve tissue. (From C. Golgi. 1903. *Opera Omnia. Volume II: Istologia Normale—1883-1902*. Milan: Ulrico Hoepli.)

BOX 1.1 Elements of the Neuron Doctrine

- The neuron is an anatomical unit—the fundamental structural and functional unit of the nervous system.
- The neuron is composed of three parts: cell body, dendrites, and axons.
- Neurons are discrete cells, which are not continuous with other cells.
- The points of connection between neurons are called synapses.
- The neuron is a physiological unit. Electrical activity flows through the neuron in one direction (from dendrites to the axon, via the cell body).
- The neuron is the developmental–genetic unit of the nervous system.

not fused but are contiguous (for example, Ramón y Cajal's 1894 Croonian lecture, partially reproduced in English in Shepard, 1991). This conclusion led to the now accepted view that neurons are truly independent, genetically derived units that are composed of (a) the cell body or soma, (b) dendrites, and (c) a single axon. With this conceptual breakthrough Ramón y Cajal also was able to figure out the brain's basic wiring diagram—axons could travel short or long distances but they always terminated at specific locations among fields of dendrites. Axon endings were contiguous with dendrites but not continuous (fused) with them. Sir Charles Sherrington (1906) subsequently named this axon–dendritic junction—the point of contiguity between axons and dendrites—the **synapse**. The functional significance of this anatomical arrangement was recognized by Ramón y Cajal in what is called the Law of Dynamic Polarization, the idea that a neuron receives signals (nerve impulses) at its dendrites and transmits them via the soma, then along the axon in one direction—away from the cell body.

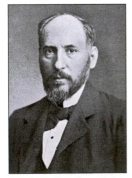

Santiago Ramón y Cajal

At the very heart of contemporary investigations of the mechanisms of memory storage is the **synaptic plasticity hypothesis**, which posits that "the strength of synaptic connections—the ease with which an action potential in one cell excites (or inhibits) its target cell—is not fixed but is plastic and modifiable" (Squire and Kandel, 1999, p. 35). However, this hypothesis was not initially universally embraced. In the 1890s there was a heated debate as to whether neurons maintained a fixed structure throughout the lifetime of an individual (see DeFelipe, 2006). Further testimony to Ramón y Cajal's brilliance was his position on this issue and his willingness to speculate from his anatomical descriptions that the points of contiguity between axons and dendrites (synapses) provide opportunities for modification by experience. In his theory of cerebral gymnastics he even proposed a model of how this could happen (DeFelipe, 2006). Thus, Ramón y Cajal is also acknowledged for the development of one of the field's most important ideas.

Behavioral Methods

The Golden Age documented important clinical phenomena that provided initial insights into memory organization and produced ideas that remain fundamental to contemporary investigations. Remarkably, this period also produced some of the essential behavioral methods that in one form or another continue to be used to study how the brain supports learning and memory. Ebbinghaus's contribution already has been discussed. His work provided the basis for the scientific study of human memory.

Neurobiologists want to understand how the brain supports learning and memory. Studies of normal people and patients with brain damage can identify interesting phenomena that can provide some insight into the organization of memory. However, there are obvious major ethical concerns that constrain the direct manipulation of the human brain. Thus, to directly manipulate and measure brain events, neurobiologists have relied extensively on methods that allow the study of learning and memory with nonhuman animals. During the Golden Age, Ivan Pavlov and Edward L. Thorndike developed methodologies that remain essential to contemporary researchers who study the learning and memory processes of animals.

Pavlov (1927) began his career shift from studying digestive physiology to investigating the integrative activity of the brain. In doing so, he developed the fundamental paradigm for studying **associative learning** and memory in animals (Figure 1.8). The essence of this methodology, called **classical** (or Pavlovian) **conditioning**, is that a neutral stimulus such as the ringing of a bell (called the conditioned stimulus or CS) was paired with a biologically

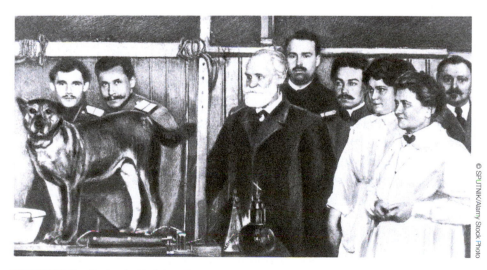

FIGURE 1.8 Pavlov in his laboratory.

© SPUTNIK/Alamy Stock Photo

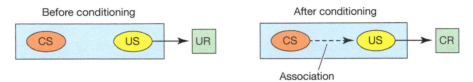

FIGURE 1.9   In the Pavlovian conditioning method, two events called the CS and US are presented together. Subsequently, the CS evokes the response called the CR. Psychologists assume that the CS evokes the CR because the CS gets associated with the US. Psychologists and neurobiologists continue to use this method to study associative learning in animals.

significant event such as food (called the unconditioned stimulus or US). The US caused the dog to salivate; this response is called the unconditioned response or UR. As a consequence of the several pairings of the bell (CS) and food (US), simply ringing the bell caused the dog to salivate. The response to the CS is called the conditioned response or CR. The ability of the CS to evoke the CR is believed to be the result of the brain associating the occurrence of the CS and US (Figure 1.9). Today no one uses dogs or measures the salivary response to study learning and memory in nonverbal animals. However, many neurobiologists still use variations of the Pavlovian conditioning methodology to study learning and memory in other nonhuman animals.

It was also during the Golden Age that Thorndike (1898) published his dissertation on animal intelligence in which he provided a methodology that permitted an objective investigation of how animals learned the consequences of their action. He invented what is referred to as Thorndike's puzzle box

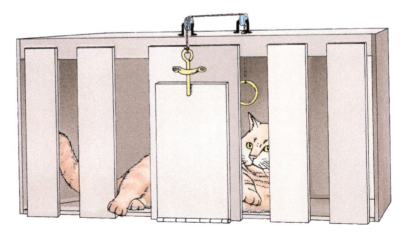

FIGURE 1.10   Edward L. Thorndike invented the methodology for studying what is now called instrumental learning. Cats, dogs, and chickens were placed into his puzzle box and had to learn how to manipulate levers to escape.

(Figure 1.10). An animal such as a cat or chicken would be placed in a wooden crate and to escape it had to learn to depress a lever to open an escape door. Thorndike's experiments provided the foundation for study of what is now called **instrumental learning**. Variations of his methods continue to be extensively employed to reveal the systems of the brain involved in how animals learn to adapt their behavior based on the consequences of their actions.

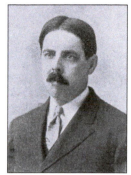

Edward L. Thorndike

Core Themes

Scientists from a wide range of disciplines have been intrigued by questions about how the brain supports learning and memory. Their efforts have generated an enormous literature that even seasoned researchers find overwhelming. No single book can begin to do justice to the current state of knowledge. However, it may be possible to provide a road map for appreciating some of the major accomplishments of this field and provide a foundation for future study. To achieve this more modest goal, this book is organized around three large themes that represent much of the field: synaptic basis of memory, molecules and memory, and neural systems and memory.

Synaptic Basis of Memory

Contemporary neuroscientists believe that the synapse is the fundamental unit of memory storage. For synapses to support memory they have to be plastic or modifiable. The last 50 years have yielded remarkable insights into the molecular processes that are engaged to support changes in the strength of synapses. Thus, the goal of a major portion of this book is to present many of the important findings and ideas that have been generated by this field.

Molecules and Memory

Memories result from behavioral experiences. The past 50 years also have witnessed the development of many useful behavioral procedures for studying memory formation in nonverbal animals. Armed with these behavioral methods, researchers have been emboldened to determine if memories are a product of some of the same cellular–molecular events that alter the strength of synaptic connections. Bringing ideas from the study of synaptic plasticity to the study of memory formation is one of the most dynamic and exciting adventures in brain–behavioral sciences. Thus, another section of this book is concerned with describing how memory researchers have been able to use what has been learned from studies of synaptic plasticity to begin to uncover the molecular basis of memory. This section also describes advances in understanding the relationship between forgetting and remembering, the nature of the engram, and what happens when memories are retrieved.

Neural Systems and Memory

The content of our experience matters to the brain. One of the important achievements of the modern era has been the realization that the brain has evolved neural systems that are specialized to capture and store the varied content generated by our experiences. This idea is generally represented by the term **multiple memory systems**. For example, different systems have been identified that enable us to keep track of the episodes that make up our personal history and to record emotionally charged events to protect us from danger. These stand apart from other brain systems that enable us to learn the consequences of our actions and acquire the routine and not so routine skills and habits that enable us to interact successfully with our environment. The last section of this book provides an introduction to some of the important developments in this domain.

Summary

This chapter has presented a number of fundamental concepts that provide a background needed to go forward as well as some of the historical foundation for the field. Many of the core phenomena, concepts, and behavioral methods that are central to the neurobiology of learning and memory emerged in what Rozin called the Golden Age of Memory, the last decade of the nineteenth century. These ideas are intimately linked to individuals (Ebbinghaus, Ribot, Korsakoff, James, Ramón y Cajal, Pavlov, and Thorndike) who have provided a context from which the central themes that guide contemporary research emerged.

References

DeFelipe, J. (2006). Brain plasticity and mental processes: Cajal again. *Nature Reviews Neuroscience, 7,* 811–817.

Ebbinghaus, H. (1913). *Uber das Gedachtnis: Untersuchungen zur Experimentellen Psychologie.* Leipzig: Dunke and Humboldt. Trans. by H. A. Ruger and C. E. Byssennine as *Memory: A Contribution to Experimental Psychology.* New York: Dover.

James, W. (1890). *Principles of Psychology.* New York: Holt.

Korsakoff, S. S. (1897). Disturbance of psychic function in alcoholic paralysis and its relation to the disturbance of the psychic sphere in multiple neuritis of nonalcoholic origins. *Vesin. Psychiatrii 4:* fascicle 2.

Pavlov, I. P. (1927). *Conditioned Reflexes.* London: Oxford University Press.

Ramón y Cajal, S. (1894). The Croonian lecture: la fine structure des centres nerveux. *Proceedings of the Royal Society of London, 55,* 444–468 (in French).

Ramón y Cajal, S. (1894–1904). *Textura del Sistema Nervioso del Hombre y de los Vertebrados.* Trans. by N. Swanson and L. W. Swanson as *New Ideas on the Structure of the Nervous System in Man and Vertebrates.* Cambridge, MA: MIT Press, 1990.

Ribot, T. (1890). *Diseases of Memory*. New York: Appleton and Company.

Rozin, P. (1976). The psychobiology of memory. In M. R. Rosenzweig and E. L. Bennett (Eds.), *Neural Mechanisms of Learning and Memory* (pp. 3–46). Cambridge, MA: MIT Press.

Shepard, G. M. (1991). *Foundations of the Neuron Doctrine*. New York: Oxford University Press.

Sherrington, C. S. (1906). *The Integrative Action of the Nervous System*. New York: Charles Scribner's Sons.

Squire, L. R. (1987). *Memory and Brain*. New York: Oxford University Press.

Squire, L. R. and Kandel, E. R. (1999). *Memory: From Mind to Molecules*. New York: W. H. Freeman and Company.

Thorndike, E. L. (1898). Animal intelligence: an experimental study of the associative processes in animals. *Psychological Review, Monograph Supplement 2, no. 8.*

PART 1
Synaptic Basis of Memory

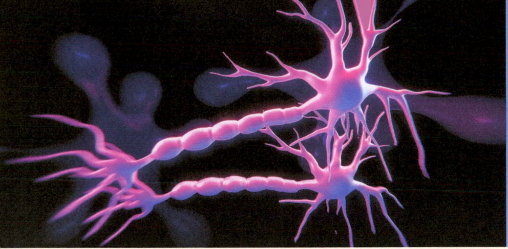

Memory and the Brain: Central Concepts

We know memories exist because most aspects of our behavior and cognitive activity are influenced by our past experiences and, by inference, their preserved representations in our brains. Not only do memories exist, psychologists and neurobiologists believe they come in different forms. Such adjectives as *episodic*, *semantic*, *declarative*, *procedural*, *primary*, *secondary*, and *working* have been used to label the different memory types that are distinguished by their properties and the functions they support. The challenge to neurobiologists is to link these abstract concepts of memory to brain processes.

To understand what is involved first requires a discussion of how to view memory from the perspective of the brain. After a discussion of the phenomenon of long-term potentiation (LTP) and an explanation of how synapses are modified, an organizing framework is provided for understanding these processes.

A Brain's View of Memory

Historically, a commonly held view was that the brain works like a warehouse for information: "Memories are items to be stored away … until … needed, whereupon some search is undertaken to retrieve those items." (Eichenbaum and Cohen, 2001, p. 6). The idea of a warehouse for memory is a metaphor. However, it could be viewed as a hypothesis that there are specific brain regions *dedicated* to storing memories and that these regions can be located. This hypothesis has not fared well. Memories are not stored as items: "…no one has found regions [of the brain] that serve as dedicated warehouse(s)…" (Eichenbaum and Cohen, 2001, p. 6).

If memories are not "items" stored in specialized areas of the brain, then what are they? What should we look for? How would we know one if we found it? Over 60 years ago Donald Hebb, a founder of the modern field of cognitive neuroscience, provided a good starting point. First, he rejected the warehouse metaphor.

> Neurologists, information theorists, and biochemists sometimes think of a memory as a sort of *thing* which can be stored in part of the brain (as a punched card can be stored in a computer). They seem even to think that a memory might be stored inside a single cell. We avoid all such improbabilities by thinking in terms of behavior, or paths in the CNS (central nervous system) that have been changed by the learning process. (Hebb, 1966, p. 122)

Elaborating on this issue, Hebb wrote:

> Fundamentally, memory is the retention of learning. As such it must be a lasting modification of transmission paths, something which concerns the relation between neurons. It cannot be in one neuron nor can memories all be stored in one part of the brain (unless all transmission paths go through that region and the changes in the path occur there only, which is unlikely). (Hebb, 1966, p. 122)

Gary Lynch and Michel Baudry (1984, p. 1057) echoed this view in their seminal paper on the biochemistry of memory: "So far as we know, the brain interacts with the environment through axon discharges and synaptic transmission and it follows that the substrates of memory are triggered and act upon these physiological events."

Hebb (1949, p. 60) also introduced another important concept—the **cell assembly**—described by Eichenbaum and Cohen (2001, p. 41) as "diffuse circuits of connected neurons that develop to represent specific percepts or concepts." He proposed that structural changes in these assemblies make lasting memories possible. He also proposed a mechanism for how this could happen.

When an axon of cell A is near enough to excite a cell B and repeatedly or persistently takes part in firing it, some growth process or metabolic change takes place in one or both cells such that A's efficiency, as one of the cells firing B, is increased. (Hebb, 1949, p. 60)

These ideas remain central to the field. Memories from the brain's view are the *changes in the connectivity* among the collection of neurons responding to a particular experience. Changes are not localized to some dedicated storage area but are distributed throughout the neural systems engaged by the memory-producing event. The duration of the changes can be very short-lived or relatively permanent, and the content of the memory will be determined by the specific sets of neuronal assemblies activated by the memory-producing experience.

In principle, we now have a road map for providing a neurobiological account of memory. All that we need to do is:

- identify the neuronal assemblies engaged by a memory-producing event;
- determine how the structure and function of components of the assembly are changed by the event;
- understand the activity-dependent cellular processes that bring about the changes; and
- understand the processes by which the changed assemblies (the memory) are retrieved to influence ongoing behavior and cognitive activity.

This framework implies a linear order of attack. However, this is not how it has unfolded. Historically, neurobiologists found it extremely difficult to actually identify specific distributed neuronal assemblies that support memories. In addition, to address each of these high-level goals requires very specialized methods and this unintentionally produced a divide-and-conquer approach, with different groups of neurobiologists focusing on different parts of the problem.

Moreover, over the last 50 years electrophysiological, histological, and molecular biological tools have developed that permitted investigations of (a) the functional and structural changes in neuronal connections (synapses) produced by neural activity and (b) the cellular–molecular processes that created them. A consequence of this situation is that our understanding of these components of the problem has advanced more rapidly than our understanding of neuronal assemblies. The story continues with a discussion of the discovery of the phenomenon of long-term potentiation (LTP).

The Phenomenon of Long-Term Potentiation

Memories are the product of strengthening connections among neurons activated by experience. As canonized in the synaptic plasticity hypothesis, this happens at the **synapse**, the point of contact between the sending (or presynaptic) neuron and the receiving (or postsynaptic) neuron. In an ideal world one would like to study how behavioral experiences modify the synapses that support their memories. This is a daunting task because it requires locating the neurons that compose the assemblies that support the **memory trace** (also called an **engram**) and their natural sensory inputs.

Fortunately, in the mid 1960s events were occurring in Oslo, Norway, that would pave the way for researchers to study how synapses in the mammalian brain can be modified by experience. Per Andersen had just returned from a two-year postdoctoral position with the Nobel Laureate, Sir John Eccles, and was setting up a new laboratory. As it so happened, Terje Lømo was visiting Oslo in search of a position and a chance encounter with Andersen led to a position in his laboratory (Lømo, 2016). Lømo was invited to follow up on one of Andersen's observations—that stimulation of afferent fibers into the hippocampus produced an unexpected enhanced excitatory response that lasted a few minutes. By varying the properties of the stimulation, Lømo was able to produce an enhancement that lasted more than an hour (Lømo, 1966).

Timothy Bliss learned of Lømo's work and subsequently joined Andersen's research group to continue work on this project. Together they produced the definitive set of experiments that established the phenomenon now called **long-term potentiation** (**LTP**) (Bliss and Lømo, 1973; see also Bliss and Gardner-Medwin, 1973). The significance of their discovery cannot be overstated. Moreover, as Roger Nicoll (2017, p. 282) noted: "There is not a single controversial finding in this paper, which is a very remarkable thing in this field." It is noteworthy that Bliss and Lømo raised the possibility that their discovery might have something to do with learning and memory.

While in Eccles's laboratory, Andersen also began to investigate the trisynaptic organization of the hippocampus (also called the **trisynaptic circuit**), which was originally discovered by Ramón y Cajal (Andersen, 1975; Andersen, 2004; Andersen et al., 1971). Before describing the essence of Bliss and Lømo's experiments, it is important to understand this circuit (Figure 2.1), which consists of three components:

1. Neurons in the **entorhinal cortex** connect to a region in the hippocampus called the **dentate gyrus** by what is called the **perforant path**.
2. Neurons in the dentate gyrus connect to the **CA3** region by what are called **mossy fibers**.
3. Neurons in CA3 connect to neurons in the **CA1** region by what are called **Schaffer collateral fibers**.

Although it was not possible to study specific neuron-to-neuron connections in the intact hippocampus, this organization of the hippocampus makes it possible to study connections linking neurons in one region or subfield to neurons in another subfield. The specific methods

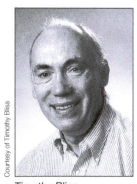

Timothy Bliss

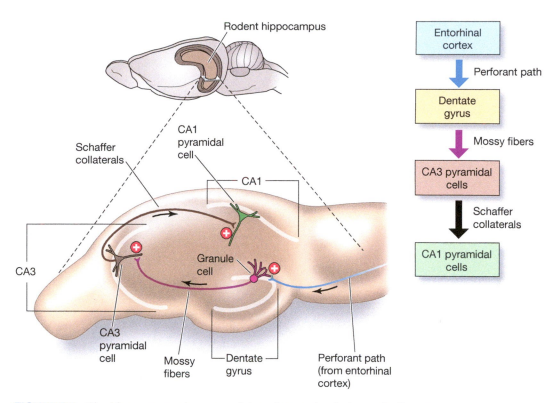

FIGURE 2.1   The hippocampus has a very interesting anatomical organization, commonly called the trisynaptic circuit. This schematic representation of the rodent hippocampus shows the direction of the flow of information.

are described in a later section of this chapter. The basic strategy is simple: you stimulate a set of fibers known to synapse onto neurons in a particular subfield and record what happens in that region when the impulse arrives. If the stimulated fibers connect to cells near the recording electrode, you will detect a response in those neurons.

Bliss and Lømo (1973) discovered LTP in the hippocampus of living rabbits. They stimulated the fibers in the perforant path and recorded synaptic activity that occurred in the dentate gyrus (Figure 2.2). The basic experiment was simple.

1. They established that a weak stimulus applied to the perforant path would evoke some synaptic activity in the dentate gyrus.

2. They next delivered a stronger stimulus to the same perforant path fibers, which evoked a much larger synaptic response.

3. They then repeatedly presented the weak stimulus and found that it now evoked a bigger response.

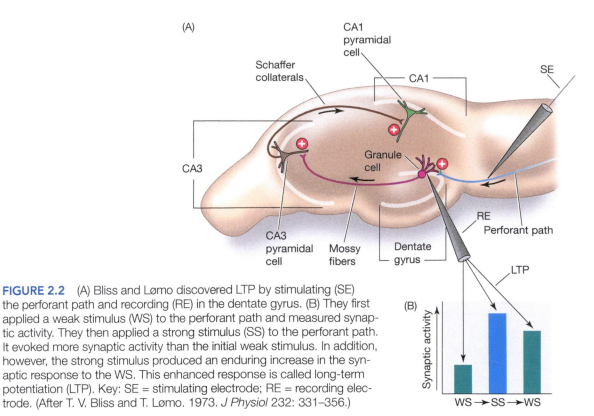

FIGURE 2.2 (A) Bliss and Lømo discovered LTP by stimulating (SE) the perforant path and recording (RE) in the dentate gyrus. (B) They first applied a weak stimulus (WS) to the perforant path and measured synaptic activity. They then applied a strong stimulus (SS) to the perforant path. It evoked more synaptic activity than the initial weak stimulus. In addition, however, the strong stimulus produced an enduring increase in the synaptic response to the WS. This enhanced response is called long-term potentiation (LTP). Key: SE = stimulating electrode; RE = recording electrode. (After T. V. Bliss and T. Lømo. 1973. *J Physiol* 232: 331–356.)

Thus, the strong stimulus potentiated the response to the weak stimulus and the potentiated response lasted a relatively long time (several hours). Hundreds of researchers have dedicated their scientific careers to the study of LTP as a model system for discovering the mechanisms that produce lasting changes in synaptic strength. To appreciate their discoveries, it is necessary to understand the conceptual basis of LTP and the methodology used to study it.

The Conceptual Basis of LTP

Although Bliss and Lømo discovered LTP in the hippocampus of a living rabbit, the most widely employed basic procedure for studying LTP is an **in vitro preparation** (Yamamoto and McIlwain, 1966), illustrated in Figure 2.3. It requires dissecting a very thin transverse slice of tissue from the hippocampus and placing it into a special chamber that contains a cocktail of chemicals in a solution that will keep the slice of tissue functional for several hours. A stimulating electrode is then positioned to deliver electrical current to a chosen set of fibers and a recording electrode is placed in the region where these fibers terminate (Skrede and Westgaard, 1971).

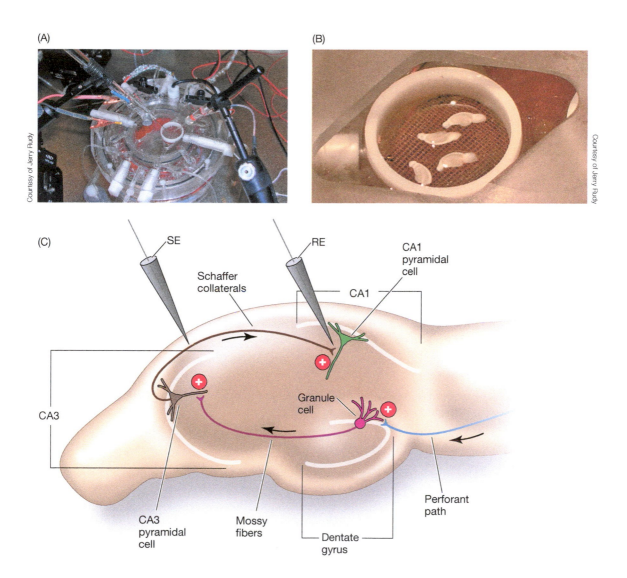

(A)

Courtesy of Jerry Rudy

(B)

Courtesy of Jerry Rudy

(C)

SE

Schaffer
collaterals

RE

CA1
pyramidal
cell

CA1

CA3

Granule
cell

Perforant
path

CA3
pyramidal
cell

Mossy
fibers

Dentate
gyrus

FIGURE 2.3 LTP can be studied in tissue slices taken from the hippocampus. This is called an in vitro preparation. (A) The recording apparatus consists of a large chamber that is filled with fluid needed to keep the slice viable, a small chamber that holds the slice being studied, the stimulating electrode used to induce LTP, and the recording electrode used to measure the field EPSP. (B) Prior to beginning the experiment, slices of hippocampal tissue are placed into the small recording chamber. (C) Many researchers use the in vitro methodology to study LTP induced in neurons in the CA1 region of the hippocampus. To do this they stimulate the Schaffer collateral fibers and record field potentials from a recording electrode placed in the CA1 region. Key: SE = stimulating electrode; RE = recording electrode.

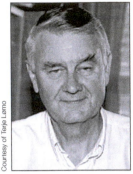

Terje Lømo

Bliss and Lømo (1973) stimulated the axonal fibers in the perforant path and recorded the synaptic response in the dentate gyrus. Many researchers choose instead to stimulate the Schaffer collateral fibers and record the response of the pyramidal cells in the CA1 subfield (see Figure 2.3). The recording electrode is placed in the extracellular space among a population of pyramidal cells in CA1. It records the extracellular **excitatory postsynaptic potential (EPSP)**, which is referred to as the **field potential** or **field EPSP** (or abbreviated further as **fEPSP**). The field potential is the dependent variable in the LTP experiment; it is what the researcher measures. To understand field potential requires a review of the basic structure and function of the neuron and how neurons communicate, as well as a discussion of membrane potential, synaptic depolarization and hyperpolarization, and synaptic strength.

STRUCTURE AND FUNCTIONS OF THE NEURONS   An idealized neuron is presented in Figure 2.4, which shows that a neuron is composed of a cell body, dendrites, an axon, and axon terminals. Neurons are connected in networks and serve many functions. A neuron is:

- an input device that receives chemical and electrical messages from other neurons;
- an integrative device that combines messages received from multiple inputs;
- a conductive–output device that sends information to other neurons, muscles, and organs; and
- a representation device that stores information about past experiences as changes in synaptic strength.

The function a particular neuron serves depends on whether it is a presynaptic "sending" neuron or a postsynaptic "receiving" neuron. As noted, the synapse (Figure 2.5) is the point of contact between the sending and receiving neuron. It is where neurons communicate and information is thought to be

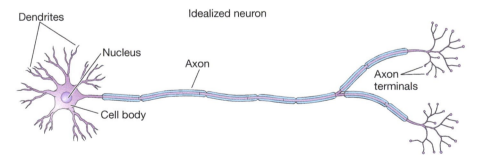

Idealized neuron

Dendrites

Nucleus

Axon

Axon terminals

Cell body

FIGURE 2.4   A neuron is composed of a cell body (which contains the nucleus), dendrites, an axon, and axon terminals.

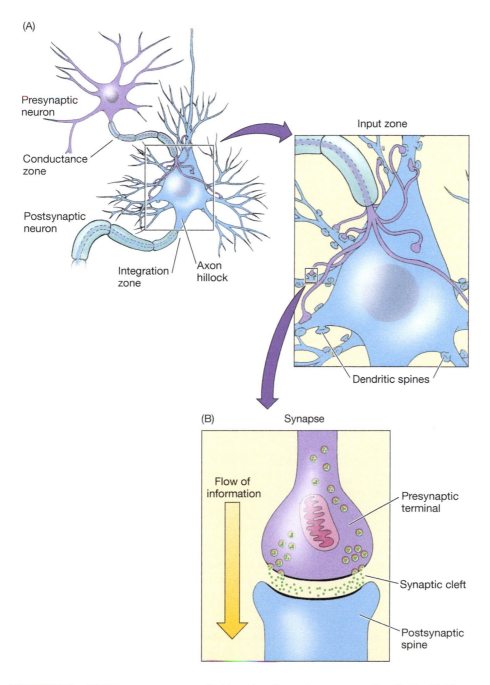

(A)

Presynaptic
neuron

Conductance
zone

Postsynaptic
neuron

Integration
zone

Axon
hillock

Input zone

Dendritic spines

(B)

Synapse

Flow of
information

Presynaptic
terminal

Synaptic cleft

Postsynaptic
spine

FIGURE 2.5 (A) Neurons are connected in networks and serve many functions. (B) The basic components of a synapse are the presynaptic terminal, a synaptic cleft, and a post-synaptic dendrite. This figure shows a presynaptic neuron synapsing onto a dendritic spine.

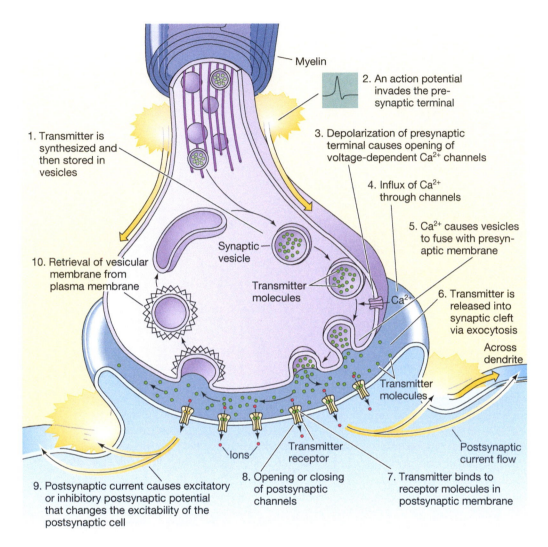

Myelin

2. An action potential invades the pre-synaptic terminal

1. Transmitter is synthesized and then stored in vesicles

3. Depolarization of presynaptic terminal causes opening of voltage-dependent Ca^{2+} channels

4. Influx of Ca^{2+} through channels

5. Ca^{2+} causes vesicles to fuse with presynaptic membrane

Synaptic vesicle

10. Retrieval of vesicular membrane from plasma membrane

Transmitter molecules

Ca^{2+}

6. Transmitter is released into synaptic cleft via exocytosis

Across dendrite

Transmitter molecules

Postsynaptic current flow

Ions

Transmitter receptor

9. Postsynaptic current causes excitatory or inhibitory postsynaptic potential that changes the excitability of the postsynaptic cell

8. Opening or closing of postsynaptic channels

7. Transmitter binds to receptor molecules in postsynaptic membrane

FIGURE 2.6 When an action potential arrives in the presynaptic axon terminal, neurotransmitter molecules are released from synaptic vesicles into the synaptic cleft where they bind to specific receptors, causing a chemical or electrical signal in the postsynaptic cell.

stored. The basic components of a synapse are the **presynaptic terminal**, the **postsynaptic dendrite**, and the **synaptic cleft**, which is a small space between the terminal and the spine that contains structures that maintain the connection.

NEURONAL COMMUNICATIONS   Information transmitted between neurons depends on a combination of electrical events that allows the presynaptic neuron to influence the postsynaptic neuron. Some of the important details of this

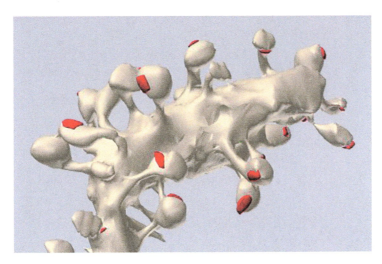

FIGURE 2.7 Dendrites are extensively populated with structures called dendritic spines. A spine is a small (submicrometer) membranous extrusion that protrudes from a dendrite. This figure illustrates a three-dimensional reconstruction of a section of a dendrite with spines of different shapes and sizes. Dendritic spines are of special interest because (a) key receptors involved in the regulation of synaptic plasticity are located in spines and (b) changes in the composition and architecture of the spine are altered by neural activity. (From Synapse Web, Kristen M. Harris, PI, https://synapseweb.clm.utexas.edu/.)

process are shown in Figure 2.6. The general story, however, is that the terminal ending of the sending neuron contains packages of molecules called **neurotransmitters**, which are packaged in **synaptic vesicles**. These molecules are called neurotransmitters because they are the primary communication agent of the sending neuron. When **action potentials** (spikes of electrical activity that travel along the axon) are generated in the axon of the sending neuron, they can cause the neurotransmitters to be released into the synaptic cleft. The receiving neuron has specialized receptors, generally located on the dendritic spines (Figure 2.7), which are designed to receive the neurotransmitter released by the sending neuron. After the neurotransmitters are released, they can bind to receptors located on the dendrites of the receiving neuron.

When enough receptors are occupied, a brief electrical event called the **postsynaptic potential** is generated in the postsynaptic neuron. To understand why requires a review of the membrane potential.

MEMBRANE POTENTIAL   There is fluid inside the neurons called intracellular fluid, and neurons are surrounded by what is called extracellular fluid. The intracellular fluid is separated from the surrounding extracellular fluid by a cell membrane. Both the intracellular and extracellular fluids contain positively and negatively charged molecules called **ions**. The **membrane potential** is the difference in the electrical charge inside the neuron's cell body compared to

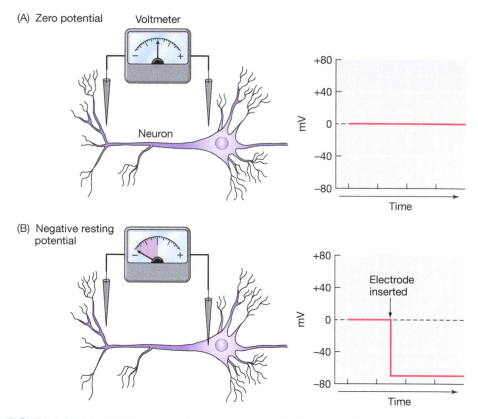

FIGURE 2.8 (A) When two recording electrodes are in the extracellular space surrounding neurons, there is zero potential between them. Likewise, the membrane potential would be zero if the ionic composition of the extracellular and intracellular fluids were exactly the same. (B) However, if one electrode is inserted into the neuron but the other electrode remains in the extracellular space, it would record the resting membrane potential as negative because in the inactive state there are more negatively charged ions in the intracellular fluid than in the extracellular fluid.

the charge outside the cell body. If the ionic composition of the intracellular and extracellular fluids were exactly the same, the membrane potential would be zero. However, the composition is not the same. There are more negatively charged ions in the intracellular fluid than in the extracellular fluid. Thus, the membrane potential in the inactive state—the **resting membrane potential**—is negatively charged with respect to the extracellular fluid. The electrical potential is measured in millivolts (mV); each millivolt is 1/1000 of a volt. The resting membrane potential is typically in the range of –50 to –80 mV where the negative sign (–) represents a negative potential (Figure 2.8).

SYNAPTIC DEPOLARIZATION AND HYPERPOLARIZATION The membrane potential is dynamic and can be driven to become either less negative or more negative. The term **depolarization** represents the case where the membrane potential becomes less negative. When depolarization occurs, the composition of the intracellular fluid becomes more like the composition of the extracellular fluid. The term **hyperpolarization** represents the case where the membrane potential becomes more negative. When hyperpolarization occurs, the composition of the intracellular fluid becomes less like the composition of the extracellular fluid. The process of depolarization drives the neuron *towards* generating action potentials, while the process of hyperpolarization drives the neuron *away* from generating action potentials (Figure 2.9).

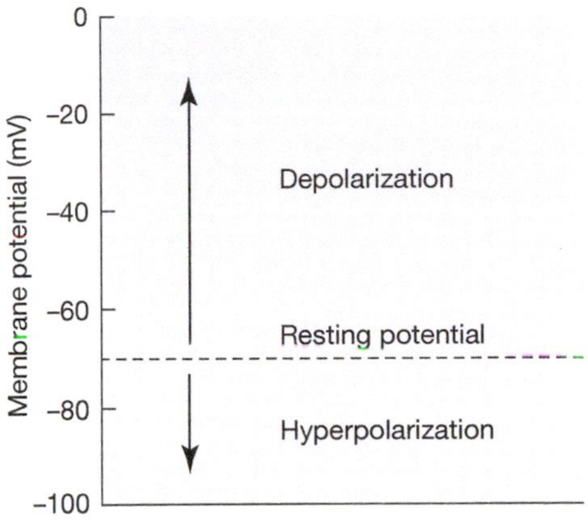

FIGURE 2.9 The resting membrane potential is negative. Depolarization occurs when the ionic composition of the intracellular fluid becomes less negative. Hyperpolarization occurs when the ionic composition of the intracellular fluid becomes more negative.

The electrical stimulation used to produce LTP in the hippocampus generates action potentials in the axons of the sending neurons. As a result, many of the synapses on the postsynaptic neurons will depolarize, that is, positive ions will flow into those neurons. This is called **postsynaptic depolarization**. In principle, postsynaptic potentials can be recorded from either a very small intracellular electrode (an electrode that penetrates the neuron) or from a larger electrode placed in the extracellular fluid in the region where the stimulated axons synapse with the receiving neurons (Figure 2.10). The intracellular electrode would detect positive ions flowing into the neuron, indicating depolarization. However, the extracellular electrode will detect a change in the potential difference between the ionic composition of the extracellular fluid at the recording electrode and another, distant and inactive electrode called the ground electrode. Normally the potential difference between the extracellular recording electrode and ground is zero. As the positive ions flow into the postsynaptic membrane, however, they will flow away from the extracellular recording electrode. This means that the potential between the recording and ground electrodes will become negative. Theoretically, as more synapses contribute to depolarization, the negative potential will increase because more positive ions, in particular sodium, will flow away from the extracellular recording electrode and into the postsynaptic neuron.

SYNAPTIC STRENGTH   The discussion of the membrane potential and field potentials provides a foundation for defining synaptic strength. In the context of the LTP experiment, **synaptic strength** is measured by the amount of postsynaptic depolarization produced by the stimulus—how many positive ions flow into the postsynaptic neurons surrounding the extracellular recording electrode. The extracellular electrode reads this as the flow of positive ions away from its tip. Thus, the size of the field potential recorded by the extracellular electrode is assumed to *indirectly measure* the strength of the synaptic connections linking the presynaptic and postsynaptic neuron.

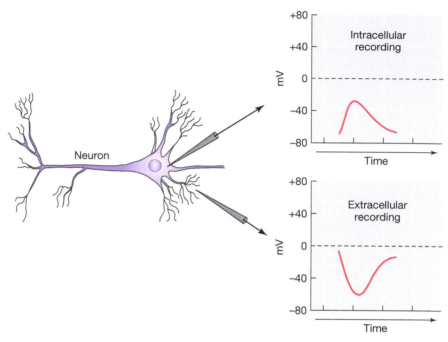

FIGURE 2.10 Postsynaptic potentials can be recorded from either an intracellular electrode that penetrates the neuron or an electrode placed in the extracellular fluid. The intracellular electrode detects positive ions flowing into the neuron, indicating depolarization. The extracellular electrode measures the electrical potential between the extracellular fluid and a ground electrode. When synapses depolarize, positive ions move away from the tip of the electrode into the neuron. This results in the electrical potential between the extracellular fluid and ground electrode becoming negative. Thus, the extracellular recording has a negative slope.

Methodology for Inducing and Measuring LTP

Figure 2.11A illustrates the delivery of a high-frequency stimulus to Schaffer collateral fibers or axons that synapse onto the CA1 pyramidal neurons. An extracellular recording is positioned to measure the field potential that is produced when synapses located on pyramidal neurons depolarize. The waveform produced by the recording electrode is complex because the electrode detects several electrical events (Figure 2.11B). One event is a stimulus artifact associated with simply triggering the current generator that produces the stimulus, another is the **fiber volley** (the action potentials generated by the electrical stimulus), and another is the critical field potential.

The fiber volley represents the fact that the electrical stimulus applied to the fibers generated action potentials that arrived at the recording site. The field potential is detected as the downward slope of the waveform, which measures the rate at which positive ions are leaving the recording field and depolarizing

(A)

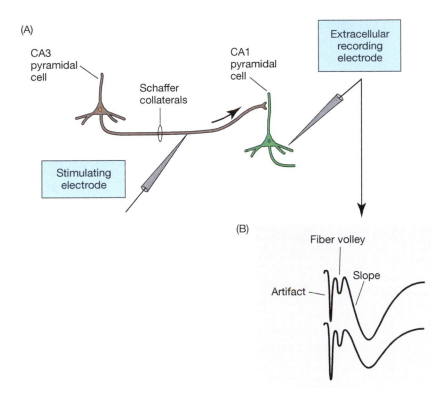

(B)

(C)

FIGURE 2.11   (A) A stimulating electrode delivers a small amount of electric current to Schaffer collateral fibers. (B) The extracellular recording electrode detects a population of depolarizing synapses in the CA1 region and generates a waveform. The steepness of the slope of the waveform represents the amount of synaptic depolarization around the recording electrode. Thus, more synaptic depolarization is recorded in the top waveform than in the bottom one. (C) A quantitative representation of the results of a typical LTP experiment.

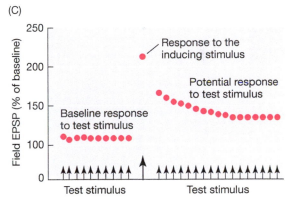

synapses. The steepness of the slope is assumed to reflect the amount of postsynaptic depolarization that occurred. A quantitative representation of the results of a typical LTP experiment is provided in Figure 2.11C.

To understand Figure 2.11 it is necessary to describe the details of the LTP experiment. A good place to start is with a discussion of how the independent variable in the LTP experiment—the intensity of the electric current used to evoke the field potential—is determined. The electrical current applied to the fibers is measured in microamperes, µA. This unit of measure is very small. You would not detect this level of current if it were applied to your finger. Nevertheless, it will generate action potentials in the fibers to which it is applied. In an LTP experiment there are two stimuli: the **test stimulus** and the **inducing stimulus**. The test stimulus is relatively weak and thus evokes a small field potential and will not produce LTP. The inducing stimulus is much stronger and evokes a larger field potential.

The intensity of the test stimulus is usually arrived at by preliminary tests in which the intensity of the stimulus is varied, from about 2.5 to 45 µA (Sweat, 2003), and the experimenter measures the amplitude of the fiber volley and the slope of the field EPSP. The goal of this preliminary stage is to find a test stimulus that evokes a field EPSP that is about 35–50% of the maximum response (Figure 2.12).

The test stimulus has two functions. First, it is repeatedly presented to establish a baseline level of synaptic activity, that is, a baseline field EPSP. Once the baseline is established, the strong, inducing stimulus is presented. Its function is to change the strength of the synaptic connections between the stimulated fibers and the receiving neurons. The second function of the test stimulus is to act as a probe to determine if the inducing stimulus changed the strength of connections between the presynaptic fibers and the postsynaptic neurons.

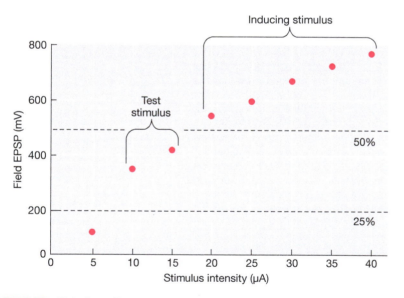

FIGURE 2.12   This figure illustrates a hypothetical relationship between the slope of the field EPSP and the intensity of the stimulus. In this example, either the 10 or 15 µA stimuli might be selected to serve as the baseline test stimulus and intensities from 20 µA to 40 µA might serve as the inducing stimulus.

Thus, after the inducing stimulus is presented, the test stimulus is repeatedly presented (about every 20 seconds). If the experiment is successful, then the test stimulus will evoke a much larger field EPSP than it did during the baseline period (see Figure 2.11C).

The dependent variable shown in Figure 2.11—field EPSP (% of baseline)—represents the difference between the field EPSP produced by the test stimulus during the baseline period prior to when the inducing stimulus is presented (T1), and the response to the test stimulus after the inducing stimulus is presented (T2). To calculate this value, simply divide the value of T2 by the value of T1 and multiply by 100:

$$\text{Field EPSP (\% of baseline)} = T2/T1 \times 100.$$

For example, if the average baseline field EPSP (T1) was 350 mV and the field EPSP evoked by the test stimulus after the inducing stimulus was presented (T2) was 500 mV, then the field EPSP (% of baseline) value would be 143%. In order to conclude that the inducing stimulus strengthened the synaptic connections between axon fibers stimulated by the test stimulus and the postsynaptic neurons—that it induced LTP—this value must exceed 100%. Note that the results presented in Figure 2.11 would lead to the conclusion that the strong inducing stimulus had produced LTP.

The inducing stimulus, which generates LTP, is stronger than the test stimulus. Its intensity is also determined from the preliminary tests (see Figure 2.12). If a weak induction protocol is desired, the stimulus might be set to evoke at least half the maximal field potential. In this protocol the stimulus would be presented at a high frequency (100 Hz = 100 times in a second) for 1 second. If a stronger protocol is desired, then the intensity of the inducing stimulus might be set to evoke the near maximal response. In the stronger protocol, the stimulus would be presented three times at 100 Hz. The three presentations would be separated by 20 seconds. Researchers often call the inducing stimulus the high-frequency stimulus (HFS).

Long-Term Depression: The Polar Opposite of LTP

Although experience can strengthen synaptic connections, embedded in the concept of synaptic plasticity is the idea that experience can also weaken synaptic connections. Synaptic plasticity is in fact bidirectional. Depending on the nature of experience-produced synaptic activity, the synaptic connection can be either strengthened or weakened. The term **long-term depression (LTD)** is used to represent the case in which synaptic activity weakens the strength of the synaptic connections. The experimenter uses a high-frequency stimulus protocol to induce LTP. The protocol used to induce LTD, however, is much different (Bear, 2003; Dudek and Bear, 1992). For example, Dudek and Bear discovered that LTD in the hippocampus could be induced by applying 900 pulses of a low-frequency stimulus (1–3 Hz), which takes about 15 minutes.

FIGURE 2.13 The delivery of a low-frequency stimulus to Schaffer collateral fibers for about 15 minutes produces a long-term depression in the dendritic field of CA1 neurons. Note that the slope of the field EPSP evoked by the test stimulus is markedly reduced. In addition, this effect is blocked when the NMDA receptor antagonist APV is applied to the slice. See Chapter 3 for an explanation of NMDA receptor antagonists. (After S. M. Dudek and M. F. Bear. 1992. *Proc Natl Acad Sci USA* 89: 4363–4367.)

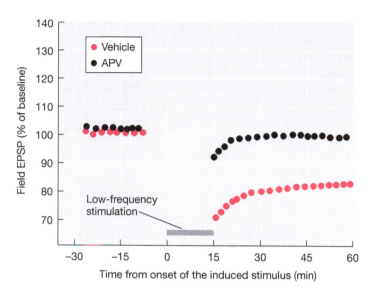

This reduced the field EPSP evoked by the test stimulus for at least an hour (Figure 2.13).

How Synapses Are Modified

The LTP methodology provides a remarkable tool for detecting changes in the ability of presynaptic sending neurons to produce synaptic potentials in the postsynaptic receiving neurons. However, changes in the field potential, measured in an LTP experiment, raise two critical questions.

1. What synaptic changes are produced by the inducing stimulus?
2. What processes are engaged to produce these changes?

In the discussion that follows it becomes clear that the basic composition and structure of dendritic spines that receive the presynaptic input change dramatically and these changes are a product of a large number of biochemical interactions. Several concepts are introduced that are essential to understanding how these answers were arrived at. A functional description of the synapse as a biochemical factory is presented, followed by a review of the key elements of signaling cascades that modify synapses.

The Synapse as a Biochemical Factory

A standard view of a synapse is that it comprises three components: (1) a presynaptic component—a terminal ending of an axon of a sending neuron, (2) a postsynaptic component of the receiving neuron, and (3) a synaptic cleft that separates the two primary components. To understand how it can be modified, however, it is useful to think of a synapse as a biochemical factory with each component containing molecules needed to accomplish specific functions. Some of the components and processes involved in the release of neurotransmitters by the presynaptic neuron already have been described (see Figure 2.5). So the primary focus here is on postsynaptic processes.

The synaptic cleft, which separates the pre and postcomponents of the synapse, is occupied by the **extracellular matrix (ECM)**, illustrated in Figure 2.14.

(A)

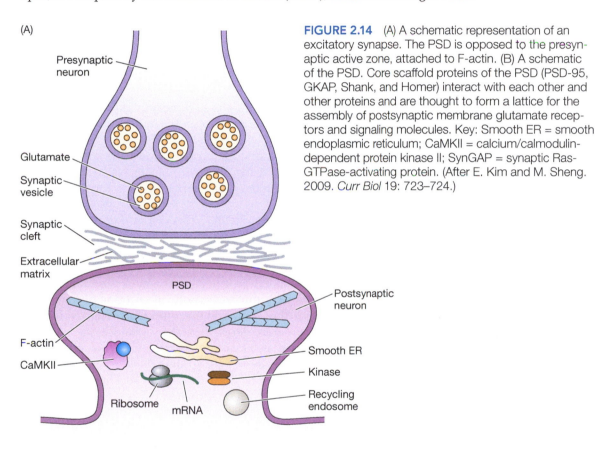

FIGURE 2.14 (A) A schematic representation of an excitatory synapse. The PSD is opposed to the presynaptic active zone, attached to F-actin. (B) A schematic of the PSD. Core scaffold proteins of the PSD (PSD-95, GKAP, Shank, and Homer) interact with each other and other proteins and are thought to form a lattice for the assembly of postsynaptic membrane glutamate receptors and signaling molecules. Key: Smooth ER = smooth endoplasmic reticulum; CaMKII = calcium/calmodulin-dependent protein kinase II; SynGAP = synaptic Ras-GTPase-activating protein. (After E. Kim and M. Sheng. 2009. *Curr Biol* 19: 723–724.)

(B)

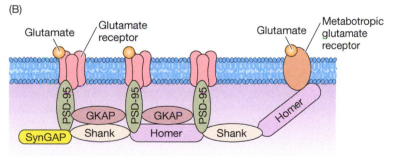

This matrix is composed of molecules synthesized and secreted by neurons and glial cells (Dityateve and Fellin, 2008). The ECM forms a bridge between the pre and postsynaptic neurons and the molecules it contains interact with the neurons to influence their function.

Changes in synaptic potentials produced by an LTP-inducing stimulus are primarily the result of modifying **excitatory synapses**—synapses whose post-synaptic component is a dendritic spine that contains membrane-spanning receptors, called glutamate receptors, that respond to the excitatory neurotransmitter **glutamate**. Synapses that contain dendritic spines are organized both to participate in synaptic transmission and to be modified by synaptic activity. Some general features of an excitatory synapse are shown in Figure 2.14.

POSTSYNAPTIC DENSITY   A major feature of excitatory synapses is a thickening of the postsynaptic membrane termed the **postsynaptic density** (**PSD**). The PSD contains several hundred proteins that include glutamate receptors, ion channels, signaling enzymes, scaffolding proteins, and adhesion molecules (see Figure 2.14). Several core, scaffolding proteins (PSD-95, GKAP, Shank, and Homer) play a key role in organizing the postsynaptic density (Kim and Sheng, 2009; Sheng and Hoogenraad, 2007).

Glutamate receptors located in dendritic spines respond to glutamate released from the presynaptic neuron. The postsynaptic density contributes to this process in two complementary ways. One of its functions is to localize both glutamate receptors and adhesion molecules in the postsynaptic membrane. In this way it facilitates the adhesion of the pre and postsynaptic components and aligns the glutamate receptors with the presynaptic neurotransmitter release zones. This alignment increases the likelihood that glutamate released into the extracellular space will bind to the receptors. Excitatory synapses are plastic—they can be modified when glutamate receptors are activated. This requires the activation of other signaling molecules by the glutamate receptors. A second function of the postsynaptic density is to position these signaling molecules near the glutamate receptors so they can be activated.

OTHER SYNAPTIC PROTEINS   Other proteins below the PSD are positioned to respond to the activation of glutamate receptors (see Figure 2.14). Many of these are structural proteins, such as **actin**, that provide scaffolding that gives the cell its structure. Actin filaments also provide a substrate for molecular motors to cargo protein to the postsynaptic density. Others are functional proteins—enzymes that catalyze reactions and modify the function of other proteins. In addition, there are other complexes such as recycling **endosomes** that transport internalized receptors to and from the plasma membrane, **ribosomes** that are responsible for translating new protein, and smooth **endoplasmic reticulum** (**ER**) that can sequester and release calcium.

In considering the above description, it is important to know that this is a static representation of a dynamic state of affairs. In reality the molecular composition of synapses constantly changes. Some believe that the entire complement of molecules—receptors, scaffolding protein, kinases, and so forth—can turn over two to three times a day (Ehlers, 2003). Where do these molecules go? Some degrade but it is often the case that they move from one spine to another adjacent spine on the same dendrite. Some of this movement is due to passive diffusion processes and some is due to active **endocytosis** and **exocytosis**—processes that deliver molecules to and from the plasma membrane. Moreover, there is *competition among spines* for these synaptic proteins. An LTP-inducing stimulus engages processes that modify and rearrange the existing molecular composition of spines.

Signaling Cascades

Excitatory synapses are modified by synaptic activity that begins when glutamate is released by the presynaptic neuron. This activity initiates a set of events—**signaling cascades** that are involved in every aspect of synaptic modification. The fundamental properties of a generic signaling cascade are illustrated in Figure 2.15, which presents the components involved in the cascade—first messenger, second messenger, and target proteins (kinases and phosphatases)—and the sequence of the cascades.

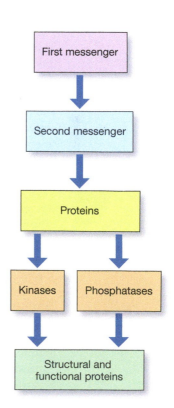

FIRST AND SECOND MESSENGERS   The signaling cascade is initiated when a **first messenger**—an extracellular substance, such as a neurotransmitter (for example, glutamate) or a hormone—binds to a cell-surface receptor and initiates intracellular activity. The second step in the cascade involves **second messengers**—molecules that relay signals from receptors on the cell surface to target molecules inside the cell. There are multiple second messengers (see Siegelbaum et al., 2000 for a detailed review), including calcium, **cyclic adenosine monophosphates (cAMP)**, and **inositol triphosphate (IP3)**.

Second messengers are not proteins, so the number of second messenger molecules can be increased rapidly when a neurotransmitter or hormone binds to membrane receptors. This rapid increase is possible because their synthesis does not depend on the relatively slower transcription and translation processes (described in detail in Chapter 5). The

FIGURE 2.15 The signaling cascade is initiated when a first messenger—an extracellular substance, such as a neurotransmitter (for example, glutamate) or a hormone—binds to a cell-surface receptor and initiates intracellular activity. The second step in the cascade involves second messengers—molecules that relay signals from receptors on the cell surface to target intracellular protein kinases and phosphatases that then target other proteins.

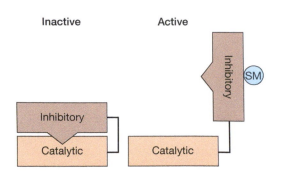

FIGURE 2.16 Kinases are composed of an inhibitory and regulatory domain. In its normal inactive state the catalytic unit is unable to phosphorylate other proteins. The binding of a second messenger (SM) to the inhibitory domain exposes the catalytic unit and puts the kinase in an active state, enabling it to carry out its phosphorylation function.

rapid production of second messenger molecules provides a way *to amplify the effect* of the first messenger inside the cell.

PROTEIN KINASES AND PHOSPHATASES   Once generated, second messengers diffuse and target two classes of proteins, **kinases** and **phosphatases**. A protein kinase is an enzyme that modifies other proteins by chemically adding phosphate groups to them. This process, called **phosphorylation**, can change the protein's cellular location, its ability to associate with other proteins, or its enzyme activity.

A prototypical protein kinase is composed of two domains—a regulatory–inhibitory domain and a catalytic domain. The catalytic domain carries out the phosphorylation function of the kinase. However, this activity is normally inhibited by the regulatory domain. Thus, a kinase can be in two states: (1) it can be inactive and unable to phosphorylate other proteins or (2) it can be active and able to phosphorylate other proteins (including other kinases). To become active the catalytic unit must be released from the inhibitory unit. Second messengers target the inhibitory domain, unfold it, and thereby expose and activate the catalytic domain (Figure 2.16). Dissociation of the second messenger can return the kinase to its inactive state. In this way, second messengers regulate the state (inactive or active) of kinases and thus their function. Second messengers also target proteins called phosphatases. These proteins are designed to remove phosphates from proteins and by doing so play an important role in regulating cellular activity.

An Organizing Framework: Three Principles

The number of molecules and biochemical interactions that contribute to altering synaptic connections is enormous, and it is far beyond the scope of this book to provide a complete account of what is known. A more modest goal is to identify some of the key outcomes and processes and provide a coherent framework for understanding how this happens. Three principles help to organize the complexities of the field.

1. The duration of LTP can vary.

2. The duration of LTP depends on the set of molecular processes engaged by synaptic activity.

3. Synapses are strengthened and maintained in a sequence of temporal, distinct but overlapping processes.

The Duration of LTP Can Vary

The duration of long-term potentiation depends on the parameters of the inducing stimulus. Generally speaking, as the intensity of the inducing stimulus increases so does the duration of LTP. For example, a **theta-burst stimulation (TBS)** protocol has been used in many important experiments to induce LTP because it models a natural pattern of neural activity occurring in the hippocampus when a rodent is exploring a novel environment (Larson et al., 1993). The invention of the TBS protocol resulted when Gary Lynch, Ursula Staubli, and John Lawson realized that the natural sniffing behavior of rodents was at virtually the same frequency as the naturally occurring hippocampal theta rhythm (Lynch, 2003).

One theta burst consists of trains of 10 × 100-Hz bursts (5 pulses per burst) with a 200-millisecond interval between bursts. Figure 2.17 illustrates a family of LTP functions that can be produced by varying the number of theta bursts. Note that the duration of LTP increases with the number of theta bursts. The data illustrated in this figure have two implications: (1) changes in synaptic

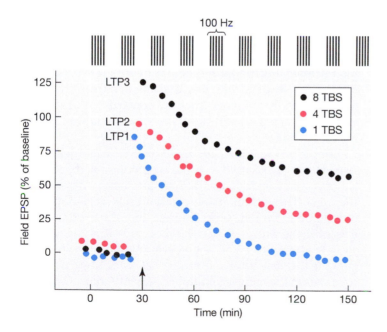

FIGURE 2.17 The number of theta-burst stimuli (TBS) determines the duration of LTP. This family of LTP functions implies that changes in synaptic strength can vary in duration and may have different molecular bases. A fundamental goal of neurobiologists is to understand these differences. (After C. R. Raymond and S. J. Redman. 2002. *J Neurophysiol* 88: 249–255.)

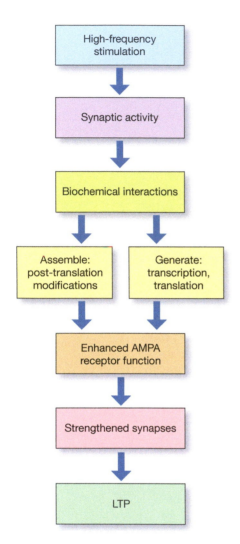

FIGURE 2.18 When high-frequency stimulation generates synaptic activity, biochemical interactions are initiated that lead to several functional outcomes that are critical to the induction of LTP. Post-translation modification processes assemble and rearrange existing proteins. Transcription and translation processes generate new proteins. A major consequence of these processes is that the contribution of AMPA receptors to synaptic depolarization is enhanced, that is, synapses are strengthened.

strength can vary in duration and (2) the molecular basis of these synaptic changes is likely different. This being the case, then an important goal is to discover the variation in the molecular processes that are associated with the variation in the duration of LTP.

Molecular Processes Determine LTP Durability

Three general categories of molecular events contribute to LTP: (1) **transcription** processes that are engaged to produce the **messenger ribonucleic acid (mRNA)** needed to make additional proteins, (2) **translation** processes that convert the mRNA into protein (Figure 2.18), and (3) **post-translation processes** that modify and rearrange existing synaptic proteins. Post-translation processes operating in spines can dramatically change the strength of synapses. However, the generation of new protein can be necessary to ensure these changes will endure. This will occur when synaptic activity is strong enough to initiate transcription processes that generate mRNA needed for creating new protein and/or the translation of mRNA into protein, also called **protein synthesis**.

Synapses Are Strengthened and Maintained in Stages

Changes in synaptic strength can occur within a minute or so following the induction stimulus. However, these potentiated synapses are not stable and will revert back to their prepotentiated state unless the inducing stimulus initiates additional molecular events (Lynch et al., 2007). This leads to the idea that the synaptic changes that support the memory trace are constructed in stages, as hypothesized by William James (see Chapter 1 and McGaugh, 2000).

Chapters 3 to 8 are organized around this idea, and these stages are referred to as the (a) generation, (b) stabilization, (c) consolidation, and (d) maintenance phases (Figure 2.19). These chapters reveal that each stage depends on unique molecular processes and that the primary targets of these processes are the reorganization of AMPA receptor trafficking and actin cytoskeleton proteins that provide the structural and functional scaffolding needed to maintain the increased number of AMPA receptors. Together, these outcomes change the structure and function of the synapses activated by stimulation that induces LTP.

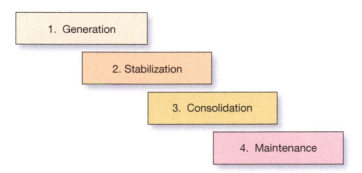

FIGURE 2.19   Changes in synaptic strength that support LTP evolve in four overlapping stages and can be identified by the unique molecular processes that support each stage.

Summary

From the brain's perspective, memories are the product of modified synaptic connections among collections of neurons (neuronal assemblies). Locating the relevant synapses that link the neurons is a difficult task. However, the discovery of LTP provided a methodology that enabled neurobiologists to study the molecular underpinnings of experience-induced changes in synaptic strength.

Neurons communicate through chemical synapses. The release of excitatory neurotransmitters by the presynaptic neuron causes receptors on the postsynaptic neuron to allow positive ions to enter the cell and produce what is called synaptic depolarization—the intracellular fluid becomes less negative compared to the extracellular fluid.

To produce LTP, the experimenter applies electrical stimulation to axon fibers to cause the release of neurotransmitters to a population of synapses on postsynaptic neurons. An extracellular electrode measures positive ions flowing out of the extracellular fluid—the field potential (fEPSP). The field potential is assumed to indirectly measure the depolarization of hundreds of synapses on neurons surrounding the recording electrode. LTP is thought to represent the strengthening of synapses activated by the inducing stimulus—an increase in the capacity of these synapses to influx positive ions in response to the test stimulus. The strength of synapses can also be weakened by synaptic activity. This is called long-term depression and is produced by applying long-lasting, low-frequency stimulation.

It is useful to think of the components of a synapse as biochemical factors, with each component containing molecules needed to accomplish specific functions. Signaling cascades can modify and rearrange the existing molecules and can generate new molecules through activating translation and transcription processes. Potentiated synapses can have different durations, which are determined by the molecular processes activated by the inducing stimulus. These processes are described in the next five chapters within a framework that assumes that the synaptic changes that support the memory trace evolve in overlapping stages—generation, stabilization, consolidation, and maintenance.

References

Andersen, P. (1975). Organization of hippocampal neurons and their interconnections. In R. L. Isaacson and K. H. Pribram (Eds.), *The Hippocampus, Volume 1* (pp. 155–175). Boston: Springer.

Andersen, P. (2004). Per Andersen. In L. R. Squire (Ed.), *The History of Neuroscience in Autobiography* (pp. 2–3). San Diego: Academic Press.

Andersen, P., Bliss, T. V., and Skrede, K. K. (1971). Lamellar organization of hippocampal excitatory pathways. *Experimental Brain Research, 13*, 222–238.

Bear, M. F. (2003). Bidirectional synaptic plasticity: from theory to reality. *Philosophical Transactions of the Royal Society of London Series B, 358*, 649–655.

Bliss, T. V. and Gardner-Medwin, A. R. (1973). Long-lasting potentiation of synaptic transmission in the dentate area of the unanaesthetized rabbit following stimulation of the perforant path. *Journal of Physiology, 232*, 357–374.

Bliss, T. V. and Lømo, T. (1973). Long-lasting potentiation of synaptic transmission in the dentate area of the anaesthetized rabbit following stimulation of the perforant path. *Journal of Physiology, 232*, 331–356.

Dityateve, A. and Fellin, T. (2008). Extracellular matrix in plasticity and epileptogenesis. *Neuron Glia Biology, 4*, 235–247.

Dudek, S. M. and Bear, M. F. (1992). Homosynaptic long-term depression in area CA1 of hippocampus and effects of N-methyl-D-aspartate receptor blockade. *Proceedings of the National Academy of Sciences USA, 89*, 4363–4367.

Ehlers, M. D. (2003). Activity level controls postsynaptic composition and signaling via the ubiquitin-proteasome system. *Nature Neuroscience, 6*, 231–242.

Eichenbaum, H. and Cohen, N. J. (2001). *From Conditioning to Conscious Recollection: Memory Systems of the Brain.* Oxford: Oxford University Press.

Hebb, D. O. (1949). *Organization of Behavior.* New York: John Wiley & Sons, Inc.

Hebb, D. O. (1966). *A Textbook of Psychology.* Philadelphia: W. B. Saunders Company.

Kim, E. and Sheng, M. (2009). The postsynaptic density. *Current Biology, 19*, 723–724.

Larson, J., Xiao, P., and Lynch, G. (1993). Reversal of LTP by theta frequency stimulation. *Brain Research, 600*, 97–102.

Lømo, T. (1966). Frequency potentiation of excitatory synaptic activity in the dentate area of the hippocampal formation. *Acta Physiologica Scandinavia, 68*, 128.

Lømo, T. (2016). Scientific discoveries: what is required for lasting impact. *Annual Review of Physiology, 78*, 1–21.

Lynch, G. (2003). Long-term potentiation in the Eocene. *Philosophical Translations of the Royal Society B, 358*, 625–628.

Lynch, G. and Baudry, M. (1984). The biochemistry of memory: a new and specific hypothesis. *Science*, *224*, 1057–1063.

Lynch, G., Rex, C. S., and Gall, C. M. (2007). LTP consolidation: Substrates, explanatory power, and functional significance. *Neuropharmacology*, *52*, 12–23.

McGaugh, J. L. (2000). Memory: a century of consolidation. *Science*, *287*, 248–251.

Nicoll, R. A. (2017). A brief history of long-term potentiation. *Neuron*, *93*, 281–290.

Sheng, M. and Hoogenraad. (2007). The postsynaptic architecture of excitatory synapses: a more quantitative view. *Annual Review of Biochemistry*, *76*, 823–847.

Siegelbaum, S. A., Schwartz, J. H., and Kandel, E. R. (2000). Modulation of synaptic transmission: second messengers. In E. R. Kandel, J. H. Schwartz, and T. H. Jessell (Eds.), *Principles of Neural Science, Fourth Edition* (pp. 229–239). New York: McGraw-Hill Companies.

Skrede, K. K. and Westgaard, R. R. (1971). The transverse hippocampal slice: a well-defined cortical structure maintained invitro. *Brain Research*, *35*, 589–593.

Sweat, J. D. (2003). *Mechanisms of Memory*. London: Academic Press.

Yamamoto, C. and McIlwain, H. (1966). Potentials evoked in vitro in preparations from the mammalian brain. *Nature*, *210*, 1055–1056.

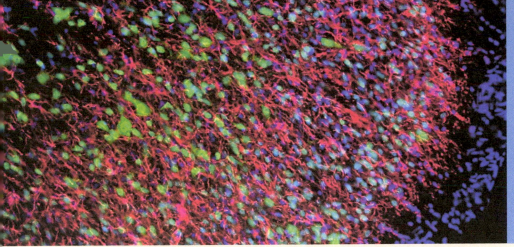

Courtesy of Heidi E. W. Day

3

Generating Long-Term Potentiation

At first glance the idea that one can understand the synaptic basis of memory by studying LTP, especially in a slice of hippocampal tissue, might seem preposterous. Thus, Gary Lynch, in recalling his response to one of the first papers reporting the use of hippocampal slices (Yamamoto and McIlwain, 1966), remarked:

> I simply couldn't picture slices of adult brain retaining their in vivo physiological properties. However, if this was the case, and the published results were certainly impressive, then it seemed that a revolution was at hand. Seen parochially, it meant that we would not have to search for a small population of synapses in a very large place but instead could stimulate multiple fiber populations converging on a defined dendritic location. (G. Lynch. 2003. *Phil Trans R Soc Lond B* 358: 625–628.)

The consensus that LTP is a suitable model for studying memory raises two questions.

1. What synaptic changes take place that produce LTP?
2. What processes bring about the change?

Regarding the first question, a heated debate centered on two general possibilities: LTP is the result of (1) presynaptic changes that increase the release of glutamate or (2) postsynaptic changes that increase the postsynaptic neuron's sensitivity to glutamate. Many years of debate were required to settle the issue. For the moment, while not denying that there can be presynaptic changes, it is safe to assume that important postsynaptic changes are essential to LTP (Nicoll, 2017; Vincent-Lamarre et al., 2018). What follows is a description of some of the key elements of the signal processes that generate these postsynaptic changes, focusing on the role of glutamate receptors and post-translation processes in generating LTP.

The Role of Glutamate Receptors

The first step toward producing LTP occurs when the inducing stimulus generates sufficient activity in the presynaptic terminal to release the first messenger glutamate, which can then bind to glutamate receptors located in dendritic spines on the postsynaptic neuron. Some glutamate receptors are called **ionotropic receptors** or ligand-gated channels. They are constructed from four or five protein subunits that come together to form a potential channel or pore (Figure 3.1). These receptors span the cell membrane; they protrude outside the cell as well as inside the cell and are positioned to interact with signaling molecules

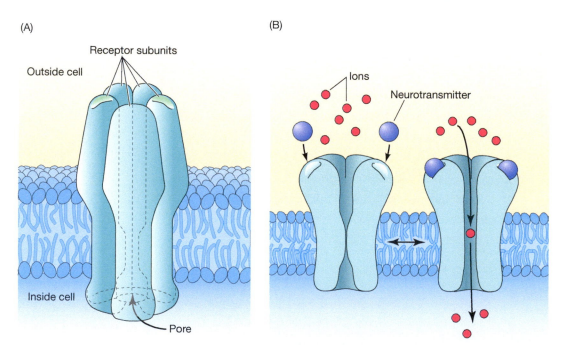

FIGURE 3.1   (A) Ionotropic receptors are located in the plasma membrane. (B) When a neurotransmitter binds to the receptor, the channel or pore opens and allows ions such as Na^+ and Ca^{2+} to enter the cell.

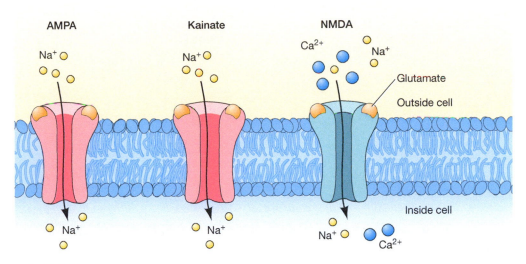

FIGURE 3.2 There are three types of glutamate receptors. AMPA and NMDA receptors, which are located in dendritic spines, play a major role in the induction and expression of LTP. When glutamate binds to these receptors their channels open and positively charged ions in the extracellular fluid (Na$^+$ and Ca^{2+}) enter the neuron.

present in both the extracellular space and the **cytosol** (the internal fluid of the neuron). They are called ionotropic receptors because, when their channels open, ions such as Na$^+$ or Ca^{2+} can enter the cell. They are called ligand-gated channels because it is the binding of a **ligand** (an ion, molecule, or molecular group) that opens the channel. Thus, glutamate is also a ligand that binds to the site on glutamate receptors and changes the conformation or shape of the receptor so that the channel is briefly open and ions can enter the cell (Figure 3.2).

Glutamate binds to three ionotropic receptors: (1) the a-amino-3-hydroxyl-5-methyl-4-isoxazole-propionate (**AMPA receptor**), (2) the N-methyl-D-aspartate (**NMDA receptor**), and (3) the kainate receptor (see Figure 3.2). However, only the AMPA and NMDA receptors are pertinent to this discussion because they are the primary contributors to long-term potentiation. In studying Figure 3.2 it is important to note that when glutamate binds to AMPA receptors the primary outcome is the influx of sodium into the cell and when it binds to NMDA receptors calcium enters.

LTP Induction Requires NMDA Receptors

Our understanding of how LTP is generated took a giant step forward when Graham Collingridge and his colleagues (Collingridge et al., 1983) used a competitive NMDA receptor **antagonist** (amino-phosphono-valeric acid, abbreviated as APV) to prevent glutamate from binding to the receptor.

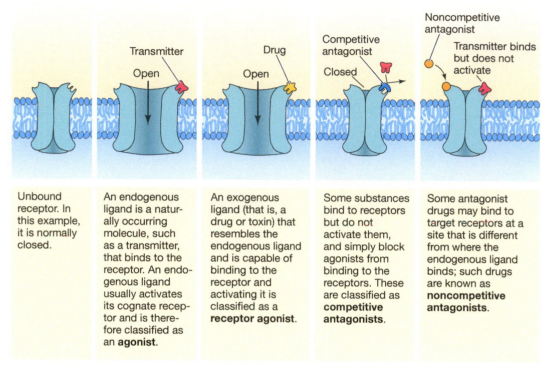

FIGURE 3.3 The agonistic and antagonistic actions of drugs.

(Figure 3.3 illustrates the agonistic and antagonistic actions of drugs on receptors.) Collingridge made two important observations: (1) applying APV before delivering the induction stimulus prevented the generation of LTP (Figure 3.4), but (2) if APV was applied during the test phase (after LTP had been induced) the test stimulus still evoked an enhanced field potential. Collingridge concluded that NMDA receptors may be necessary for the *induction* of LTP but they are *not* necessary for the *expression* of LTP. (Recall that expression of LTP is measured as the enhanced field potential compared to baseline.) Both conclusions are now widely accepted as correct. The phrase "NMDA receptor-dependent LTP" is often used to denote the special importance of the NMDA receptor to the induction–generation of LTP.

At roughly the same time, Gary Lynch (Lynch et al., 1983, p. 719) discovered that LTP depended on the presence of calcium in the postsynaptic neuron and concluded "…that LTP is caused by a modification of the postsynaptic neuron and that its induction depends on the level of free calcium." Shortly thereafter it was reported that NMDA receptors are highly permeable to calcium (Ascher and Nowak, 1988; MacDermott et al., 1986). Thus, the NMDA receptor is a gateway to LTP because it can allow the second messenger calcium to enter the dendritic spines.

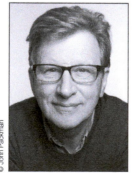

Graham Collingridge

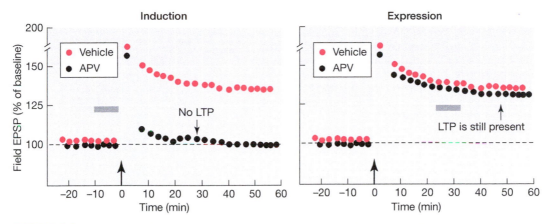

FIGURE 3.4   APV, an NMDA receptor antagonist, prevents the induction of LTP but has no effect on its expression. The bar in each figure represents the application of the drugs—APV or the vehicle. (After G. L. Collingridge et al. 1983. *J Physiol* 34: 334–345.)

Two Events Open the NMDA Channel

An additional observation completed the basic story. Specifically, activating the NMDA receptor is *voltage dependent*. Not only must glutamate bind to the receptor, the postsynaptic membrane must depolarize (Malenka et al., 1989). This step is necessary because at the resting membrane potential the magnesium ion (Mg^{2+}) occupies the NMDA receptor and the membrane must depolarize to remove the Mg^{2+} block and allow the influx of calcium (Figure 3.5).

In summary, the induction of LTP begins when extracellular calcium enters the spine via the NMDA calcium channels. Opening the calcium channel requires two events: (1) the binding of glutamate and (2) the depolarization of the postsynaptic membrane. Although the opening of the NMDA receptor channel is critical for the induction of LTP, the positive calcium ions it influxes contribute little or nothing to the expression of LTP.

Increase in AMPA Receptors Supports LTP Expression

Given that NMDA receptors do not contribute to the expression of LTP, then other receptors must be critical. There is agreement that LTP is expressed by the binding of glutamate to AMPA receptors (Nicoll, 2017). This conclusion is based in part on the observation that pharmacological agents that antagonize AMPA receptors prevent the expression of LTP (Dunwiddie et al., 1978; Kauer et al., 1988; Muller et al., 1988). This makes sense because LTP, as measured by field potential, reflects the rate at which Na^+ is leaving the extracellular fluid (and entering the postsynaptic neuron via AMPA receptors). Consequently, one can conclude: (a) the expression of LTP reflects an increase in the sensitivity of the postsynaptic neuron to glutamate release and (b) this increase in some way centers on a change in the contribution of AMPA receptors.

FIGURE 3.5 (A) The NMDA receptor binds to glutamate. It also binds to Mg^{2+} (sometimes called the magnesium plug) because Mg^{2+} binds to the NMDA channel. (B) The opening of the NMDA receptor requires two events: (1) glutamate must bind to the receptor and (2) the cell must depolarize. When this happens, the magnesium plug is removed and Ca^{2+} can enter the cell.

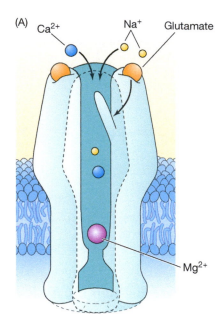

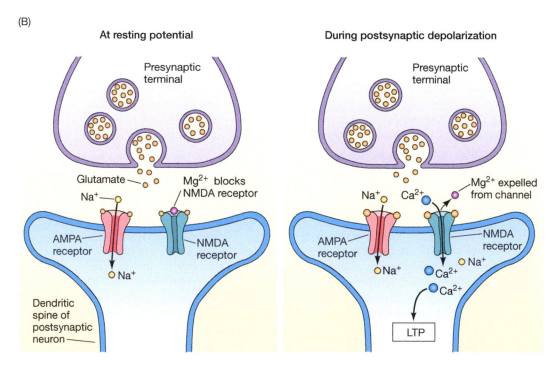

In principle this change could reflect two outcomes: (1) the properties of existing AMPA receptors change so that in response to glutamate their channels open longer and thus allow more Na⁺ to enter the spine or (2) processes are engaged that increase the number of AMPA receptors in dendritic spines. It is noteworthy that more than 30 years ago, Gary Lynch and Michel Baudry (1984) proposed that LTP (and memory storage) was the result of an increase in the number of glutamate receptors in the spine (AMPA receptors had not been identified at that time). This general idea proved to be correct (Figure 3.6). Two prominent researchers, Robert Malenka and Mark Bear, concluded: "It now appears safe to state that a major mechanism for the expression of LTP involves increasing the number of AMPA receptors in the plasma membrane at synapses via activity-dependent changes in AMPA receptor trafficking" (Malenka and Bear, 2004, p. 7). Thus, the fundamental challenge is to understand the biochemical–molecular processes that regulate AMPA receptor trafficking.

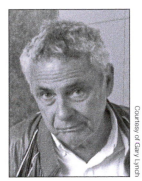

Gary Lynch

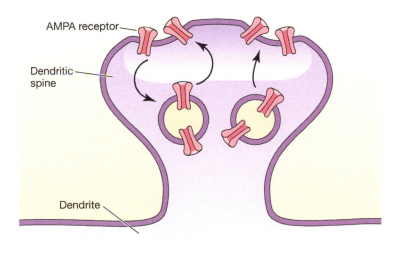

FIGURE 3.6 The complementary ideas that an LTP-inducing stimulus can rapidly increase the number of AMPA receptors in the spines and that this is the fundamental outcome that supports the expression of LTP are now central principles of the field. AMPA receptors traffic into and out of dendritic spines. AMPA trafficking is regulated constitutively (double arrows) and by synaptic activity (single arrow). Constitutive trafficking routinely cycles AMPA receptors into and out of dendritic spines, while synaptic activity is thought to deliver new AMPA receptors to them.

Post-Translation Processes

The molecular machinery needed to generate LTP is available in dendritic spines (see previous Figure 2.14) and only requires the modification and rearrangement of existing proteins. No new proteins need to be generated. When calcium enters the spine via NMDA receptors, signaling cascades are set in motion to produce two major outcomes: (1) AMPA receptors are rapidly delivered to the postsynaptic density and (2) the actin cytoskeleton in the spine head is temporarily degraded.

AMPA Receptor Trafficking

The concept of AMPA receptor trafficking is relatively new. An earlier view was that receptors were immobile at central synapses. This view changed when neuroscientists understood that the fluid composition of neurons would permit diffusion of membrane proteins (such as receptors and scaffolding proteins) and it was discovered that AMPA receptors randomly diffuse laterally around the extrasynaptic region of dendritic spines (Choquet, 2018). During this period, Xiaping Xie (Xie et al., 1997) suggested that in unpotentiated synapses AMPA receptors are widely distributed and many are located beyond the range where they can receive an effective concentration of released glutamate. According to this view, the consequence of LTP induction is lateral diffusion of AMPA receptors so that they cluster and more closely align with presynaptic sites where glutamate is released (Xie et al., 1997). Daniel Choquet (Borgdorff and Choquet, 2002) confirmed this view by tracking the movement of AMPA receptors. These experiments and many others (Choquet, 2018) produced the understanding of AMPA receptor trafficking described below.

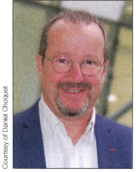

Courtesy of Daniel Choquet

Daniel Choquet

CONSTITUTIVE TRAFFICKING   AMPA receptor trafficking is continuous and regulated by what are called **constitutive trafficking** processes—cycling of AMPA receptors into and out of dendritic spines (illustrated in Figure 3.7). AMPA receptors are found both in the cell and on the plasma membrane. Some of these receptors are present in the postsynaptic density (PSD) where they are best positioned to respond to glutamate. Others are not in the PSD and are referred to as nonsynaptic or extrasynaptic receptors. In close proximity to the PSD is a region called the **endocytotic zone** (Petrini et al., 2009) that contains complex molecules designed to capture AMPA receptors leaving the PSD and to repackage them in **endosomes** for recycling to the membrane. The role of synaptic activity produced by an LTP-inducing stimulus is to reorganize the constitutive processes to increase the number of AMPA receptors immobilized in the PSD (see Figure 3.7).

Constitutive processes deliver AMPA receptors to the PSD in three steps (Derkach et al., 2007; Opazo et al., 2010).

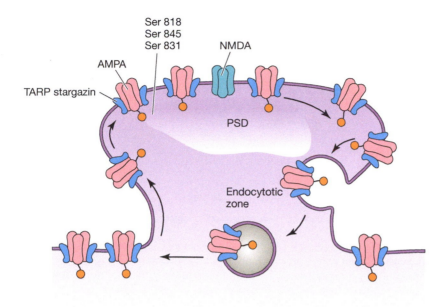

FIGURE 3.7   AMPA receptors are in constant random motion laterally diffusing along the plasma membrane where they enter and leave the PSD. Extrasynaptic receptors are more mobile than those in the PSD. Receptors cycling through the PSD might be captured in the endocytotic zone and packaged for recycling.

1. Intracellular vesicles containing AMPA receptors (endosomes) are mobilized to deliver the receptors to the perisynaptic region, a region near the PSD.

2. These receptors then diffuse somewhat randomly but laterally along the membrane to enter the PSD.

3. Some receptors are trapped in the PSD and immobilized for some period of time and others leave the PSD and are captured in the endocytotic zone for recycling.

The job of constitutive trafficking processes is to ensure that synapses have the necessary supply of AMPA receptors to support synaptic transmission and increase synaptic strength. AMPA receptors can be composed of different subunits (GluA1, GluA2, GluA3, GluA4). Under basal conditions they contain GluA2 subunits. The initial induction of LTP, however, is primarily the result of increasing the number of AMPA receptors composed of GluA1 subunits (sometimes referred to as GluA2-lacking AMPA receptors). Such GluA1 AMPA receptors have phosphorylation sites (Ser 818, Ser 831, Ser 845) that contribute

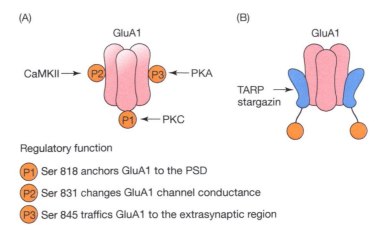

(A)

GluA1

CaMKII → P2 | P3 ← PKA

P1 ← PKC

Regulatory function

P1 Ser 818 anchors GluA1 to the PSD

P2 Ser 831 changes GluA1 channel conductance

P3 Ser 845 traffics GluA1 to the extrasynaptic region

(B)

GluA1

TARP → stargazin

FIGURE 3.8 (A) AMPA receptors have serine sites that when phosphorylated by different kinases make different contributions to receptor trafficking and channel conductance. Protein kinase A (PKA) phosphorylates the Ser 845 site to traffic the receptor to the extrasynaptic region. Protein kinase C (PKC) phosphorylates the Ser 818 site and helps to anchor the receptor to the postsynaptic density. CaMKII phosphorylates the Ser 831 site and changes the channel, allowing it to influx calcium as well as sodium. (B) Transmembrane AMPA receptor regulatory proteins (TARPs) also co-assemble with AMPA receptors. TARPs called stargazin are critical to trapping AMPA receptors in the PSD.

to this outcome (Figure 3.8A). Transmembrane AMPA receptor regulatory proteins, called **TARPs**, also co-assemble with AMPA receptors and are critical to trapping them in the PSD (Figure 3.8B).

How does the LTP-inducing stimulus increase the number of these AMPA receptors trapped or immobilized in the PSD? There is a two-part answer to this question. One answer centers on the capture of additional receptors that are laterally diffusing around the plasma membrane; the other centers on recycling endosomes.

LATERAL DIFFUSION   Opazo et al. (2010) have described this process. It requires the interaction of three molecules: (1) an important and unusual kinase, calcium/calmodulin-dependent protein kinase II (called **CaMKII**, see Box 3.1), discovered by Mary Kennedy (Kennedy et al., 1983); (2) a TARP called **stargazin**; and (3) PSD-95 scaffolding proteins. In their proposal, PSD-95 scaffolding proteins form potential "slots" for trapping AMPA receptors that are laterally diffusing through the PSD. For the slots to capture the receptors requires that CaMKII phosphorylate serine residues of the AMPA/stargazin complex (Opazo et al., 2010). This releases stargazin from the membrane and facilitates its binding to PSD-95. It is this binding of stargazin to PSD-95 that traps additional AMPA receptors in the postsynaptic density (Bats et al., 2007). As CaMKII phosphorylates more of the stargazin serine residues, the receptors become more stable. In support of the essential role

BOX 3.1 CaMKII Autophosphorylates

(A)

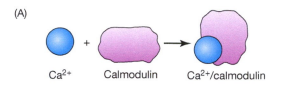

Ca^{2+} Calmodulin   Ca^{2+}/calmodulin

The protein **calmodulin** serves as a surrogate for second-messenger calcium and undergoes a conformational change when it binds to calcium. This new shape enables it to bind to other proteins that do not have Ca^{2+} binding sites. A primary target is CaMKII.

(B)

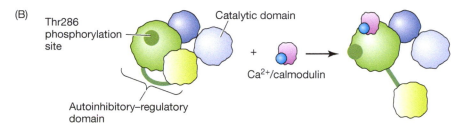

Thr286 phosphorylation site

Catalytic domain

Ca^{2+}/calmodulin

Autoinhibitory–regulatory domain

The CaMKII subunit consists of two domains, an autoinhibitory–regulatory domain and a catalytic domain. The regulatory domain contains a phosphorylation site Thr286 that is unexposed when the kinase is in an inactive state. Ca^{2+}/calmodulin serves as a second messenger and activates the kinase. This exposes both the catalytic domain and the Thr286. Phosphorylation of this site will also keep the kinase in an active state even when the second messenger dissociates from the regulatory domain.

(C)   CaMKII subunit

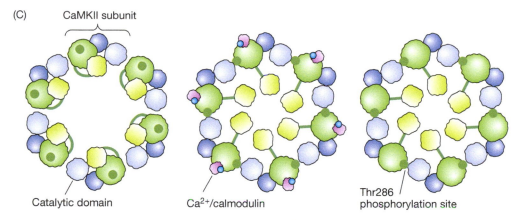

Catalytic domain   Ca^{2+}/calmodulin   Thr286 phosphorylation site

Subunits of the kinase assemble into a ring-like complex called a holoenzyme. When Ca^{2+}/calmodulin binds to the autoinhibitory–regulatory domain of all subunits, the subunits become active and the Thr286 phosphorylation site on the regulatory unit is exposed. Because of the ring-like structure of the holoenzyme, a subunit can now phosphorylate its neighbor. This process of autophosphorylation enables the subunits to remain active even when Ca^{2+}/calmodulin is no longer present. Thus, the holoenzyme can remain in a perpetually active state.

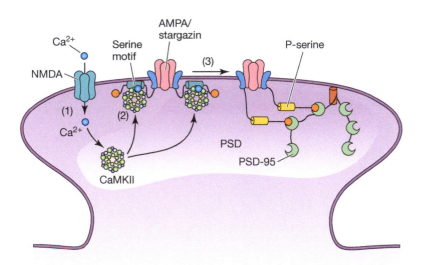

FIGURE 3.9 AMPA receptors become trapped in the PSD when (1) the influx of calcium into the spine via NMDA receptors (2) activates CaMKII. This kinase phosphorylates serine (P-serine) residues on the terminal of the TARP stargazin. This activity releases the terminal from the membrane and (3) facilitates its binding to PSD-95 complexes, thereby trapping the receptor in the PSD. The stability of the trap increases as CaMKII phosphorylates more of the stargazin serine residues.

of the stargazin–PSD-95 coupling in trapping AMPA receptors, it has been reported that, upon binding to glutamate, AMPA receptors dissociate from stargazin with the result of more rapid diffusion of the receptors (Constals et al., 2015; Figure 3.9).

CaMKII not only participates in increasing the contribution of AMPA receptors to synaptic potentials through its trapping role, it also changes the channel properties of the GluA1 AMPA receptors by phosphorylating the Ser 831 site on the receptor. This event allows the channel to influx Ca^{2+} as well as Na^+. For this reason, GluA1 receptors are often also referred to as *calcium-permeable* AMPA receptors. The net result of these effects is a strongly potentiated synapse—one whose ability to influx Na^+ and Ca^{2+} has been significantly but temporarily enhanced.

RECYCLING ENDOSOMES   Michael Ehlers and his colleagues (Wang et al., 2008) reveal that a second process that centers on the regulation of recycling endosomes also is critical to the delivery of AMPA receptors. The initial generation of LTP depends on the rapid trapping in the PSD of already present AMPA receptors randomly diffusing around the extra-synaptic regions of the plasma membrane. Although these receptors are initially trapped, endocytotic processes work to remove them from the

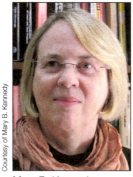

Mary B. Kennedy

PSD. This action could result in the loss of LTP. However, additional *intracellular pools of AMPA receptors* are contained in *recycling endosomes,* and the influx of calcium through NMDA receptors interacts with myosin motor proteins (myosin Vb) so they can attach to an effector complex (Rab11) on the endosome. These motor proteins travel along actin filaments to cargo the endosome containing the receptor to the extrasynaptic regions where the AMPA receptors can then more slowly enter the PSD (Figure 3.10).

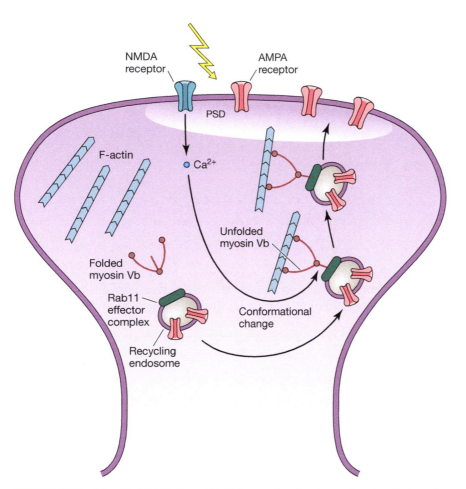

FIGURE 3.10   Neuronal activation of NMDA receptors leads to a localized influx of Ca^{2+} at dendritic spines. This influx induces a Ca^{2+}-dependent conformational change in the motor protein, myosin Vb. The unfolding of myosin Vb exposes a cargo-binding domain, which mediates the recruitment of the motor to the membrane-associated Rab11 effector complex on the recycling endosome. The activated myosin then delivers AMPA receptors to synaptic sites, leading to the localized increase in AMPA receptor density characteristic of LTP. (After E. Perlson and E. Holzbaur. 2008. *Cell* 135: 414–415.)

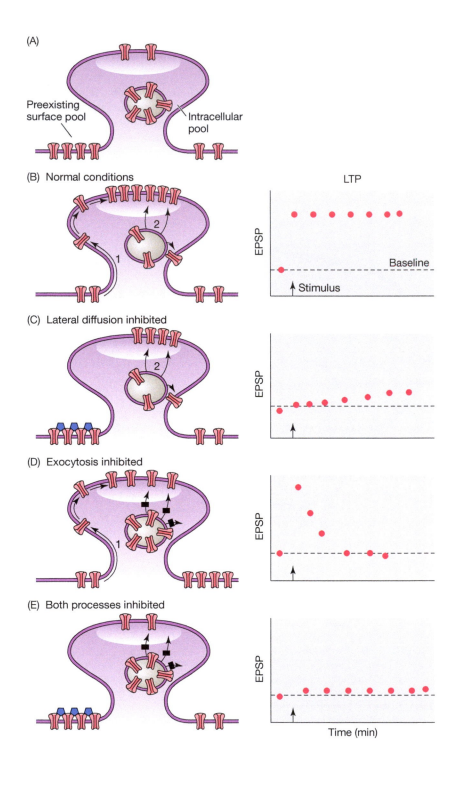

(A)

Preexisting surface pool

Intracellular pool

(B) Normal conditions

LTP

EPSP

Baseline

Stimulus

(C) Lateral diffusion inhibited

EPSP

(D) Exocytosis inhibited

EPSP

(E) Both processes inhibited

EPSP

Time (min)

◀ **FIGURE 3.11**   When LTP is induced, two independent processes deliver AMPA receptors to the PSD. (A) Prior to LTP induction there are preexisting surface pools and intracellular pools of AMPA receptors. (B) Under normal conditions the induction of LTP (1) first initiates the lateral diffusion of receptors in the surface pool into the PSD and (2) then delivers receptors from the intracellular pool by motor proteins (see Figure 3.10) into the PSD and to the surface. This produces LTP that can endure for at least 30 minutes. (C) If lateral diffusion is prevented, then LTP gradually emerges as the AMPA receptors from the intracellular pool are delivered. (D) Inhibiting the delivery of the intracellular pool results in the rapid reduction of LTP, which returns to baseline in about 10 minutes. (E) If both delivery processes are inhibited, the LTP will not be generated. (After A. C. Penn et al. 2017. *Nature* 549: 384–388.)

One conclusion from this discussion is that calcium engages two independent processes to increase the complement of AMPA receptors in the PSD: (1) a rapid trapping of existing AMPA receptors diffusing around the plasma membrane, and (2) a slower acting exocytosis of additional pools of AMPA receptors (contained in endosomes) to the plasma membrane. Recent research has supported this conclusion. Penn et al. (2017) found that if the diffusion of AMPA receptors was prevented at the time of the induction stimulus, the early phase of LTP was prevented, but within about 10 minutes LTP emerged. In contrast, if the delivery of new AMPA receptors contained in the endosomes was prevented, a strong LTP rapidly emerged but it quickly returned to its baseline state. When both lateral diffusion and exocytosis were prevented there was no LTP (Figure 3.11).

Actin Cytoskeleton Degradation

The rapid insertion of AMPA receptors into synapses requires not only the reorganization of AMPA receptor trafficking but also the rapid degradation of the network of actin proteins that construct the cytoskeleton architecture of the spine (see Gu et al., 2010; Lynch and Baudry, 1984; Lynch et al., 2007; Ouyang et al., 2005). Actin filaments form a meshlike structure that poses a barrier to the plasma membrane. Thus, it is important that the actin cytoskeleton be degraded (Figure 3.12) so that AMPA receptors and other proteins can be inserted rapidly into the postsynaptic density (Gu et al., 2010; Ouyang et al., 2005).

The regulation of actin dynamics is the subject of the next chapter where it is discussed in more detail. It is sufficient here to note that Lynch and Baudry (1984) proposed that NMDA-dependent Ca^{2+} is critical to the induction of LTP because it activates a signaling cascade that degrades the actin cytoskeleton. This cascade involved **calpains**, which belong to a class of enzymes called **proteases**, that can degrade proteins. One of the targets is an actin-binding protein, **spectrin**, that links the actin cytoskeleton to the plasma member. The Lynch–Baudry actin degradation hypothesis was supported when it was confirmed that calpain degrades spectrins (Simon et al., 1984) and that high-frequency stimulation used to induce LTP initiated calpain activation and spectrin degradation (Lynch et al., 1982). Thus, a $Ca^{2+} \rightarrow$ calpain $\rightarrow$ spectrin degradation signaling cascade degrades the actin network to allow rapid insertion of AMPA receptors into the PSD (Lynch et al., 2007; see Figure 3.12).

FIGURE 3.12 (A) Filament actin in the spine head is crosslinked with spectrins. (B) The protease calpain is activated when calcium enters the spine through the NMDA receptors. Calpain degrades spectrins and facilitates the disassembling of actin. (C) This activity contributes to the rapid insertion of additional AMPA receptors in the PSD.

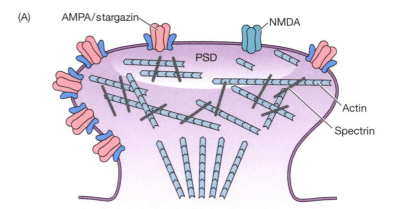

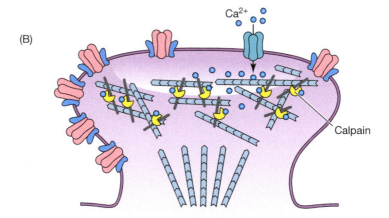

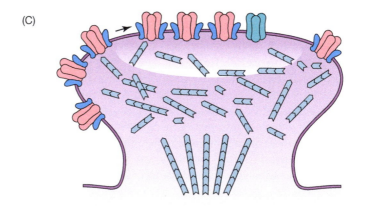

Summary

The initial generation of LTP is the result of synergistic signaling cascades that reorganize (a) constitutive AMPA receptor membrane trafficking processes and (b) actin cytoskeleton proteins. These cascades are initiated by the binding of glutamate to NMDA and AMPA receptors to open NMDA calcium channels. Ca^{2+} and its surrogate, calmodulin, target key kinases (such as CaMKII) that phosphorylate serine sites on the GluA1 receptor complex, including stargazin. These processes deliver and trap the GluA1 receptor complex to existing PSD-95 scaffolding proteins and thus disrupt the normal lateral diffusion of these receptors out of the synapse. This is followed by the delivery of additional intracellular pools of AMPA receptors located in recycling endosomes to the plasma membrane.

References

Ascher, P. and Nowak, L. (1988). The role of divalent cations in the N-methyl-D-aspartate responses of mouse central neurones in culture. *Journal of Physiology, 399,* 247–266.

Bats, C., Groc, L., and Choquet, D. (2007). The interaction between stargazin and PSD-95 regulates AMPA receptor surface trafficking. *Neuron, 5,* 719–734.

Borgdorff, A. J. and Choquet, D. (2002). Regulation of AMPA receptor lateral movements. *Nature, 417,* 649–653.

Choquet, D. (2018). Linking nanoscale dynamics of AMPA receptor organization to plasticity of excitatory synapses and learning. *Journal of Neuroscience, 38,* 9318–9329.

Collingridge, G. L., Kehl, S. J., and McLennan, H. (1983). Excitatory amino acids in synaptic transmission in the Schaffer collateral commissural pathway of the rat hippocampus. *Journal of Physiology, 334,* 33–46.

Constals, A., Penn, A. C., Compans, B., Toulme, E., Phillipat, A., Marais, S., Retailleau, N., Hafner, A. S., Coussen, F., Hosy, E., and Choquet, D. (2015). Glutamate-induced AMPA receptor desensitization increases their mobility and modulates short-term plasticity through unbinding from stargazin. *Neuron, 85,* 787–803.

Derkach, V. A., Oh, M. C., Guire, E. S., and Soderling, T. R. (2007). Regulatory mechanisms of AMPA receptors in synaptic plasticity. *Nature Reviews Neuroscience, 8,* 8101–8113.

Dunwiddie, T., Madison, D., and Lynch, G. (1978). Synaptic transmission is required for initiation of long-term potentiation. *Brain Research, 14,* 413–417.

Gu, J., Lee, C. W., Fan, Y., Komlos, D., Tang, X., Sun, C., Yu, K., Hartzell, H. C., Chen, G., Bamburg, J. R., and Zheng, J. Q. (2010). ADF/cofilin-mediated actin dynamics regulate AMPA receptor trafficking during synaptic plasticity. *Nature Neuroscience, 13,* 1208–1216.

Kauer, J. A., Malenka, R. C., and Nicoll, R. A. (1988). A persistent postsynaptic modification mediates long-term potentiation in the hippocampus. *Neuron, 1,* 911–917.

Kennedy, M. B., Bennett, M. K., and Erondu, N. E. (1983). Biochemical and immunochemical evidence that the "major postsynaptic density protein" is a subunit of a calmodulin-dependent protein kinase. *Proceedings of the National Academy of Sciences USA, 80,* 7357–7361.

Lynch, G. (2003). Long-term potentiation in the Eocene. *Philosophical Transactions of the Royal Society B Biological Sciences, 358,* 625–628.

Lynch, G. and Baudry, M. (1984). The biochemistry of memory: a new and specific hypothesis. *Science, 224,* 1057–1063.

Lynch, G., Halpain, S., and Baudry, M. (1982). Effects of high-frequency synaptic stimulation on glutamate receptor binding studied with a modified in vitro hippocampal slice preparation. *Brain Research, 244,* 101–111.

Lynch, G., Larson, J., Kelso, S., Barrionuevo, G., and Schottler, F. (1983). Intracellular injections of EGTA block induction of hippocampal long-term potentiation. *Nature, 305,* 719–721.

Lynch, G., Rex, C. S., and Gall, C. M. (2007). LTP consolidation: substrates, explanatory power, and functional significance. *Neuropharmacology, 52,* 12–23.

MacDermott, A. B., Mayer, M. L., Westbrook, G. L., Smith, S. J., and Barker, J. L. (1986). NMDA-receptor activation increases cytoplasmic calcium concentration in cultured spinal cord neurones. *Nature, 321,* 519–522.

Malenka, R. C. and Bear, M. F. (2004). LTP and LTD: an embarrassment of riches. *Neuron, 44,* 5–21.

Malenka, R. C., Kauer, J. A., Perkel, D. J., and Nicoll, R. A. (1989). The impact of postsynaptic calcium on synaptic transmission—its role in long-term potentiation. *Trends in Neuroscience, 12,* 444–450.

Muller, D., Joly, M., and Lynch, G. (1988). Contributions of quisqualate and NMDA receptors to the induction and expression of LTP. *Science, 242,* 1694–1697.

Nicoll, R. (2017). A brief history of long-term potentiation. *Neuron, 93,* 281–290.

Opazo, P., Labrecque, S., Tigaret, C. M., Frouin, A., Wiseman, P. W., De Koninck, P., and Choquet, D. (2010). CaMKII triggers the diffusional trapping of surface AMPARs through phosphorylation of stargazin. *Neuron, 67,* 239–252.

Ouyang, Y., Wong, M., Capani, F., Rensing, N., Lee, C-S., Liu, Q., Neusch, C., Martone, M. E., Wu, J. Y., Yamada, K., Ellisman, M. H., and Choi, D. W. (2005). Transient decrease in F-actin may be necessary for translocation of proteins into dendritic spines. *European Journal of Neuroscience, 22,* 2995–3005.

Penn, A. C., Zhang, C. L., Georges, F., Royer, L., Breillat, C., and Choquet, D. (2017). Hippocampal LTP and contextual learning require surface diffusion of AMPA receptors. *Nature, 549,* 384–388.

Perlson, E. and Holzbaur, E. L. F. (2008). Myosin learns to recruit AMPA receptors. *Cell*, *135*, 414–415.

Petrini, E. M., Lu, J., Cognet, L., Lounis, B., Ehlers, M. D., and Choquet, D. (2009). Endocytic trafficking and recycling maintain a pool of mobile surface AMPA receptors required for synaptic potentiation. *Neuron*, *63*, 92–105.

Simon, R., Baudry, M., and Lynch, G. (1984). Brain fodrin: substrate for calpain I, an endogenous calcium-activated protease. *Proceedings of the National Academy of Sciences USA*, *81*, 3572–3576.

Vincent-Lamarre, P., Lynn, M., Béïque, J-C. (2018). The eloquent silent synapse. *Trends in Neuroscience*, *41*, 557–559.

Wang, Z., Edwards, J. G., Riley, N., Provance, J. D., Karcher, R., Li, X., Davison, I. G., Ikebe, M., Mercer, J. A., Kauer, J. A., and Ehlers, M. (2008). Myosin Vb mobilizes recycling endosomes and AMPA receptors for postsynaptic plasticity. *Cell*, *135*, 535–548.

Xie, X., Liaw, J-S., Baudry, M., and Berger, T. W. (1997). Novel expression mechanism for synaptic potentiation: alignment of presynaptic release site and postsynaptic receptor. *Proceedings of the National Academy of Sciences USA*, *94*, 6983–6988.

Yamamoto, C. and McIlwain, H. (1966). Electrical activities in thin sections from the mammalian brain maintained in chemically-defined media in vitro. *Journal of Neurochemistry*, *13*, 1333–1343.

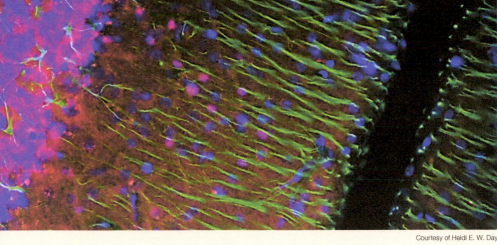

Courtesy of Heidi E. W. Day

Stabilizing Long-Term Potentiation

People who have suffered a head injury often have amnesia for events experienced within a few minutes of the accident but no loss of memory for events that occurred earlier. Such observations are the foundation for two central ideas that guide memory research.

1. The memory trace evolves in stages (see Chapter 2).
2. During the initial stages the trace is vulnerable to disruption but over time it become less fragile and resistant to disruption.

LTP also evolves in stages. It can be observed within about a minute after the inducing stimulus, but as with memory traces the supporting synaptic changes are unstable and easily disrupted (Figure 4.1). For example, the initial potentiation can be reversed if low-frequency stimulation is applied to the stimulating pathway within 5 minutes after LTP is initially induced but not if it is applied 30 minutes later (Barrionuevo et al., 1980; Larson et al., 1993; Staubli and Chun, 1996; Zhou and Poo, 2005). The implication of this finding cannot be overstated: "LTP must have a consolidation period during which it becomes resistant to disruption and is converted into a persistent form" (Lynch, 2003, p. 627).

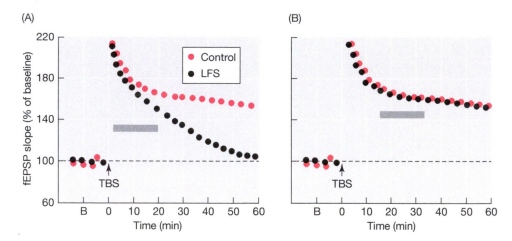

FIGURE 4.1   (A) The delivery of a low-frequency stimulus (represented by the bar) prevents the development of a lasting LTP when occurring within a minute of the TBS-inducing stimulus. (B) Low-frequency stimulation does not prevent the emergence of a durable LTP when it is delivered at least 10 minutes after TBS stimulation. These findings indicate that the synaptic changes that support LTP are not initially stable, but within about 10 minutes additional processes work to stabilize them and decrease their vulnerability to disruption. (After U. Staubli and D. Chun. 1996. *J Neurosci* 16: 853–860.)

A fundamental problem is that constitutive endocytotic processes want to remove the recently added AMPA receptors from the PSD and return potentiated synapses to their baseline state. If potentiated synapses are going to endure longer than 30 minutes or so, additional processes must be engaged *to create a dendritic spine environment* that will (a) limit the depotentiating effects of endocytotic processes and (b) ensure delivery of a steady supply of relevant synaptic proteins required to maintain the new environment (for example, AMPA receptors, kinases, and scaffolding proteins). Remarkably, over about a 30-minute period, additional processes can be recruited that will change the architecture of the spine and create such an environment. This period is called the stabilization phase and features a remarkable remodeling of the dendritic spines, which host the newly increased complement of AMPA receptors.

Structural Changes in Dendritic Spines Support LTP

Dendritic spines come in a wide variety of shapes and sizes (Figure 4.2) and constantly extend out from and retract back into dendrites (Matus, 2000). A spine's size determines how long it will endure; large spines endure much longer than small spines (Holtmaat et al., 2005). Moreover, spine size is highly correlated with the number of AMPA receptors in the postsynaptic density. Modern two-photo microscopy imaging has revealed that large spines can endure for days in living animals (Holtmaat and Svoboda, 2009).

(A)

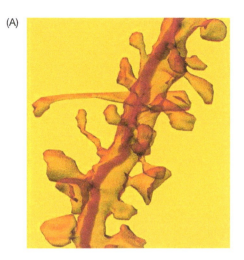

FIGURE 4.2 (A) Spines come in a wide variety of shapes and sizes. (B) Images of a dendritic branch in a living mouse, captured over six consecutive days. Note the persistent spines are large (yellow arrows) and the transient spines are small (blue arrows). (A from Synapse Web, Kristen M. Harris, PI, https://synapseweb.clm. utexas.edu/; B after A. J. Holtmaat et al. 2005. *Neuron* 20: 279–291.)

(B)

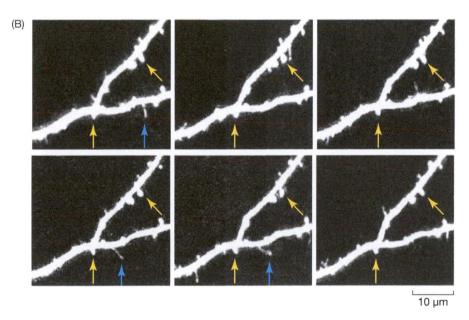

10 μm

    The preferential stability of large spines suggests that the processes that create them are critical to the stability of synapses that support LTP and memories. This turns out to be the case. For example, **theta-burst stimulation (TBS)** that produces enduring LTP also increases spine size. Moreover, these spines have a dense concentration of newly polymerized actin (Lin et al., 2005). Changes in spine size and stability are the result of many signaling cascades that orchestrate a remodeling of the actin cytoskeleton. Thus, it is necessary to understand the basics of actin management.

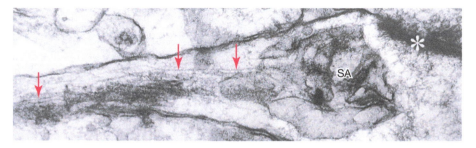

FIGURE 4.3 Actin filaments help form the spine cytoskeleton. Red arrows point to micro-filaments of actin running in parallel in the dendritic spine neck. Key: SA = spine apparatus. (From Synapse Web, Kristen M. Harris, PI, https://synapseweb.clm.utexas.edu/.)

Actin is the major cytoskeletal component of dendritic spines (Figure 4.3). A network of long- and short-branching actin filaments is present in the spine neck, and short-branched fibers are present in the spine head (Hotulainen and Hoogenraad, 2010). Actin molecules exist in two states: globular actin (G-actin) and filament actin (F-actin). G-actin are monomers that serve as building blocks for F-actin, a two-stranded helical polymer. A **polymer** is a large organic molecule formed by combining many smaller molecules (monomers); this process is called **polymerization**. F-actin is in a continuous state of turnover, with new subunits added to the barbed end of the strand and older units being removed from the pointed end. The addition and subtraction of the subunits is similar to the action of a treadmill (Figure 4.4).

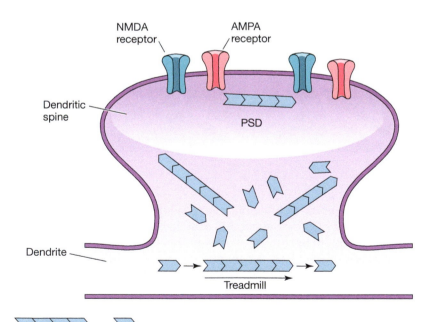

FIGURE 4.4 Actin exists in two states. Single arrow tips represent the monomer state, G-actin. Strings of arrows represent filament actin (F-actin), its polymer state. Actin is in a continuous state of turnover similar to a treadmill. Old units are removed from the pointed end and new units are added to the barbed end.

An intracellular protein called **cofilin (actin depoly-merization factor/cofilin** or **ADF/cofilin**) is an important regulator of the monomer versus filament state of actin. Cofilin can be in two states. In its active unphosphorylated state, *cofilin depolymerizes F-actin* (removes monomers from the filament) and *severs actin filaments into smaller units.* When phosphorylated on its Ser 3 site, however, cofilin's depolymerizing properties turn off and actin polymerization rapidly increases to add available F-actin strands (Figure 4.5). However, phosphatases called **slingshot** can dephosphorylate cofilin and return it to its normal state in which it severs actin filaments and limits polymerization. Under normal conditions, limiting actin polymerization is essential to neurons and disrupting this process can lead to long rods of actin filaments that may be a source of neurodegenerative diseases such as Alzheimer disease (Bamburg and Bernstein, 2016). However, the temporary disruption of these constitutive functions is essential to producing a stable form of LTP.

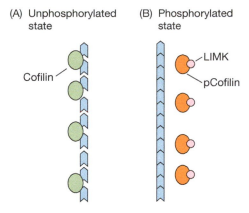

(A) Unphosphorylated state

(B) Phosphorylated state

FIGURE 4.5 The state of cofilin regulates actin polymerization. (A) In its normal unphosphorylated state, cofilin severs and depolymerizes actin filaments. (B) When phosphorylated cofilin (pCofilin) no longer interferes with actin polymerization.

Stabilizing LTP Requires Actin Polymerization

The importance of actin regulation for LTP emerged over 25 years ago when it was discovered that drugs (latrunculin or cytochalasin) that prevent actin polymerization also prevent the emergence of the enduring form of LTP. However, when the drugs were delivered prior to the TBS induction, they did not interfere with the generation of LTP, illustrated in Figure 4.6A (Kim and Lisman, 1999; Krucker et al., 2000). Remarkably, if the same drugs were delivered about 10–15 minutes following TBS, they had no effect on the duration of LTP (Figure 4.6B). These results indicated that LTP can be generated in the absence of newly polymerized actin, but to stabilize the synaptic changes requires newly polymerized actin filaments. Moreover, the stabilization phase can occur in about 15 minutes.

These early studies provided evidence that the regulation of actin dynamics is central to stabilizing LTP, and it is now generally believed that the creation of enlarged spines with a stable actin cytoskeleton is fundamental to this outcome. *So what happens during the initial 30 minutes or so following the induction stimulus to create stable spines?* This question is answered in two ways. First, the current view of some of the key events that stabilize the actin–spine architecture is described. Second, some of the experimental evidence that supports this view is presented. In both cases, no attempt is made to be comprehensive. However, there are a number of excellent review papers that serve this purpose (Bertling and Hotulainen, 2017; Borovac et al., 2018; Konietzny et al., 2017; Okamoto et al., 2009; Rácz and Weinberg, 2012). In overview, the creation of large enduring

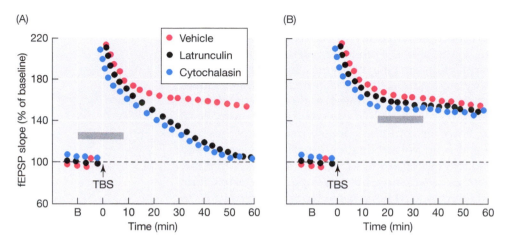

FIGURE 4.6 (A) When drugs such as latrunculin and cytochalasin that prevent actin polymerization are applied before TBS (represented by the bar), they do not prevent the generation of LTP, but it rapidly decays. (B) LTP is maintained if these drugs are applied 15 minutes after LTP is induced. Thus, actin polymerization is necessary to stabilize LTP. (After T. Krucker et al. 2000. *Proc Natl Acad Sci USA* 6: 6856–6861.)

dendritic spines takes place in two stages. Initially the existing actin cytoskeleton is disassembled; in the second stage it is expanded and rebuilt.

Phase 1: Actin Filaments Are Unbundled and Severed

At the time LTP is induced the spine head typically contains a dense network of short, cross-linked, branched actin filaments, while the spine neck contains loosely arranged bundles of F-actin (Figure 4.7A) that are held together by inactive CaMKII complexes (Khan et al., 2019; Okamoto et al., 2007).

When LTP is induced, calcium enters the spine and activates a number of intracellular events that unbundle and sever much of the existing actin organization.

- Calcium binds to **calmodulin** and the Ca^{2+}/calmodulin complex leads to the activation (autophosphorylation) of CaMKII.

- Now activated, CaMKII complexes detach from F-actin strands, unbundling them (Figure 4.7B). Note that these activated CaMKII complexes are now free to carry out catalytic functions needed to reconfigure AMPA receptor trafficking and other important functions (Okamoto et al., 2007).

- This unbundling exposes the liberated filaments to other actin-binding proteins that sever long actin strands into more numerous smaller strands.

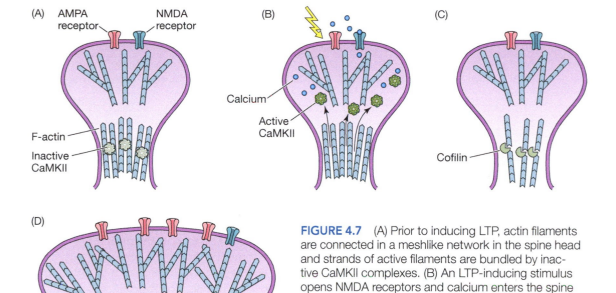

(A) AMPA receptor   NMDA receptor

F-actin

Inactive CaMKII

(B)

Calcium

Active CaMKII

(C)

Cofilin

(D)

FIGURE 4.7 (A) Prior to inducing LTP, actin filaments are connected in a meshlike network in the spine head and strands of active filaments are bundled by inactive CaMKII complexes. (B) An LTP-inducing stimulus opens NMDA receptors and calcium enters the spine where, via calmodulin, it activates CaMKII, which then disengages from actin bundles. (C) Now unbundled actin filaments are exposed to severing by proteins such as cofilin. This results in multiple strands of small actin filaments. (D) Cofilin is phosphorylated and this allows the rapid polymerization of long strands of actin, which promotes the expansion of the spine. Additional synaptic proteins then reorganize the actin into a stable framework (see text for details).

Several important events contribute to severing actin filaments (Figure 4.7C).

- Unphosphorylated cofilin is transported to the spine region where it binds to F-actin and can both sever and depolymerize the filament (Bosch et al., 2014). Cofilin severing of F-actin is facilitated by its binding with actin-interacting protein, which caps the fragments (Ono, 2003) and prevents the actin fragments from rejoining. This results in increasing the number of actin fragments available to be polymerized.

- Additional shorter actin filaments also can be produced by actin phosphorylation that accompanies LTP induction (Bertling and Hotulainen, 2017).

- In parallel with the effects of these actin-binding proteins, mechanical forces associated with the activation of myosin IIb motor proteins result in the shearing of actin bundles into smaller strands of F-actin, described in greater detail later in the TBS section (Rex et al., 2010).

Phase 2: The Actin–Spine Architecture Is Reconstructed

Severing processes produce a large number of small nascent filaments. However, should severing continue unabated, it would be impossible to construct a large and stable spine. A number of events bring these severing processes to a halt.

- Cofilin is phosphorylated. In this state it no longer severs or depolymerizes actin filaments. This outcome is the result of a calcium-initiated signaling cascade that leads to the activation of LIM kinase (**LIMK**), which in turn phosphorylates cofilin (see Figure 4.5).
- Phosphatases dephosphorylate actin and myosin IIb motors, terminating their severing activity.

With the shutdown of severing processes and increase in the number of small F-actin strands, there is a shift in the direction of actin regulation processes *from disassembling to rebuilding* (Figure 4.7D). These new small F-actin strands are rapidly polymerized. This occurs because cofilin is phosphorylated (pCofilin) and profilin, another actin-binding protein, enters the spine to promote polymerization. However, this is only temporary because the phosphatase slingshot will soon dephosphorylate cofilin. Thus, a number of other actin-binding proteins are called into play to reorganize these new strands of F-actin into a network that both enlarges the spine and provides some protection against cofilin. These proteins support (a) actin branching (Arp2/3), which promotes expansion of the spine head, (b) crosslinking filaments (α-actinin), (c) actin bundling (inactive CaMKII), and (d) linking the actin cytoskeleton to the plasma membrane (spectrin). Thus, in about 30 minutes following the induction of LTP the actin–spine architecture is essentially destroyed and then rebuilt into an enlarged stable spine that will help provide resistance to the endocytotic processes that otherwise would remove AMPA receptors and return the spine to its prepotentiated state. In addition, these large stable spines will ensure delivery of a steady supply of relevant synaptic proteins required to maintain the new environment.

Experimental Evidence

Our current understanding of how actin dynamics are regulated and contribute to LTP is based on an enormous literature (Bertling and Hotulainen, 2017; Borovac et al., 2018; Konietzny et al., 2017; Lynch et al., 2007; Okamoto et al., 2007; Rácz and Weinberg, 2012). Thus, a review of the supporting evidence has to be selective. Two general lines of work are considered. In one case, advances in our knowledge of the temporal dynamics gained from technical advances that enabled researchers to *image single dendritic spines in real time* are described (see Bosch and Hayashi, 2012). In the second case, lessons from studying TBS-induced changes in populations of small spines are discussed.

Single Spine Imaging

Beginning in the 1970s, Eva Fifková and her colleagues (Fifková and Van Harreveld, 1977; Van Harreveld and Fifková, 1975) developed methods that allowed changes in spine morphology to be observed at the electron microscopic level (see Figure 4.3 as an example). This work was initiated very shortly after LTP was discovered. Fifková and her colleagues reported that within about 2 minutes after LTP induction, spines on stimulated neurons enlarged and this change lasted up to 23 hours. This work thus revealed that the morphology of dendritic spines could be modified by an LTP-inducing stimulus. However, such studies left unanswered questions about whether existing spines were modified or whether LTP stimulated the growth of new spines (Bosch and Hayashi, 2012). To gain this level of understanding required the development of methods that enabled researchers to image individual spines in real time.

A major advance came when Haruo Kasai's group (Matsuzaki et al., 2004) employed a two-photon-induced glutamate uncaging technique to control the release of a very small amount of glutamate directly over target spines (Figure 4.8). By *injecting the neuron with a vector for green fluorescent protein* (GFP), they were able to image changes in spine volume in real time. This is possible because GFP fluoresces when stimulated rapidly by light. This led to a number of important discoveries.

- Within 10 seconds after glutamate uncaging, spine enlargement was detected.

- Long-lasting changes in spine size is dependent on original spine size; the change in the volume of initially small spines endured for hours but this was not true for initially large spines.

- Spine enlargement was blocked by NMDA antagonists and CaMKII inhibitors.

- Inhibiting actin polymerization with latrunculin had no effect on initial spine volume increases but prevented enduring changes. This indicated that LTP in single spines was regulated by the same calcium-initiated events operating in conventional LTP preparations.

- Spine growth also was accompanied by an increase in the AMPA receptor currents, which was attributed to the insertion of AMPA receptors into the PSD.

Building on this work, Haruo Kasai's group (Honkura et al., 2008) fused GFP to actin and through photo activation of fused GFP (which caused it to fluoresce) were able to directly observe actin movement in individual spines in real time. This work confirmed that the spine enlargement observed by Matsuzaki et al. (2004) was the outcome of actin dynamics initiated by uncaging glutamate. In addition, this work revealed that in

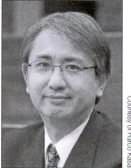

Haruo Kasai

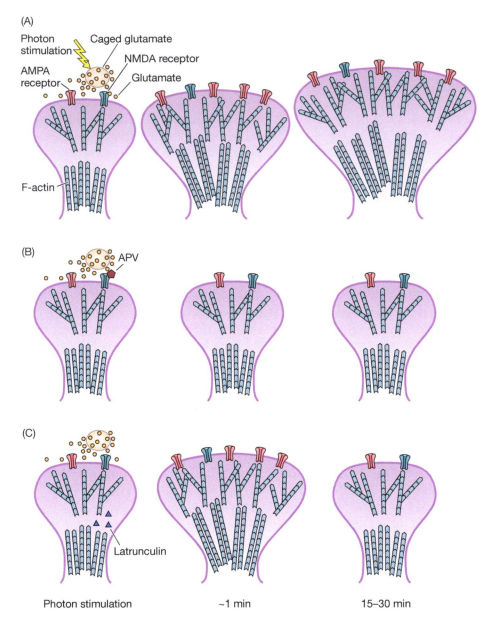

FIGURE 4.8   (A) Photon uncaging of glutamate directly over a single spine rapidly initiates the expansion of the actin cytoskeleton. (B) Inhibiting NMDA receptors by APV prevents the expansion of the spine. (C) The actin polymerization inhibitor latrunculin does not block initial spine expansion but prevents it from enduring.

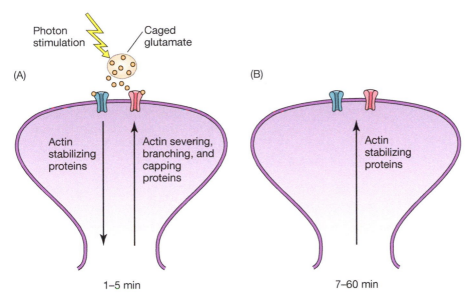

FIGURE 4.9   Following uncaging glutamate there is a rapid turnover of actin-related proteins. (A) During the initial 5 minutes, actin stabilizing proteins vacate the spine while actin severing, branching, and capping proteins invade the spine. (B) This is followed by the gradual return of actin stabilizing proteins.

expanded spines actin is organized into three different pools of F-actin. Of special interest was the discovery that uncaged glutamate rapidly produced an enlargement pool of actin fibers with a slow turnover rate, which they proposed produced an enlarged stable spine.

Subsequently, Miquel Bosch and his colleagues (Bosch et al., 2014) used these same general procedures to image in real time the trafficking of a large number of actin-binding proteins in and out of spines. This work revealed that during the first few minutes following glutamate uncaging the spine was enriched with proteins that modify F-actin by severing (cofilin), branching (Arp2/3), or capping (Aip1) it. At the same time, proteins known to stabilize F-actin (CaMKII and α-actinin) temporarily vacated the spine. During a second phase that occurred 7–60 minutes following uncaging, actin stabilizing proteins returned to their baseline concentration (Figure 4.9). Unless cofilin is phosphorylated, one would predict that its severing activity would continue and prevent spine enlargement. Consistent with this prediction, when the activity of LIMK, which phosphorylates cofilin, was reduced the spines did not enlarge.

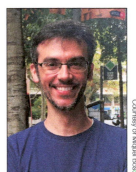

Miquel Bosch

TBS Induces Actin Regulation

Measuring a single spine's response to glutamate in real time provided many insights into the temporal dynamics of the processes that regulate actin dynamics.

(A)

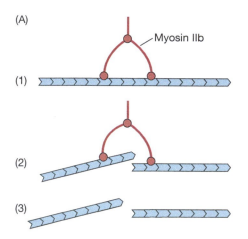

(1)

(2)

(3)

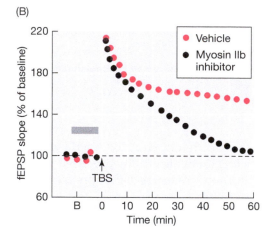

(B)

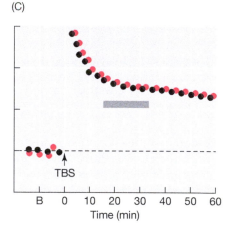

(C)

FIGURE 4.10 (A) Myosin IIb exerts a shearing action (1) and (2) that breaks actin filaments into smaller units (3) that can be reassembled elsewhere in the spine. (B) Applying drugs (represented by the bar) that inhibit myosin IIb prior to TBS prevents the stabilization of LTP but does not interfere with its induction. (C) Inhibiting myosin IIb at least 10 minutes after the induction does not reverse LTP. (B, C after C. S. Rex et al. 2010. *Neuron* 63: 603–617.)

However, it is important to consider key insights provided from studies based on LTP induced by TBS because such experiments tell us how spines respond to glutamate and other neurotransmitters released *by natural patterns of neural activity*.

Christine Gall, Gary Lynch, and their colleagues have provided much of what we know about how TBS engages the critical processes involved in rapid polymerization (Chen et al., 2007; Lin et al., 2005; Rex et al., 2009).

- Within about 2–7 minutes of TBS there is almost a 10-fold increase in the number of spines containing pCofilin and pPAK, its upstream regulator.

- This is accompanied by a rapid polymerization of actin in a reasonably small number of spines in the dendritic region of stimulation.

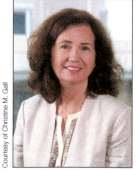

Christine Gall

- However, after about 15 minutes theses markers are no longer present.
- These outcomes are blocked by inhibiting NMDA receptor function and by preventing actin polymerization.

As described earlier, actin severing processes are critical to building large spines. TBS stimulation results in actin severing by engaging the motor protein **myosin IIb**. Myosin motor proteins are strongly associated with actin filaments, which provide tracks along which these proteins move (Figure 4.10). As the myosin IIb motors move they exert a shearing force on long actin filaments, breaking them into smaller units that can then be further severed and then rapidly polymerized (Medeiros et al., 2006).

Myosin IIb is activated by a TBS-induced, NMDA-dependent Ca^{2+} signal cascade and has been clearly associated with stabilizing synapses (Rex et al., 2010). For example, inhibiting the activity of myosin IIb prevents the enduring form of LTP but has no effect on its induction. However, inhibiting myosin IIb 10 minutes after TBS has no effect on enduring LTP. Note, the temporal pattern of results associated with inhibiting myosin IIb are the same as those produced by preventing polymerization with the drug latrunculin, and both treatments reduce actin filament levels in spines (Rex et al., 2010).

The state of cofilin is a major determiner of the temporal dynamics of actin regulation. In its active state cofilin is a severing and depolymerizing agent, but when it is phosphorylated these properties are terminated. Thus, for TBS to generate an expanded and enduring actin network in dendritic spines, cofilin must be phosphorylated. The signaling pathways initiated by calcium–CaMKII that do this go through small proteins with enzymatic properties known as **GTPases** (Hedrick and Yasuda, 2017). For example, in Figure 4.11, a GTPase (such as Rho) activates an effector kinase (for example, ROCK), which phosphorylates LIMK, which then phosphorylates cofilin. Several GTPases (Rho, Rac, Cdc42) have been shown to influence actin polymerization. Rex et al. (2010) determined that the Rac–PAK cascade plays an important role in orchestrating the reorganization of the actin cytoskeleton to ensure its stability.

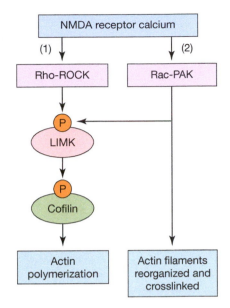

FIGURE 4.11 Calcium entering the synapse through NMDA receptors activates two signaling cascades that regulate actin. Both pathways activate LIMK, a kinase that phosphorylates cofilin and allows actin polymerization. The second pathway, the Rac-PAK cascade, also activates processes that reorganize and crosslink actin filaments to make them resistant to depolymerization.

Cell Adhesion Molecules Help Stabilize the Trace

Many of these intracellular signaling cascades that influence actin dynamics operate through calcium–CaMKII signaling and spine enlargement.

However, stabilization also depends on TBS activating cell adhesion molecules—proteins that are located on the cell surface and bind with other cells or with the extracellular matrix. Some of these molecules help cells stick to each other and their surrounds. Many classes of cell adhesion molecules have been identified in synapses (see McGeachie et al., 2011). The discussion below, however, focuses on only two classes—**integrin receptors** and **neural cadherins** (abbreviated as **N-cadherins**). Both of these have been clearly linked to stabilizing LTP.

INTEGRIN RECEPTORS   Integrin receptors connect the extracellular matrix to the actin cytoskeleton. Integrins are heterodimer cell adhesion molecules. They are formed from two different subunits called α and β. Integrin receptors respond to molecules in the extracellular matrix and to intracellular signals such as calcium (McGeachie et al., 2011). Integrins also are responsive to synaptic activity and regulate actin (Chun et al., 2001; Kramár et al., 2006; Shi and Ethell, 2006).

For integrins to contribute to the regulation of actin dynamics, synaptic activity must increase the contribution of these receptors. Although the precise mechanisms are not yet understood, there is evidence that intracellular integrin receptors can be trafficked into synaptic regions. Recall that the rapid trapping of GluA1 AMPA receptors in the PSD supports the early phase of LTP and that these receptors have special properties—they influx both calcium and sodium. Lin et al. (2005) provided evidence that calcium entering the spine through GluA1 receptors plays an important role in trafficking integrins into the synaptic region. Other sources of calcium (discussed in Chapter 3) might also be important for driving integrins into the synaptic region. However, the general point here is that calcium-dependent signaling cascades enhance the contribution of integrins by increasing their numbers in the synaptic membrane (Figure 4.12).

Integrins respond to ligands contained in the extracellular matrix. However, neutralizing the response of β integrins to these ligands prevents enduring LTP normally produced by TBS, but has no effect on the initial induction phase (see Figure 4.12D). TBS that normally produces an enduring LTP also significantly increases the number of spines that contain filament actin. Interfering with the function of β integrins, however, also completely prevents actin filament formation. Thus, integrins provide another path, perhaps via GTPases (Brakebusch and Fässler, 2003) by which cofilin can be phosphorylated. Kramár et al. (2006) proposed that integrins might participate in the reorganization of actin filaments by attaching crosslinking proteins such as spectrin that increase the resistance of actin filaments to depolymerization.

NEURAL CADHERINS   Synapses require the coupling of the presynaptic and postsynaptic components so that the postsynaptic component is positioned

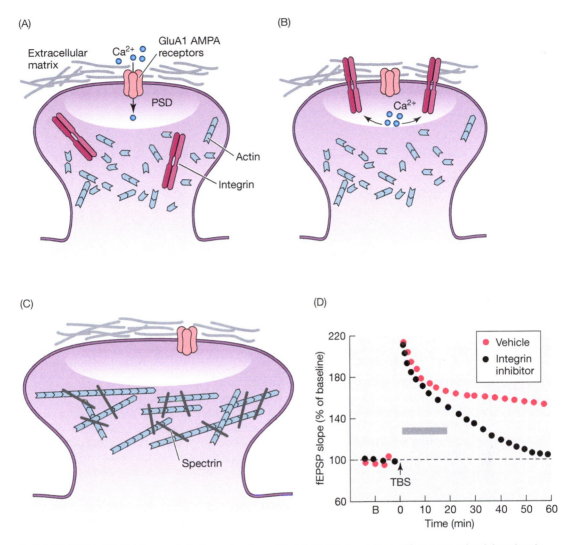

FIGURE 4.12 (A) Calcium enters the spine from GluA1 AMPA receptors. (B) Increased calcium levels traffic integrin receptors in the PSD region, where they bind to ligands in the extracellular matrix (ECM). (C) As a result of activation of the integrin receptors, actin filaments are reorganized to increase their resistance to depolymerization. (D) Inhibiting integrin receptors prevents the late phase of LTP but does not prevent induction. (D after E. A. Kramár et al. 2006. *Proc Natl Acad Sci USA* 103: 5579–5584.)

to respond to glutamate released from the presynaptic neuron. N-cadherins help to couple the pre and postsynaptic components. N-cadherins are calcium-dependent, cell adhesion molecules; they are strands of proteins held together by Ca^{2+} ions. N-cadherins are anchored in the plasma membrane of both the presynaptic terminal and postsynaptic spine. They can exist as either

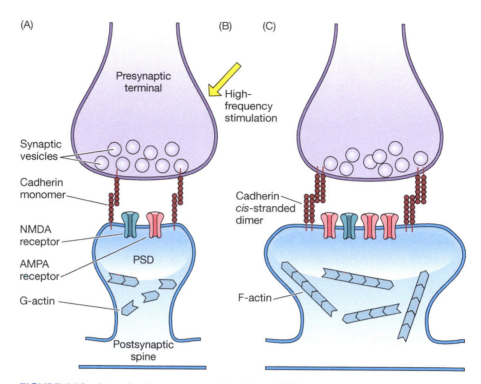

FIGURE 4.13 N-cadherins are reorganized by an LTP-inducing stimulus. (A) Illustration of an unpotentiated synapse with the presynaptic terminal and postsynaptic spine weakly bonded by cadherin monomers. (B) A high-frequency stimulation is delivered to this synapse to induce LTP. (C) The high-frequency stimulus promotes cadherin dimerization so the now-enlarged spine containing additional AMPA receptors is tightly coupled to the presynaptic terminal and well positioned to receive glutamate released from the presynaptic terminal. (After G. W. Huntley et al. 2002. *Neuroscientist* 8: 221–233.)

monomers or *cis*-stranded dimers (Figure 4.13). The monomer form is weakly adhesive but the *cis*-stranded or bonded dimers are strongly adhesive. Thus, when a dimer from the presynaptic domain contacts an identical dimer from the postsynaptic domain they form what is sometimes called an "adhesive zipper" that couples the two domains into a stable relationship (Huntley et al., 2002).

N-cadherin complexes respond to synaptic activity (Bozdagi et al., 2000). Several facts point to a critical role of N-cadherins in spine stability. First, TBS selectively promotes the formation of N-cadherin clusters in stimulated spines. This effect requires calcium to enter on NMDA receptors (Mendez et al., 2010; see Figure 4.14A). Second, spines with N-cadherin clusters are enlarged compared to those without clusters. Third, N-cadherins are not required for the

(A)

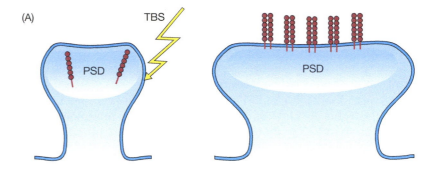

(B)

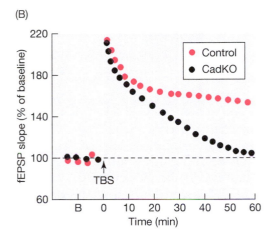

FIGURE 4.14 (A) Spines activated by TBS become larger and contain clusters of N-cadherins. (B) TBS induces LTP in slices from mice genetically modified to knock out the gene for N-cadherins (CadKO). However, these slices cannot sustain LTP. (A after P. Mendez et al. 2010. *J Cell Biol* 189: 589–600; B after O. Bozdagi et al. 2010. *J Neurosci* 30: 9984–9989.)

initial induction of LTP but they are critical to enduring LTP (Bozdagi et al., 2010; see Figure 4.14B) and for spines to maintain their size.

N-cadherins are important because (a) they are indirectly anchored to actin filaments and could provide sites for capturing newly generated actin polymers (Honkura et al., 2008), and (b) the larger spines associated with LTP may have an expanded surface and require additional adhesion molecules to keep the pre and postsynaptic components tightly coupled (Murthy et al., 2001). More tightly coupling the presynaptic and modified postsynaptic components of the synapse could ensure that glutamate released by the presynaptic neuron would be optimally received by receptors on dendritic spines. Thus, this alignment would help to increase the likelihood that the postsynaptic neuron would depolarize in response to a fixed amount of glutamate released by the presynaptic neuron. This coupling could also contribute to increasing the durability of the synapse (see Figure 4.13).

Summary

This chapter has covered many of the events that contribute to the production of enduring large spines and consequently stabilizing LTP. However, two important general points should not be missed.

First, the processes that stabilize LTP are not required for its generation. Many results support this conclusion. Each of the following treatments prevented the stabilization of LTP without interfering with its generation.

- Low-frequency stimulation
- Inhibiting actin polymerization
- Inhibiting the calcium–GTPase pathways needed to phosphorylate cofilin
- Inhibiting the activation of myosin IIb motors
- Inhibiting integrin receptors
- Genetic deletion of N-cadherins

Second, LTP is stabilized in a short period of time because when these treatments were delayed for at least 10 minutes they had no effect.

LTP is stabilized in three somewhat overlapping phases. Initially, actin-severing events are engaged, while actin stabilizers are neutered. This results in the creation of multiple small nascent strands of F-actin which provide seeds for the second phase during which GTPase signaling leads to phosphorylating cofilin and the rapid polymerization of actin and a large stable pool of F-actin. During the third phase, actin-stabilizing proteins return to rebundle actin filaments, crosslink them and bind them, to the plasma membrane. This third phase also involves the recruitment of integrin receptors to the PSD where they interact with ligands in the extracellular matrix to help reorganize the actin filaments. During this period there also is a reorganization of N-cadherins to tightly couple the pre and postsynaptic components and position the glutamate receptors to receive glutamate released from its presynaptic terminal.

References

Bamburg, J. R. and Bernstein, B. W. (2016). Actin dynamics and cofilin–actin rods in Alzheimer disease. *Cytoskeleton, 73,* 477–497.

Barrionuevo, G., Schottler, S., and Lynch, G. (1980). The effects of repetitive low frequency stimulation on control and "potentiated" synaptic responses in the hippocampus. *Life Sciences, 27,* 2385–2391.

Bertling, E. and Hotulainen, P. (2017). New waves in dendritic spine actin cytoskeleton: from branches and bundles to rings, from actin binding proteins to post-translational modifications. *Molecular Cellular Neuroscience, 84,* 77–84.

Borovac, J., Bosch, M., and Okamoto, K. (2018). Regulation of actin dynamics during structural plasticity of dendritic spines: signaling messengers and actin-binding proteins. *Molecular and Cellular Neuroscience, 91,* 122–130.

Bosch, M., Castro, J., Saneyoshi, T., Matsuno, H., Sur, M., and Hayashi, Y. (2014). Structural and molecular remodeling of dendritic spine substructures during long-term potentiation. *Neuron, 82,* 444–459.

Bosch, M. and Hayashi, Y. (2012). Structural plasticity of dendritic spines. *Current Opinion in Neurobiology, 22,* 283–288.

Bozdagi, O., Shan, W., Tanaka, H., Benson, D. L., and Huntley, G. W. (2000). Increasing numbers of synaptic puncta during late-phase LTP: N-cadherin is synthesized, recruited to synaptic sites, and required for potentiation. *Neuron, 28,* 245–259.

Bozdagi, O., Wang, X., Nikitczuk, J. S., Anderson, T. R., Bloss, E. B., Radice, G. L., Benson, D. L., and Huntley, G. W. (2010). Persistence of coordinated long-term potentiation and dendritic spine enlargement at mature hippocampal CA1 synapses requires N-cadherin. *Journal of Neuroscience, 30,* 9984–9989.

Brakebusch, C. and Fässler, R. (2003). The integrin–actin connection, an eternal love affair. *EMBO Journal, 22,* 2324–2333.

Chen, L. Y., Rex, C. S., Casale, M. S., Gall, C. M., and Lynch, G. (2007). Changes in synaptic morphology accompany actin signaling during LTP. *Journal of Neuroscience, 27,* 5363–5372.

Chun, D., Gall, C. M., Bi, X., and Lynch, G. (2001). Evidence that integrins contribute to multiple stages in the consolidation of long-term potentiation. *Neuroscience, 105,* 815–829.

Fifková, E. and Van Harreveld, A. (1977). Long-lasting morphological changes in dendritic spines of dentate granular cells following stimulation of the entorhinal area. *Journal of Neurocytology, 6,* 211–230.

Hedrick, N. G. and Yasuda, R. (2017). Regulation of Rho GTPase proteins during spine plasticity for the control of local dendritic plasticity. *Current Opinion in Neurobiology, 45,* 193–201.

Holtmaat, A. and Svoboda, K. (2009). Experience-dependent structural synaptic plasticity in the mammalian brain. *Nature Reviews Neuroscience, 10,* 647–658.

Holtmaat, A. J., Trachtenberg, J. T., Wilbrecht, L., Shepherd, G. M., Zhang, X., Knott, G. W., and Svoboda, K. (2005). Transient and persistent dendritic spines in the neocortex in vivo. *Neuron, 20,* 279–291.

Honkura, N., Matsuzaki, M., Noguchi, J., Ellis-Davies, G. C., and Kasai, H. (2008). The subspine organization of actin fibers regulates the structure and plasticity of dendritic spines. *Neuron, 57,* 719–729.

Hotulainen, P. and Hoogenraad, C. C. (2010). Actin in dendritic spines: connecting dynamics to function. *Journal of Cell Biology, 189,* 619–629.

Huntley, G. W., Gil, O., and Bozdagi, O. (2002). The cadherin family of cell adhesion molecules: multiple roles in synaptic plasticity. *Neuroscientist, 8,* 221–233.

Khan, S., Downing, K. H., and Malloy, J. E. (2019). Architectural dynamics of CaMKII–actin networks. *Biophysical Journal, 116,* 104–119.

Kim, C. H. and Lisman, J. E. (1999). A role of actin filament in synaptic transmission and long-term potentiation. *Journal of Neuroscience, 19,* 4314–4324.

Konietzny, A., Bar, J., and Mikhaylova, M. (2017). Dendritic actin cytoskeleton: structure, functions, and regulations. *Frontiers in Cellular Neuroscience, 11,* Article 147.

Kramár, E. A., Lin, B., Rex, C. S., Gall, C. M., and Lynch, G. (2006). Integrin-driven actin polymerization consolidates long-term potentiation. *Proceedings of the National Academy of Sciences USA, 103,* 5579–5584.

Krucker, T., Siggins, G. R., and Halpain, S. (2000). Dynamic actin filaments are required for stable long-term potentiation (LTP) in area CA1 of the hippocampus. *Proceedings of the National Academy of Sciences USA, 6,* 6856–6861.

Larson, J., Xiao, P., and Lynch, G. (1993). Reversal of LTP by theta frequency stimulation. *Brain Research, 600,* 97–102.

Lin, B., Kramár, E. A., Bi, X., Brucher, F. A., Gall, C. M., and Lynch, G. (2005). Theta stimulation polymerizes actin in dendritic spines of hippocampus. *Journal of Neuroscience, 25,* 2062–2069.

Lynch, G. (2003). Long-term potentiation in the Eocene. *Philosophical Translations of the Royal Society London B, 358,* 625–628.

Lynch, G., Rex, C. S., and Gall, C. M. (2007). LTP consolidation: substrates, explanatory power, and functional significance. *Neuropharmacology, 52,* 12–23.

Matsuzaki, M., Honkura, N., Ellis-Davies, G. C., and Kasai, H. (2004). Structural basis of long-term potentiation in single dendritic spines. *Nature, 429,* 761–766.

Matus, A. (2000). Actin-based plasticity in dendritic spines. *Science, 290,* 754–758.

McGeachie, A. B., Cingolani, L. A., and Goda, Y. (2011). Stabilizing influence: integrins in regulation of synaptic plasticity. *Neuroscience Research, 70,* 24–29.

Medeiros, N. A., Burnette, D. T., and Forscher, P. (2006). Myosin II functions in actin-bundle turnover in neuronal growth cones. *Nature Cell Biology, 8,* 215–226.

Mendez, P., DeRoo, M., Poglia, L., Klauser, P., and Muller, D. (2010). N-cadherin mediates plasticity-induced long-term spine stabilization. *Journal of Cell Biology, 189,* 589–600.

Murthy, V. N., Schikorski, T., Stevens, C. F., and Zhu, Y. (2001). Inactivity produces increases in neurotransmitter release and synapse size. *Neuron, 32,* 673–682.

Okamoto, K., Bosch, M., and Hayashi, Y. (2009). The roles of CaMKII and F-actin in the structural plasticity of dendritic spines: a potential molecular identity of a synaptic tag? *Physiology, 24,* 357–366.

Okamoto, K., Narayanan, R., Lee, S. H., Murata, K., and Hayashi, Y. (2007). The role of CaMKII as an F-actin-bundling protein crucial for maintenance of dendritic spine structure. *Proceedings of the National Academy of Sciences USA, 104,* 6418–6423.

Ono, S. (2003). Regulation of actin filament dynamics by actin depolymerizing factor/cofilin and actin-interacting protein 1: new blades for twisted filaments. *Biochemistry, 42*, 13363–13370.

Rácz, B. and Weinberg, R. (2012). Microdomains in forebrain spines: an ultrastructural perspective. *Molecular Neurobiology, 47*, 77–89.

Rex, C. S., Chen, L. Y., Sharma, A., Liu, J., Babayan, A. H., Gall, C. M., and Lynch, G. (2009). Different rho GTPase-dependent signaling pathways initiate sequential steps in the consolidation of long-term potentiation. *Journal of Cell Biology, 186*, 85–97.

Rex, C. S., Gavin, C. F., Rubio, M. D., Kramár, E., and Rumbaugh, G. (2010). Myosin IIb regulates actin dynamics during synaptic plasticity and memory formation. *Neuron, 67*, 603–617.

Shi, Y. and Ethell, I. M. (2006). Integrins control dendritic spine plasticity in hippocampal neurons through NMDA receptor and Ca^{2+}/calmodulin-dependent protein kinase II-mediated actin reorganization. *Journal of Neuroscience, 26*, 1813–1822.

Staubli, U. and Chun, D. (1996). Factors regulating the reversibility of long-term potentiation. *Journal of Neuroscience, 16*, 853–860.

Van Harreveld, A. and Fifková, E. (1975). Swelling of dendritic spines in the fascia dentata after stimulation of the perforant fibers as a mechanism of post-tetanic potentiation. *Experimental Neurology, 49*, 736–749.

Zhou, Q. and Poo, M. M. (2005). Reversal and consolidation of activity-induced synaptic modifications. *Trends in Neuroscience, 27*, 378–383.

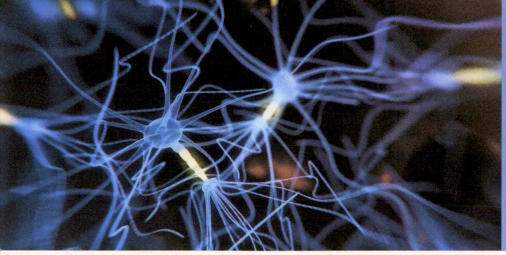

Consolidating LTP: Translation and Transcription

Over 100 years ago, Müller and Pilzecker (1900) proposed the consolidation hypothesis—that new memories require a long period of time to become resistant to disruption. Initially, this hypothesis had no impact on memory research. It became front and center for neurobiologists, however, when it was reported that inhibitors of protein synthesis had no effect on short-term memory but prevented the formation of long-term memories (Flexner et al., 1963; McGaugh, 2000; Roberts and Flexner, 1969). This result led to the ***de novo* protein synthesis (DNPS) hypothesis**—the idea that for memories to endure, the learning experience must produce new proteins, that is, *proteins not present at the time of the learning event*. This hypothesis became almost inextricably linked to the consolidation perspective and has dominated thinking about the persistence of memory ever since.

But what gets consolidated? The original consolidation hypothesis recognized that building a persistent memory requires time, but *neither it nor the DNPS hypothesis specified what does the building or what gets built*. This is not surprising because when the DNPS hypothesis was originally proposed, LTP had not been discovered and no one had any idea of the complex postsynaptic cellular–molecular events that could be engaged to change the structure of spines. The synaptic processes that generate and stabilize LTP are fairly recent discoveries. Importantly, researchers now understand that the disruption of actin regulation processes that build large spines is catastrophic to the *endurance* of LTP but not for its *generation*. This observation supports the hypothesis that the fundamental consolidating event is the *construction of an enlarged, stable actin cytoskeleton that is strongly linked to the extracellular matrix and to its presynaptic partner* (Lynch and Baudry, 1984; Lynch et al., 2015; Lynch et al., 2007; Rudy, 2015).

Chapter 4 provides overwhelming evidence for this hypothesis. It only takes 15–30 minutes to stabilize potentiated spines and any treatment that interferes with actin dynamics during this period is catastrophic for LTP. Ironically, from the DNPS view, no new proteins are needed; this all takes place in advance of the synthesis of new proteins. Without this outcome new proteins would be irrelevant and, in fact, the synthesis of new synaptic proteins depends on actin polymerization.

The construction of large stable spines may be the consolidating event. Nevertheless, there is evidence that synaptic events that produce an enduring LTP initiate the **transcription** and **translation** of **messenger ribonucleic acid (mRNA)** into new proteins that can be important for synaptic changes to endure. In this chapter and the next, the *consolidation phase* is identified as the time period during which these new proteins are generated.

The *De Novo* Protein Synthesis Hypothesis

The basic claim of this hypothesis is that for LTP to endure synaptic activity, it also needs to initiate (1) genomic signaling to activate transcription processes to produce mRNA (genes) and (2) translation processes that convert the mRNA into proteins (**protein synthesis**). Unlike the post-translation processes, which are short lived, the processes involved in producing new protein can last for hours.

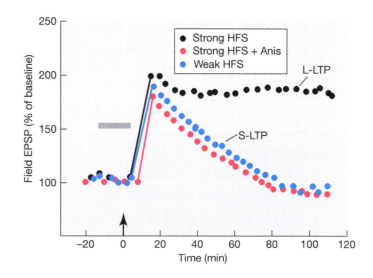

FIGURE 5.1 A weak high-frequency stimulus (HFS) induces a short-lasting LTP (S-LTP), whereas a strong HFS produces a long-lasting LTP (L-LTP). However, pretreatment (gray bar) with anisomycin, a protein synthesis inhibitor, prevents the strong stimulus from producing L-LTP but leaves the early-phase, short-lasting component intact. This result indicates that S-LTP produced by the weak stimulus depends only on post-translation modifications and rearrangements of existing protein, but the consolidation of the synaptic changes that support L-LTP requires new protein. Key: Anis = anisomycin.

FIGURE 5.2   Long-lasting LTP depends on parallel effects of the LTP-inducing stimulus. It initiates both local translation and genomic signaling cascades (synapse-to-nucleus and soma-to-nucleus signals) that transcribe new mRNA that can then be translated.

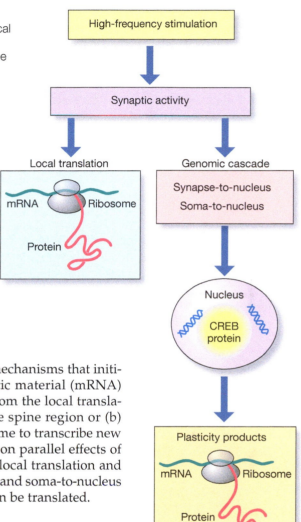

The relevance of the DNPS hypothesis for producing enduring LTP was recognized when it was discovered that protein synthesis inhibitors (such as anisomycin) block the development of a **long-lasting LTP** (**L-LTP**) but not a **short-lasting LTP** (**S-LTP**) (for example, Frey et al., 1988; Krug et al., 1984). This general finding, illustrated in Figure 5.1, makes the point that when protein synthesis is prevented, the resulting LTP resembles that produced by a weak inducing stimulus—the synapses revert back to their original unpotentiated state. Thus, the implication of these results is that enduring synaptic change depends on the generation of new protein.

The generation of new protein depends on mechanisms that initiate protein synthesis—the translation of genetic material (mRNA) into protein. New protein can (a) be derived from the local translation of mRNAs already present in the dendrite spine region or (b) result from synaptic activity signaling the genome to transcribe new mRNA (Figure 5.2). Long-lasting LTP depends on parallel effects of the LTP-inducing stimulus. It can initiate both local translation and genomic signaling cascades (synapse-to-nucleus and soma-to-nucleus signals) that transcribe new mRNA that can then be translated.

Local Protein Synthesis

The standard view of protein synthesis is that mRNA is translated as it passes through a membrane system that surrounds the nucleus. However, translation machinery (endoplasmic reticulum, Golgi elements, ribosomal assemblies) is also present locally in the vicinity of dendritic spines (Steward and Schuman, 2001). Moreover, relevant mRNAs are also distributed within the dendrite as well as the cell body of the neuron or soma (Miyashiro et al., 1994). They include mRNAs for proteins that are needed to induce LTP, such as CaM-KII and AMPA receptors (Figure 5.3). It also has been reported that the induction of LTP is associated with the movement of ribosomes into dendritic spines (Ostroff et al., 2018). The presence of translation

FIGURE 5.3 Messenger RNA and protein translation machinery, such as endoplasmic reticulum (ER) and ribosomes, are present locally in the dendritic spine region. Synaptic activity can activate this machinery and translate this mRNA.

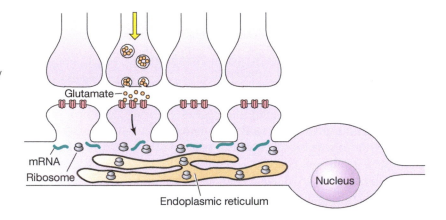

Glutamate

mRNA
Ribosome
Endoplasmic reticulum
Nucleus

machinery and mRNA in the local dendritic region suggests that proteins are translated locally from already existing mRNA (**local protein synthesis**).

Two research strategies have revealed that local protein synthesis plays an important role in the consolidation of synaptic changes (Sutton and Schuman, 2006). The first involves separating dendrites in the CA1 region of the hippocampus from their cell bodies, making it impossible for proteins that have been newly synthesized in the soma from a genomic cascade to influence synaptic strength (Figure 5.4). Studies with this preparation have observed L-LTP that is dependent on protein synthesis (Kang and Schuman, 1996; Vickers et al., 2005).

The second strategy involves applying protein synthesis inhibitors selectively to the cell bodies and dendritic fields of CA1 pyramidal cells. Bradshaw

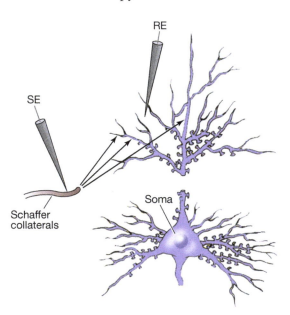

RE

SE

Soma

FIGURE 5.4 In this preparation, the dendritic field is surgically separated from the soma. This prevents the delivery to the stimulated synapses of new proteins that were the product of a genomic signaling cascade. Nevertheless, stimulation delivered to the Schaffer collateral fibers can produce a relatively long-lasting LTP. Key: SE = stimulating electrode; RE = recording electrode.

Schaffer collaterals

et al. (2003) took advantage of the fact that pyramidal neurons in this region have both apical and basal dendrites and receive input from different Schaffer collateral fibers (Figure 5.5). Applying the protein synthesis inhibitor emetine selectively to the soma of these cells did not influence L-LTP. In contrast, the application of emetine to the apical dendrites blocked L-LTP in those dendrites but did not block L-LTP in the basal dendrites, while selectively applying emetine to the basal dendrites blocked L-LTP in those dendrites but did not affect L-LTP in the apical dendrites. The observation that a dose of emetine selectively delivered to the soma did not influence L-LTP but did so when delivered to

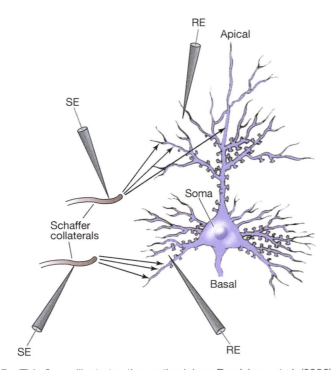

FIGURE 5.5   This figure illustrates the methodology Bradshaw et al. (2003) used to demonstrate the contribution dendritic protein synthesis makes to L-LTP. By stimulating one set of Schaffer collateral fibers they could produce L-LTP in synapses located on dendrites in the apical region of the neuron. By stimulating another set of Schaffer collaterals they could produce L-LTP in synapses located on dendrites in the basal region of the neuron. When the protein synthesis inhibitory emetine was applied to the entire slice, it prevented L-LTP in both dendritic fields. However, when emetine was applied to just the apical dendrites, it blocked L-LTP only in those dendrites, and when applied to just the basal dendrites, it blocked L-LTP only in the basal dendrites. It did not block L-LTP in either region of the dendrites when it was applied to just the soma. These results mean that L-LTP depended on proteins that were translated in the dendrites in response to the LTP-inducing stimulus. Key: SE = stimulating electrode; RE = recording electrode. (After K. D. Bradshaw et al. 2003. *Eur J Neurosci* 18: 3150–3152.)

the dendritic fields strongly implicates a role for local protein synthesis in the generation of L-LTP. The mechanisms that produce local protein synthesis are discussed in detail in Chapter 6.

Genomic Signaling

Not all mRNAs required for producing L-LTP are present locally. They become available later because synaptic activity and neuronal depolarization generate a genomic signaling cascade that results in the transcription of new mRNA. In this case the signaling molecules enter the nucleus to phosphorylate **transcription factors**—proteins that interact with DNA to produce mRNA. This results in the production of mRNAs that subsequently are translated into new proteins (see Figure 5.2).

All parts and functions of a cell depend on ongoing constitutive transcription and translation processes. The distinguishing feature of the genomic signaling hypothesis is that it assumes that transcripts (mRNA) needed to sustain LTP are *produced as a direct consequence of neural activity associated with the stimulus that induces LTP*. The new mRNA and proteins generated as a result of this neural activity are sometimes called **plasticity products** (**PPs**) because they are involved in modifying synapses.

The genomic signaling hypothesis gained support when Nguyen et al. (1994) reported that inhibitors of transcription blocked the development of enduring LTP, but did not interfere with its initial development and stabilization. The hypothesis that L-LTP depends on transcription also gained more specificity when it became known that a transcription factor called **cAMP-responsive, element-binding** (**CREB**) protein was implicated in both synaptic plasticity and long-term memory (see Figure 5.2 and Nguyen and Woo, 2003; Silva et al., 1998; and Yin and Tully, 1996 for reviews). It is important to know how CREB protein is activated. Adams and Dudek (2005) have described two general models of how the signals reach the nucleus: **synapse-to-nucleus signaling** and **soma-to-nucleus signaling** (Figure 5.6).

Synapse-to-Nucleus Signaling

The synapse-to-nucleus signaling model is complex. However, the general outline of the process is relatively simple. The stimulation of a postsynaptic neuron first activates second messengers that then activate protein kinases. Second messengers or their kinase targets translocate into the nucleus where they phosphorylate CREB protein and transcription is initiated. There are multiple intracellular pathways that converge to phosphorylate CREB protein (Figure 5.7). This convergence suggests that CREB protein activation will reflect the combined influence of several sources.

There is no need to discuss all of the possible signaling pathways (see Lim et al., 2017 for a detailed review). However, it is instructive to describe some key ones. One such signaling cascade also involves the activation of **protein**

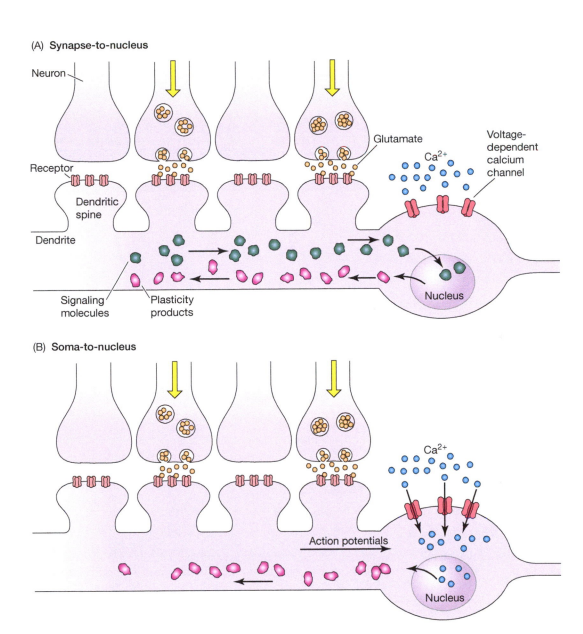

(A) Synapse-to-nucleus

Neuron

Receptor

Dendritic spine

Dendrite

Glutamate

Ca²⁺

Voltage-dependent calcium channel

Signaling molecules   Plasticity products

Nucleus

(B) Soma-to-nucleus

Ca²⁺

Action potentials

Nucleus

FIGURE 5.6 Synaptic activity can signal the nucleus in two ways. (A) The synapse-to-nucleus signaling model assumes that synaptic activity initiates a cascade that produces signaling molecules that eventually translocate to the nucleus to initiate transcription. (B) The soma-to-nucleus signaling model assumes that, as a result of action potentials produced by synaptic activity, Ca²⁺ enters the soma through voltage-dependent calcium channels (vdCCs) where it can more directly initiate transcription. Note that both of these hypotheses could be true.

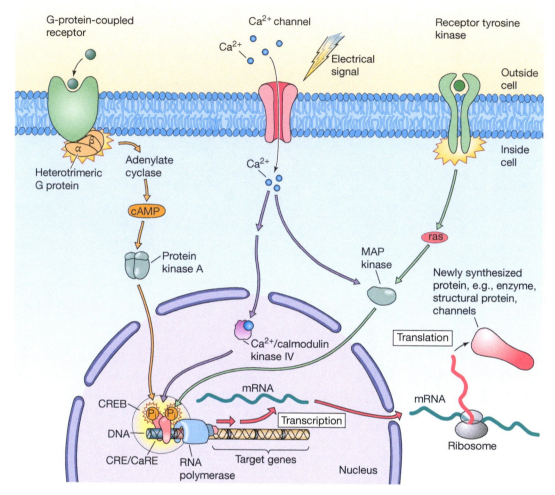

FIGURE 5.7 Transcription occurs in the nucleus where a portion of DNA (deoxyribonucleic acid) is converted into RNA (ribonucleic acid). Transcription then is the transfer of information contained in DNA into mRNA. Ribosomes translate mRNA into protein. This is also called protein synthesis. There are many synapse-to-nucleus signaling pathways that can lead to the phosphorylation of CREB protein and to the production of new mRNA and new proteins that are critical for L-LTP.

kinase A (PKA). When activated by cAMP, PKA can translocate to the nucleus to phosphorylate CREB protein and initiate transcription. Moreover, PKA inhibitors can block the development of long-lasting LTP, and this is accompanied by a reduction in genes controlled by CREB protein (Nguygen and Woo, 2003).

Another signaling cascade involves the activation of the extracellular-regulated kinase (ERK)–mitogen-activated protein (MAP) kinase (**ERK–MAPK**).

When activated, both PKA and ERK–MAPK are thought to translocate to the nucleus where they engage transcription factors, including CREB protein, and induce transcription of plasticity-related mRNAs. Stimulation that leads to the induction of long-lasting LTP induces the transcription of CREB-dependent mRNAs. Inhibitors of PKA and ERK–MAPK activation block the transcription of these mRNAs. Moreover, inhibitors of these kinases also block the development of enduring LTP.

Calcium signals originating in the spine can also be transmitted from activated postsynaptic compartments to the nucleus through the propagation of regenerative calcium waves released from internal calcium stores in the **endoplasmic reticulum** (**ER**). The propagation of this calcium wave is possible because the ER surrounds the nucleus and also extends into axons and dendrites (see the discussion of extracellular and intracellular sources of calcium below).

Soma-to-Nucleus Signaling

According to the soma-to-nucleus signaling model, the action potentials produced when a cell depolarizes also can generate a signal. Repetitive action potentials are assumed to open **voltage-dependent calcium channels** (**vdCCs**) that are located on the plasma membrane of the soma. When these channels open, calcium enters the soma. **Calmodulin** already exists in the nucleus. Thus, when activated by Ca^{2+} it could induce the activation of nuclear enzymes such as CaMKIV that can phosphorylate CREB protein. Activated calmodulin outside of the nucleus also might translocate to the nucleus. This source of Ca^{2+} might also stimulate ERK to translocate to the nucleus to participate in the phosphorylation of CREB protein.

Two arguments support an action-potential, soma-to-nucleus model (Adams and Dudek, 2005). First, the amount of signal generated at single synapses that reaches the nucleus may not be enough to initiate transcription. Second, signaling molecules activated by synaptic processes have a long journey to reach the nucleus. So the time it takes for them to translocate to the nucleus may be too long to allow them to participate in the immediate transcription of genes needed to support L-LTP.

There also is experimental support for the soma-to-nucleus model. A strong prediction from this model is that soma-to-nucleus signaling can substitute for synapse-to-nucleus signaling to produce L-LTP. Dudek and Fields (2002) provided support for this prediction. Recall that a weak stimulus protocol will generate only S-LTP but that a strong stimulus will generate L-LTP (see Figure 5.1). A strong stimulus also is likely to produce the action potentials needed to open the calcium channels.

Dudek and Fields reasoned that if action potentials are the critical event for L-LTP, then it should be possible to convert S-LTP into L-LTP by initiating action potentials without strongly stimulating synapses. To do this they weakly stimulated Schaffer collateral input to CA1 neurons and then initiated action potentials in the CA1 cells antidromically (by stimulating from axon to soma in these cells). These action potentials were sufficient to prevent the decay of LTP normally produced by weak stimulation. The action potentials alone also were sufficient to phosphorylate ERK and CREB protein (Figure 5.8).

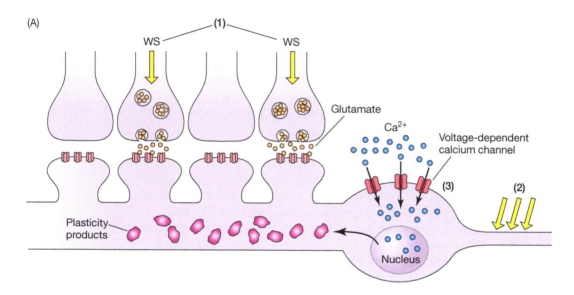

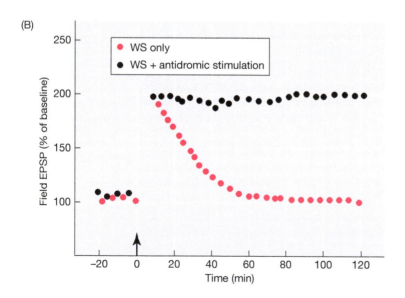

FIGURE 5.8   (A) This figure illustrates how Dudek and Fields (2002) tested the soma-to-nucleus signaling hypotheses. They applied a weak stimulus (WS) to the Schaffer collateral fiber pathway (1). In some slices this was followed by electrical stimulation applied to the axons (called antidromic stimulation) of the CA1 pyramidal cells (2) to produce action potentials in those neurons and allow the influx of Ca^{2+} into the soma and nucleus (3). (B) This figure shows that weak stimulation produced only a short-lasting LTP, but when it was followed by antidromic stimulation L-LTP was induced. (A, B after S. M. Dudek and R. D. Fields. 2002. *Proc Natl Acad Sci USA* 99: 3962–3967; B © 2002 National Academy of Sciences.)

Translation Requires Increased Calcium Levels

The above discussion indicates that new protein becomes available in two waves. The initial wave is the result of local synthesis and the second is the result of protein translated from mRNA generated by the genomic signal (Figure 5.9). It is important to note that increased calcium levels are required for both waves.

Calcium entering the neuron through NMDA receptors is critical for the production of LTP but this source of calcium alone may not be sufficient to produce any form of LTP (Morgan and Teyler, 1999; Raymond and Redman, 2006; Sabatini et al., 2001). To mount the signaling cascades needed to produce long-lasting synaptic changes, calcium provided by NMDA receptors needs to be amplified by different sources of Ca^{2+}. Thus, it is important to understand calcium sources and some of the complexities associated with their regulation by synaptic activity.

Two sources of calcium, one extracellular and one intracellular, can influence the induction and duration of LTP (Figure 5.10; see Baker et al., 2013 for a review). Calcium is contained in the *extracellular* fluid that surrounds the neuron. It can enter the cell through activated NMDA receptors and through the voltage-dependent calcium channels located on the plasma membrane that surrounds the soma. The vdCCs open and close in response to the depolarizing stimulation associated with action potentials. When they are open, they allow extracellular Ca^{2+} to enter the neuron, thus producing a transient increase in intracellular Ca^{2+} in the soma.

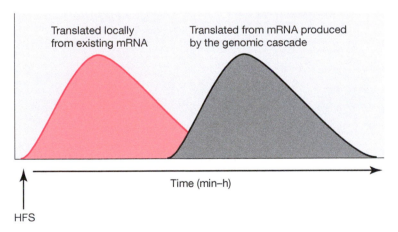

FIGURE 5.9 Strong high-frequency stimulation (HFS) can result in two waves of protein synthesis that may be important for L-LTP. The first wave occurs locally in the dendrites. The second wave occurs when new protein is synthesized from the new mRNA produced by the genomic signaling cascade. These proteins could be subsequently synthesized in either the soma or dendritic regions.

Sources of calcium

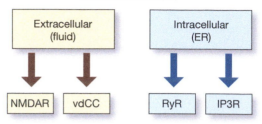

FIGURE 5.10 There are two general sources of calcium that influence LTP. One source is the Ca^{2+} in the extracellular fluid surrounding the neuron. This Ca^{2+} enters the dendritic spines through NMDA receptors (NMDAR) and enters the soma through vdCCs. The other calcium source is intracellular Ca^{2+}, which is stored in the endoplasmic reticulum (ER). It can be released when it binds to the RyRs located on the ER in the spine or when IP3 binds to IP3Rs located on ER in the dendrite.

Intracellular Ca^{2+} resides in the neuron, stored in the ER. For some time, the ER has been recognized as important to Ca^{2+} signaling (Berridge, 1998). The ER network extends continuously throughout the neuron (Droz et al., 1975; Terasaki et al., 1994), even extending into the dendritic spines (Figure 5.11). Because it is continuous within the neuron and responds to signaling events in the cytosol, Berridge (1998) characterized the ER network as the neuron within the neuron. He has proposed that these two membranes, the plasma membrane and the ER, work together to regulate many neuronal processes such as transmitter release, synaptic plasticity, and gene regulation. The ER is important in the context of synaptic plasticity because (1) it is a calcium sink that can rapidly sequester or store free Ca^{2+}, and (2) it is a calcium source that can release Ca^{2+} in response to second messengers.

To understand how these different calcium sources influence the processes that support LTP it is useful to think of the neuron as composed of three compartments: (1) spine compartment, (2) dendritic

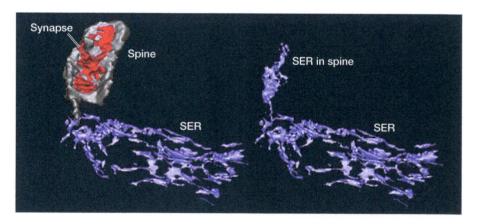

FIGURE 5.11 This figure presents a three-dimensional reconstruction of the endoplasmic reticulum (purple) in a rat hippocampal CA1 dendritic segment. The membrane of the dendrite is not visible, but in the left side of the figure the membrane of the attached spine is present. Note that the smooth endoplasmic reticulum (SER) in the dendrite is contiguous with the SER entering the thin neck of a large dendritic spine (gray). Berridge (1998) has called the endoplasmic reticulum the neuron within the neuron because it is contiguous with the neuron and responds to signaling molecules. (From Synapse Web, Kristen M. Harris, PI, https://synapseweb.clm.utexas.edu/.)

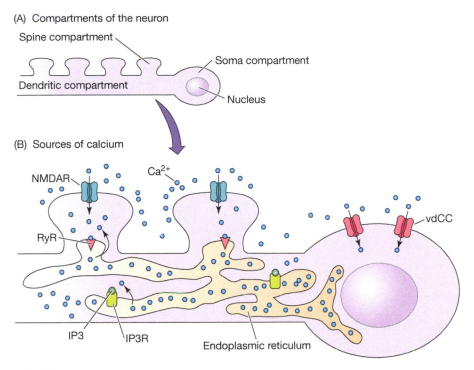

(A) Compartments of the neuron

Spine compartment

Soma compartment

Dendritic compartment

Nucleus

(B) Sources of calcium

NMDAR

Ca²⁺

vdCC

RyR

IP3

IP3R

Endoplasmic reticulum

FIGURE 5.12 (A) A neuron consists of three compartments: the soma compartment, the dendritic compartment, and the spine compartment. (B) Calcium is present in the extracellular fluid as well as stored intracellularly in the ER. Ca^{2+} levels can increase in each of the three distinct compartments of the neuron. Extracellular Ca^{2+} can enter a spine through NMDA receptors (NMDAR) and can enter the soma through vdCCs. Intracellular Ca^{2+} stored on the ER can be released into spines when Ca^{2+} binds to RyRs located in spines or can be released into the dendritic compartment when IP3 binds to IP3Rs located in the dendrite.

compartment, and (3) soma or cell body compartment (Figure 5.12A). Ca^{2+} levels can increase in each of the three distinct compartments of the neuron.

Spine and Dendritic Compartments

NMDA receptors are located on the plasma membrane of the spine compartment, and ER that protrudes into the spine contains **ryanodine receptors (RyRs)**, which bind to calcium. This spatial proximity of NMDA receptors and RyRs provides the opportunity for what is called **calcium-induced calcium release (CICR)**. It occurs when a small amount of extracellular Ca^{2+} enters through the NMDA receptor and binds to RyRs to release additional Ca^{2+} from the ER (Berridge, 1998). This process—the binding of calcium to RyRs—provides a way to amplify the extracellular Ca^{2+} entering the spine compartment through NMDA receptors and triggers some of the post-translation modifications that are necessary to induce LTP, as discussed in Chapter 3 (Figure 5.12B).

FIGURE 5.13 Metabotropic receptors activate G proteins in the plasma membrane, which may either alter the opening of a G-protein-gated ion channel (A) or stimulate an effector enzyme that either synthesizes or breaks down a second messenger (B).

(A)

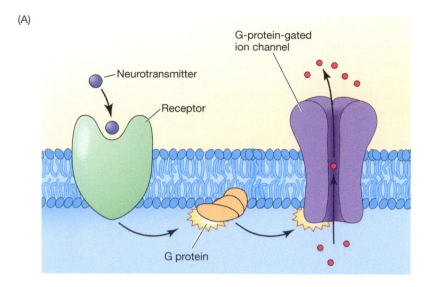

(B)

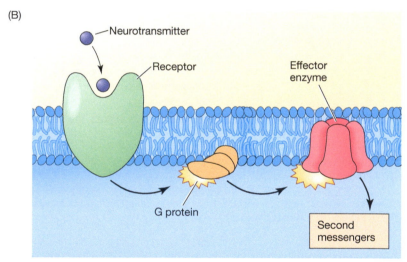

Endoplasmic reticulum in the dendritic compartment is populated with **IP3Rs (inositol triphosphate receptors)**. These receptors respond to both calcium and the second messenger **IP3 (inositol triphosphate)**, which is synthesized when the first messenger glutamate binds to a subtype of **metabotropic receptor** called **mGluR1**, located in the plasma membrane near dendritic spines. In contrast to ionotropic receptors, metabotropic receptors do not form an ion channel pore. Instead, they activate **G proteins**, which may either alter the opening of a G-protein-gated ion channel or stimulate an effector enzyme that either synthesizes or breaks down a second messenger (Figure 5.13). When second messenger IP3 binds to IP3Rs, calcium is released from the ER in the dendritic compartment. This increase in calcium in the dendritic compartment contributes to the local translation that produces the first wave of new proteins.

Soma Compartment

The plasma membrane surrounding the soma is populated with vdCCs, and extracellular calcium can enter the soma when action potentials open these channels. As noted above, calcium entering through these channels provides a way to rapidly initiate transcription (see soma-to-nucleus hypothesis) and new mRNA that ultimately is translated to yield the second wave of new protein.

The number of theta-burst stimulation (TBS) trains controls the duration of LTP (Figure 5.14A). A single TBS train produces a short-lasting form, LTP1;

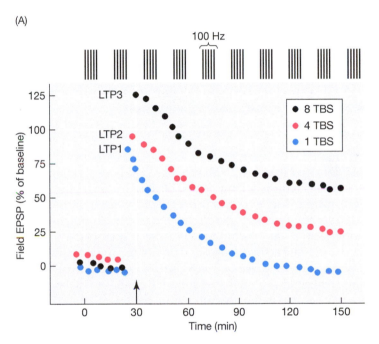

(A)

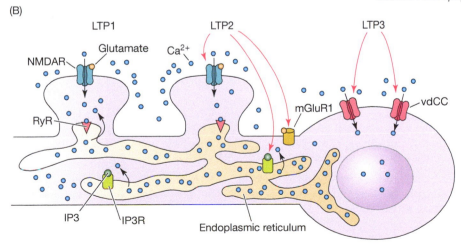

(B)

FIGURE 5.14 (A) The number of theta-burst stimuli (TBS) determines the duration of LTP. (B) This figure illustrates how different sources of Ca^{2+} contribute to different forms of LTP. LTP1 is induced when glutamate produced by a weak stimulus (1-train TBS) binds to the NMDA receptor (NMDAR). This results in a modest influx of Ca^{2+} into the spine. Acting as a second messenger, Ca^{2+} binds to the RyRs and causes the ER to release additional Ca^{2+} into the spine. LTP2 is induced when glutamate resulting from stronger stimulation (4-train TBS) binds both to NMDA receptors and to mGluR1s and results in local protein synthesis. LTP3 is produced when the strongest stimulation (8-train TBS) repeatedly opens the vdCCs, and the level of Ca^{2+} in the soma is increased to the point where it can translocate to the nucleus to initiate transcription of genes necessary for the expression of LTP3. (A after C. R. Raymond and S. J. Redman. 2002. *J Neurophysiol* 88: 249–255.)

four trains produce a moderately lasting form, LTP2; and eight trains produce a very long-lasting form, LTP3. Research by Raymond and Redman (2002, 2006) has revealed that the duration of LTP depends on the number of calcium sources recruited by TBS.

- LTP1 depends only on RyRs releasing ER calcium in the spine compartment.
- LTP2 depends on IP3 receptors releasing calcium from ER in the dendritic compartment.
- LTP3 depends on calcium entering the soma through vdCCs.

The general point of these observations is that as the number of TBS trains increases more calcium sources are engaged and they activate transcription and translation processes that increase the stability and consolidation of synaptic changes that support LTP. A summary of how calcium sources influence the induction and persistence of LTP is provided in Figure 5.14B.

Summary

Over 100 years ago, Müller and Pilzecker (1900) proposed the consolidation hypothesis—that new memories require a long period of time to consolidate and become resistant to disruption. This hypothesis became identified with the *de novo* protein synthesis hypothesis when it was discovered that inhibiting protein synthesis disrupted long-term memories but not short-term memory. The processes that consolidate an enlarged actin cytoskeleton do not require new protein. However, there is a subsequent *consolidation phase* during which new proteins are generated that may be needed to ensure that synaptic changes will endure.

Translation machinery is located in the dendritic spine region and there is evidence that synaptic activity can induce the synthesis of new proteins from mRNA available in this region. New proteins can also be generated by genomic signaling cascades that produce mRNA that can then be translated into proteins. To engage translation and transcription processes requires that the induction stimulus recruit multiple sources of calcium. Calcium sources localized to the spine compartment (the CICR cascade) only support short-lasting LTP. Longer-lasting forms of LTP require (a) IP3 to release calcium from the ER in the dendritic compartment and (b) extracellular calcium to enter the soma through vdCCs.

References

Adams, J. P. and Dudek, S. M. (2005). Late-phase long-term potentiation: getting to the nucleus. *Nature Reviews Neuroscience, 6*, 737–743.

Baker, K. D., Edwards, T. M., and Rickard, N. S. (2013). Intracellular calcium stores in synaptic plasticity and memory consolidation. *Neuroscience and Biobehavioral Reviews, 37*, 1211–1239.

Berridge, M. J. (1998). Neuronal calcium signaling. *Neuron, 21*, 13–26.

Bradshaw, K. D., Emptage, N. J., and Bliss, T. V. (2003). A role for dendritic protein synthesis in hippocampal late LTP. *European Journal of Neuroscience, 18*, 3150–3152.

Droz, B., Rambourt, A., and Koenig, H. L. (1975). The smooth endoplasmic reticulum: structure and role in the renewal of axonal membrane and synaptic vesicles by fast axonal transport. *Brain Research, 93*, 1–13.

Dudek, S. M. and Fields, R. D. (2002). Somatic action potentials are sufficient for late-phase LTP-related cell signaling. *Proceedings of the National Academy of Sciences USA, 99*, 3962–3967.

Flexner, J. B., Flexner, L. B., and Stellar, E. (1963). Memory in mice as affected by intracerebral puromycin. *Science, 141*, 57–59.

Frey, U., Krug, M., Reymann, K. G., and Matthies, H. (1988). Anisomycin, an inhibitor of protein synthesis, blocks late phases of LTP phenomena in the hippocampal CA1 region in vitro. *Brain Research, 452*, 57–65.

Kang, H. and Schuman, E. M. (1996). A requirement for local protein synthesis in neurotrophin-induced hippocampal synaptic plasticity. *Science, 273*, 1402–1406.

Krug, M., Lössner, B., and Ott, T. (1984). Anisomycin blocks the late phase of long-term potentiation in the dentate gyrus of freely moving rats. *Brain Research Bulletin, 13*, 39–42.

Lim, A. F., Lim, W. L. and Ch'ng, T. H. (2017). Activity-dependent synapse to nucleus signaling. *Neurobiology of Learning and Memory, 138*, 78–84.

Lynch, G. and Baudry, M. (1984). The biochemistry of memory: a new and specific hypothesis. *Science, 224*, 1057–1063.

Lynch, G., Kramár, E. A., and Gall, C. M. (2015). Protein synthesis and consolidation of memory-related synaptic changes. *Brain Research, 1621*, 62–72.

Lynch, G., Rex, C. S., and Gall, C. M. (2007). LTP consolidation: Substrates, explanatory power, and functional significance. *Neuropharmacology, 52*, 12–23.

McGaugh, J. L. (2000). Memory—a century of consolidation. *Science, 287*, 248–251.

Miyashiro, K., Dichter, M., and Eberwine, J. (1994). On the nature and differential distribution of mRNAs in hippocampal neurites: implications for neuronal functioning. *Proceedings of the National Academy of Sciences USA, 91*, 10800–10804.

Morgan, S. L. and Teyler, T. J. (1999). VDCCs and NMDARs underlie two forms of LTP in CA1 hippocampus in vivo. *Journal of Neurophysiology, 82*, 736–740.

Müller, G. E. and Pilzecker, A. (1900). Experimentelle beiträge zur lehre vom gedächtniss. *Zeitschrift für Psychologie*, 1–300.

Nguyen, P. V., Abel, T., and Kandel, E. R. (1994). Requirement of a critical period of transcription for induction of a late phase of LTP. *Science, 265*, 1104–1107.

Nguyen, P. V. and Woo, N. H. (2003). Regulation of hippocampal synaptic plasticity by cyclic AMP-dependent protein kinases. *Progress in Neurobiology, 71*, 401–437.

Ostroff, L. E, Watson, D. J., Cao, G., Parker, P. H., Smith, H., and Harris, K. M. (2018). Shifting patterns of polyribosome accumulation at synapses over the course of hippocampal long-term potentiation. *Hippocampus, 6,* 416–430.

Raymond, C. R. and Redman, S. J. (2002). Different calcium sources are narrowly tuned to the induction of different forms of LTP. *Journal of Neurophysiology, 88,* 249–255.

Raymond, C. R. and Redman, S. J. (2006). Spatial segregation of neuronal calcium signals encodes different forms of LTP in rat hippocampus. *Journal of Physiology, 570,* 97–111.

Roberts, R. B. and Flexner, L. B. (1969). The biochemical basis of long-term memory. *Quarterly Review of Biophysics, 2,* 135–173.

Rudy, J. W. (2015). Variation in the persistence of memory: An interplay between actin dynamics and AMPA receptors. *Brain Research, 1621,* 29–37.

Sabatini, B. L., Maravall, M., and Svoboda, K. (2001). Ca^{2+} signaling in dendritic spines. *Current Opinion Neurobiology, 11,* 349–356.

Silva, A. J., Giese, K. P., Fedorov, N. B., Frankland, P. W., and Kogan, J. H. (1998). Molecular, cellular, and neuroanatomical substrates of place learning. *Neurobiology of Learning and Memory, 70,* 44–61.

Steward, O. and Schuman, E. M. (2001). Protein synthesis at synaptic sites on dendrites. *Annual Review of Neuroscience, 24,* 299–325.

Sutton, M. A. and Schuman, E. M. (2006). Dendritic protein synthesis, synaptic plasticity, and memory. *Cell, 127,* 49–58.

Terasaki, M., Slater, N. T., Fein, A., Schmidek, A., and Reese, T. S. (1994). Continuous network of endoplasmic reticulum in cerebellar Purkinje neurons. *Proceedings of the National Academy of Sciences USA, 91,* 7510–7514.

Vickers, C. A., Dickson, K. S., and Wyllie, D. J. (2005). Induction and maintenance of late-phase long-term potentiation in isolated dendrites of rat hippocampal CA1 pyramidal neurons. *Journal of Physiology, 568,* 803–813.

Yin, J. and Tully, T. (1996). CREB and the formation of long-term memory. *Current Opinion in Neurobiology, 2,* 264–268.

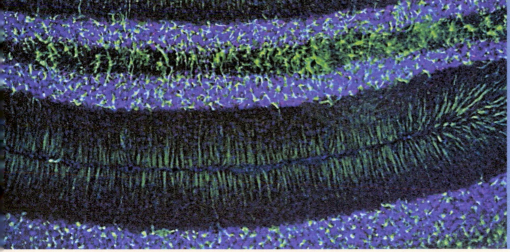

Courtesy of Heidi E. W. Day

Consolidating LTP: Specific Mechanisms

A single neuron can receive signals at several thousand independent synapses. Yet the strength of the response to the signal can be regulated at the level of single spines. How is such specificity possible? The previous chapters provide one answer—the spines responding to glutamate released by an LTP-inducing stimulus selectively undergo a rapid enlargement of the actin cytoskeleton. A second answer is that proteins can be translated locally in the dendritic spine. Consider the general problem solved by local synthesis. All components of neurons depend on a more or less continuous supply of mRNAs that must be translated into the needed protein. The classic central dogma is that all proteins are translated in the somatic space close to the nucleus (Holt and Schuman, 2013). This means that the proteins would have to be sorted and shipped out to the right places, at the right time, and in enough quantity to meet the current requirements of the neuron.

The discovery that protein synthesis can occur locally revolutionized thinking about this issue. Following transcription, mRNAs are transported and localized to specific compartments (dendrites and spines) where, in response to specific signals, they can be translated as needed. In this way an efficient and flexible *protein-on-demand system* is created that provides new proteins at the right time and place. Efficiency also derives in part because a single mRNA molecule can be translated into multiple proteins. In the case of LTP, local protein synthesis allows for relatively precise allocation of proteins to the synapses that respond to the inducing stimulus and ensures the long-term persistence of the synaptic changes.

Local protein synthesis depends on the orchestration of a large number of processes. Messenger RNA must be delivered to the dendritic spine region and synaptic activity must engage the BDNF–TrkB pathway to initiate protein synthesis. In parallel, the ubiquitin–proteasome system must be engaged to degrade proteins that inhibit transcription and translation. The immediate early gene *Arc* will be translated and will mediate consolidation produced by the BDNF–TrkB pathway (see Chapter 14 for a discussion of immediate early genes). Newly synthesized proteins then will be captured by clusters of synapses that were stimulated when LTP was generated. All of these processes are described in detail in the sections that follow. The story begins with the processes that ensure mRNAs are present locally—in the dendritic spine region.

Local Dendritic mRNA Dynamics

To arrive at specific dendritic locations, mRNAs depend on RNA-binding proteins (RNA-BPs), which bind to elements within the mRNA and attach those elements to cytoskeleton motor proteins. These motor proteins (called kinesins and dyneins) then use microtubule cytoskeleton to cargo the RNA-BPs to their primary destinations (Figure 6.1)—for example, to the dendritic spine region. During transport the translation of mRNA is prevented by repressor proteins (Buxbaum et al., 2014).

The mRNAs for many of the familiar synaptic proteins (such as CaMKII, BDNF, actin, and AMPA receptors) are present in dendrites. Robert Singer's group (Yoon et al., 2016) provided insight into the dynamics of dendritic mRNA by imaging actin mRNA in cultured neurons to model the processes. Some of the findings of this remarkable set of experiments include the following (Yoon et al., 2016).

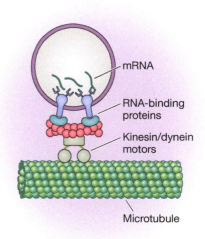

- mRNA
- RNA-binding proteins
- Kinesin/dynein motors
- Microtubule

FIGURE 6.1 Motor proteins use microtubules to transport vesicles containing mRNA from the soma to the dendritic spine region.

- Under steady-state conditions almost all of the individual mRNAs changed positions, cycling between a *stationary* phase of about 7 minutes during which they did not move and a *mobile* phase of a few seconds when they moved to a new location.

- Uncaging glutamate onto spines rapidly changed the distribution of mRNAs to the stimulated spine where, in contrast to their steady-state activity, they remained for at least 2 hours. Thus, the stimulated spines captured the mRNAs.

- The relocation of the mRNAs depended on NMDA receptor activation because inhibiting these receptors prevented redistribution.

- The persistent redistribution also depended on the polymerization of nascent actin filament because inhibiting actin dynamics prevented redistribution. Thus, a dynamic rapid remodeling of the actin network was essential for spines to capture mRNAs.

- Notably, however, blocking protein synthesis had no effect on mRNA redistribution.

- Glutamate uncaging resulted in the synthesis of new protein that was primarily restricted to spines activated by glutamate.

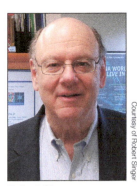

Robert Singer

Given that protein synthesis depends on ribosomes, one might expect that polyribosomes (complexes composed of three or more ribosomes) would also relocate in response to glutamate release. Consistent with this hypothesis, using electron microscopy, Kristen Harris and her colleagues (Ostroff et al., 2018) reported that the induction of LTP was accompanied by a rapid shift in the distribution of polyribosomes from the dendritic shaft to the spine base and spine head where they remained for about 2 hours.

In summary, from these results a general picture emerges (Figure 6.2). Motor proteins cargo mRNAs to appropriate dendritic regions. The mRNAs cycle between stationary and movement phases, as if they were sampling the local synaptic environment. Glutamate released onto spines causes a redistribution of mRNAs so that stimulated spines capture them. In parallel, the ribosomal translation machinery is redistributed to stimulated spines and can synthesize the protein in the specific locations where it is needed. The redistribution of the mRNA and existing proteins (for example, ribosomes) does not require the translation of new protein. However, it does require the actin management processes that generate new actin filament to produce enlarged spines.

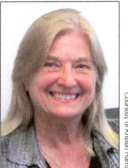

Kristen Harris

Initiation of Local Protein Synthesis

Messenger RNAs for synaptic proteins (such as actin PSD-95, Arc, GluA1, CaMKII, and AMPA receptors) are present in the local dendritic region (Schratt et al., 2004). The translation of these proteins, however, depends on the assembly of fully functional ribosomal complexes, which are composed, in part, of a basic ribosomal subunit and a number of associated proteins that are derived from a category of mRNAs called **TOPs** (**terminal oligopyrimidine tracts**), also known as **translation factors**. These mRNAs code for ribosomal proteins such as initiation factors (IFs) and elongation factors

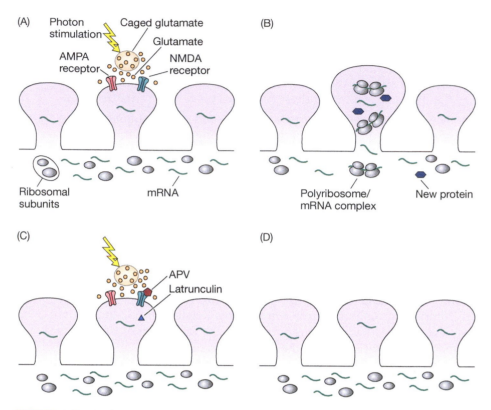

FIGURE 6.2 (A) Once transported to the dendritic spine region, mRNA continues to cycle between nearby spines. (B) Uncaging glutamate rapidly changes the spatial distribution of mRNA; functional ribosomes form polyribosome complexes that translate mRNA into new protein that is captured by stimulated spines. (C) and (D) Inhibiting NMDA receptors by APV or interfering with actin polymerization by latrunculin prevents the redistribution of mRNAs and ribosomal complexes. (After Y. J. Yoon et al. 2016. *Proc Natl Acad Sci USA* 113: E6877–E6886.)

(EFs). There are many of them. Local protein synthesis depends on a coordinated regulation of these translation factors by signaling events initiated by synaptic activity. This leads to the translation of TOPs, allowing them to join small ribosomal subunits *to create functional ribosomal complexes* that can translate other proteins.

Note the implication of this general scheme. Some functional ribosomal complexes are present in the dendritic spine region but the steady-state capacity for translation is relatively low. Synaptic activity, however, can quickly increase translation capacity in a particular dendritic spine region by initiating the translation of TOP mRNAs that can join ribosomal subunits to increase the

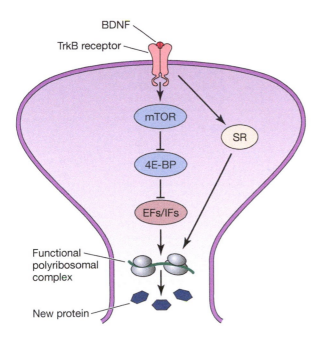

FIGURE 6.3 Local protein synthesis is initiated when BDNF binds to TrkB receptors. This results in the removal of the inhibitory influence of the TOP protein 4E-BP, so that small ribosomal (SR) subunits can combine with other TOPs—such as elongation factors (EFs) and initiation factors (IFs)—to produce competent polyribosomal complexes that translate mRNA into protein. (After A. Govindarajan et al. 2006. *Nature Rev Neurosci* 7: 575–583.)

number of polyribosomes (Tsokas et al., 2005, 2007). In this way proteins can be translated on demand where they are needed.

Signaling Pathways

Translation begins when ribosomes are recruited to TOP mRNAs. Translation, however, is repressed by one of the TOP mRNAs called eukaryotic initiating factor 4E-binding protein (4E-BP). It functions by interfering with interactions between other TOPs and thus prevents translation. The initiation of local protein synthesis requires signaling events that phosphorylate 4E-BP and disrupt its interfering function.

Two major signaling pathways can lead to phosphorylating 4E-BP. One goes through the **mitogen-activated protein kinase** (**MAPK**) and the other goes through the **mammalian target of rapamycin complex** (**mTOR**). To keep the story manageable, however, the focus here is on activating the mTOR pathway. The key signaling events are **BDNF** (**brain-derived neurotrophic factor**), **TrkB** (a tyrosine kinase receptor), and mTOR (Figure 6.3).

BDNF is a member of a family of neurotrophic factors involved in regulating the survival and differentiation of neuronal populations during development (Huang and Reichardt, 2001). It is synthesized, stored, and released from the same neurons that release glutamate (Lessmann et al., 2003), but it can be released from dendrites. Thus, the exact source of extracellular BDNF is difficult

FIGURE 6.4 Interfering with TrkB function shortly after the induction of LTP (blue bar) has no effect on the generation of LTP but prevents LTP from enduring. Interfering with TrkB function 80 minutes after LTP is induced (black bar) has no effect on either the generation or endurance of LTP. These results indicate that local protein synthesis requires less than 80 minutes. (After Y. Lu et al. 2011. *J Neurosci* 31: 11762–11771.)

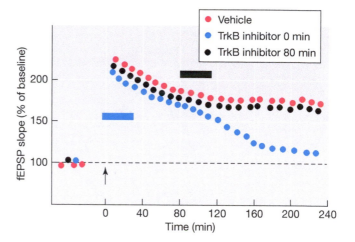

to determine. However, Jia et al. (2010) provided a strong case for presynaptic BDNF release in LTP found in the striatum. They speculated that the co-release of glutamate and BDNF from axon terminals might be a ubiquitous requirement for enduring LTP.

TrkB receptors respond to BDNF and initiate events that result in the activation of the mTOR complex, which phosphorylates the translation repressor protein 4E-BP2 to allow the assembly of functional ribosomal complexes and the rapid translation of mRNAs (Panja and Bramham, 2014). Critically, treatments that prevent BDNF from activating TrkB receptors will interfere with the translation of TOP mRNAs and development of long-lasting LTP (Kang and Schuman, 1996). As illustrated in Figure 6.4, preventing BDNF from binding to TrkB receptors within 40 minutes of TBS prevents long-lasting LTP but has no effect when applied later (Korte et al., 1995, 1998; Lu et al., 2011). These treatments have no impact on the generation phase of LTP.

Erin Schuman and her colleagues (Tang et al., 2002) were the first to report that the activation of the **mTOR– TOP pathway** is critical for synaptic changes supporting LTP. Their study showed that rapamycin—a drug that prevents the activation of mTOR (which is why this kinase is called the target of

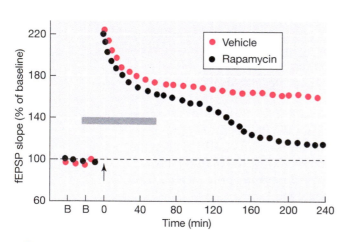

FIGURE 6.5 Application of rapamycin (represented by the bar) blocks the activation of mTOR kinase and prevents the very late-phase LTP. (After P. Tsokas et al. 2005. *J Neurosci* 25: 5833–5843 © 2005 Society for Neuroscience.)

rapamycin)—selectively impairs the late phase of LTP without influencing the initial induction. Other laboratories have linked this impaired LTP to the failure of synaptic activity to translate TOP mRNAs (Tsokas et al., 2005, 2007). These findings (Figure 6.5) indicate that lasting forms of LTP depend on signaling cascades that activate the mTOR pathway.

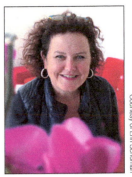

Erin Schuman

Protein Degradation

For over 50 years the idea that consolidation depends on the synthesis of new proteins has been central to the thinking about how synapse memories are consolidated. However, it is now clear that a complementary set of processes *that degrade existing protein* is just as important to LTP as the synthesis of new protein (Bingol et al., 2010; Cajigas et al., 2010; Fonseca et al., 2006; Hegde, 2010).

The Ubiquitin–Proteasome System

There are a number of specific processes devoted to protein degradation (see Bingol et al., 2010; Tai and Schuman, 2008). However, it is the **ubiquitin–proteasome system (UPS)** that is most important to the regulation of synaptic plasticity. The signaling cascades that regulate this system are complex (for example, Hegde, 2010) but the general operating principles are easily understood (Figure 6.6). The system is composed of small proteins called ubiquitin and larger protein complexes called proteasome. Ubiquitin identifies proteins that need to be degraded and proteasome is responsible for their degradation. A process called **ubiquitination** accomplishes this goal. It begins when post-translation modifications bond a single ubiquitin

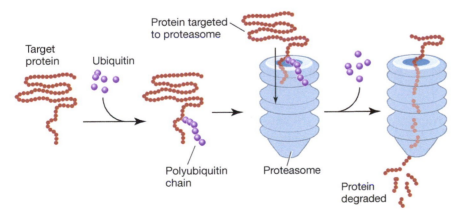

FIGURE 6.6 This figure illustrates the general principles of the ubiquitin–proteasome system (UPS). Post-translation modifications bond a ubiquitin molecule to a protein (ubiquitination). A polyubiquitin chain marks the protein for delivery to the proteasome and protein degradation.

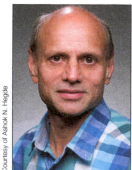

Ashok Hegde

molecule to a protein. Additional ubiquitin molecules then can be added, and this process yields a **polyubiquitin chain** (see Tai and Schuman, 2008). Proteins tagged with a polyubiquitin chain are directed to proteasomes for degradation.

The general importance of the UPS was recognized in the award of the 2004 Nobel Prize in Chemistry to Aaron Ciechanover, Avram Hershko, and Irwin Rose. Ashok Hegde (Hegde, 2010; Hegde et al., 1993) was the first to discover a role for the UPS system in synaptic plasticity. Contemporary researchers have revealed that protein degradation regulates several stages of LTP.

Components of the UPS are localized in dendrites, synapses (Ehlers, 2003; Patrick et al., 2003), and the nucleus. Glutamate transmission activates the ubiquitination processes (Bingol and Schuman, 2006; Ehlers, 2003; Guo and Wang, 2007) and the activation of CaMKII plays a critical role in recruiting proteasome molecules into dendritic spines (Bingol et al., 2010). Moreover, stimulation that induces LTP activates this system and results in protein degradation (Ehlers, 2003; Karpova et al., 2006; Lee et al., 2008).

To study the UPS pathway, researchers apply drugs such as β-lactone that prevent proteasome molecules from degrading protein. Under these conditions, even if it is tagged with ubiquitin, protein will not be degraded. If a proteasome inhibitor alters a functional outcome (such as enhancing the duration of LTP), the conclusion would be that the normal function depends on the UPS degrading protein.

Protein Degradation and LTP

Much of what is known about the contribution the UPS makes to LTP comes from a series of experiments from Hegde and his colleagues (for example, Dong et al., 2008; Hegde, 2010). The basic findings are summarized in Figures 6.7 and 6.8. Prior to the induction of LTP the hippocampal slice was treated with a proteasome inhibitor (β-lactone) or a control solution. Note that, paradoxically, relative to the control, inhibiting the proteasome function enhanced the early expression of LTP but prevented it from enduring (see Figure 6.7). As illustrated in Figure 6.8, however, rapamycin, which interferes with mTOR function, prevented the initial enhancement of LTP.

Why does inhibiting the UPS initially enhance LTP? As previously discussed, mTOR regulates local protein synthesis by interacting with TOP mRNAs. Some of the TOP mRNAs are translation activators (elF4E and eEF1A) and thus they enhance the translation of other synaptic proteins that support LTP. In other experiments Hegde's group reported that these activators were overexpressed in slices treated with β-lactone prior to LTP induction. In addition, applying molecules that interfere with the interaction of these translation activators prevented β-lactone from enhancing the initial expression of LTP and drastically reduced the expression of other proteins (Dong et al., 2014). The general point is that local protein synthesis resulting from activating the

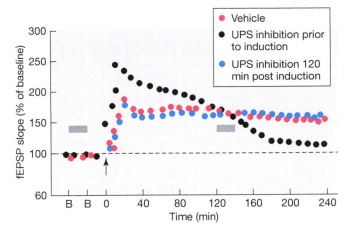

FIGURE 6.7 Inhibiting the proteasome function prior to induction enhances the early phases of LTP but prevents LTP from enduring. However, inhibiting the proteasome function 120 minutes after induction does not prevent LTP from enduring. These results suggest that (1) initially the UPS functions to limit the translation of synaptic proteins through which LTP is expressed and (2) it functions to support the enduring phase of LTP by degrading proteins that repress translation and transcription processes needed to produce new synaptic proteins. The gray bars indicate when the proteasome inhibitor was applied. (After C. Dong et al. 2008. *Learn Mem* 15: 335–347.)

BDNF → TrkB → mTOR pathway must be tightly regulated so that synaptic proteins are not overproduced. The UPS ensures this is the case by limiting the expression of translation activators.

Why does inhibiting the proteasome function prevent LTP from enduring? The answer is that in the presence of this inhibition, 4E-BP and other translation repressor proteins accumulate over time so that the local translation of mRNAs needed to sustain LTP is prevented and LTP decays down to baseline. In addition, transcription is also under the control of repressor proteins and the application of β-lactone prevents the degradation of ATF4, a CREB repressor, and this prevents transcription of relevant mRNAs.

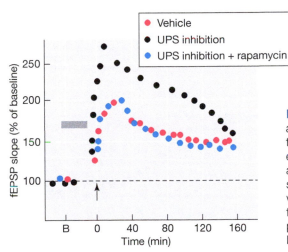

FIGURE 6.8 The initial enhancement of LTP associated with inhibiting proteasome function was prevented if the slice was also treated with rapamycin. This indicates that the activation of the mTOR pathway is responsible for the initial enhancement of LTP that was unmasked by interfering with the UPS function. The gray bar indicates when the proteasome inhibitor was applied. (After C. Dong et al. 2008. *Learn Mem* 15: 335–347.)

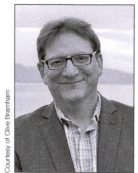

Clive Bramham

Arc Protein Synthesis

The upregulation of local protein synthesis machinery is a first step toward consolidation of LTP that is dependent on protein synthesis. Many of these proteins are familiar (AMPA receptors, PSD-95, CaMKII). *But what important new functional–structural proteins does this now active translation machinery synthesize?* Clive Bramham and his colleagues have made a strong case that **Arc** (activity-regulated, cytoskeleton-associated protein) is one such protein (for example, Bramham, 2008; Bramham et al., 2010; Bramham and Messaoudi, 2005).

Arc protein is derived from an immediate early gene *Arc*—a gene that is transcribed rapidly in response to strong synaptic activity because its transcription does not require the prior translation of some other protein. *Arc* mRNA is quickly transported precisely to the regions of synaptic activity that initiated the transcription signal (see Dynes and Steward, 2012). *Arc* mRNA thus becomes available in local regions at the time the local translation machinery is active.

Arc Antisense Blocks Long-Lasting LTP

John Guzowski and his colleagues (2000) were the first to identify a contribution of *Arc* protein to the consolidation of LTP. They used an **antisense oligonucleotide** (a synthesized strand of nucleic acid that will bind to mRNA and prevent its translation) to prevent the translation of *Arc* mRNA into protein. Blocking the translation of *Arc* mRNA had no effect on the induction of LTP but prevented it from enduring. Consistent with the idea that *Arc* protein is required for the consolidation of LTP, Messaoudi et al. (2007) reported that *Arc* antisense rapidly reverses LTP when applied up to 160 minutes after induction, but not when applied after 280 minutes (Figure 6.9). Thus, it appears that consolidation requires a sustained contribution of *Arc* translation for several hours following the induction signal.

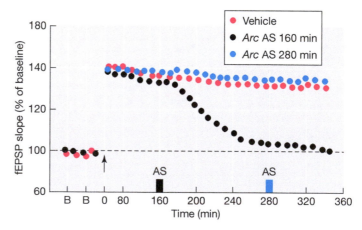

FIGURE 6.9 *Arc* antisense (AS) reverses a well-established LTP when applied about 160 minutes after the inducing stimulus but not when applied 280 minutes after. This indicates that the synaptic changes have been consolidated by 280 minutes. (After E. Messaoudi et al. 2007. *J Neurosci* 27: 10445–10455.)

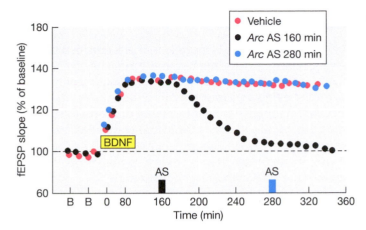

FIGURE 6.10 BDNF alone potentiates synapses. This effect of BDNF depends on the translation of *Arc* because *Arc* antisense (AS) reverses this potentiation when applied 160 minutes after BDNF. *Arc* antisense does not reverse potentiation when applied 280 minutes after BDNF. This indicates that the synaptic changes have been consolidated 280 minutes after BDNF was applied. (After E. Messaoudi et al. 2007. *J Neurosci* 27: 10445–10455.)

BDNF–TrkB Consolidation Depends on Arc Protein Synthesis

As previously described, the **BDNF–TrkB** pathway is critical for consolidating the synaptic changes supporting LTP. In fact, applying exogenous BDNF to brain tissue will produce a long-lasting LTP similar to that produced by multiple TBS (Messaoudi et al., 2007). This effect, however, depends on the synthesis of Arc protein because applying antisense to *Arc* eliminates BDNF-induced potentiation (Figure 6.10). This finding thus potentially links the **BDNF → TrkB → mTOR → TOP** signaling cascade to the synthesis of Arc protein and to consolidating synaptic changes that support potentiated synapses. However, BDNF together with NMDA-dependent calcium also activates **ERK** (extracellular-regulated kinase), which is also critical for the transcription of *Arc* mRNA. Thus, the dependency of BDNF-induced LTP on Arc expression also reflects the importance of BDNF to the transcription of *Arc* mRNA (see Bramham et al., 2010).

Arc Protein Sustains Actin Regulation

Arc protein is a key contributor to consolidating the synaptic changes supporting LTP. Preventing its synthesis within 160 minutes following LTP reverses LTP. This result is associated with two other outcomes. In the absence of Arc protein there is (1) a large reduction in phosphorylated cofilin and (2) a corresponding large loss of new actin filaments (Messaoudi et al., 2007). Thus, the regulation of actin dynamics by phosphorylating cofilin that was initiated almost immediately by the induction stimulus must be sustained for several hours for synaptic changes to be consolidated. Moreover, these processes may depend on the continued transcription and translation of Arc. Although Arc is associated with the regulation of actin via the phosphorylation of cofilin and the generation of nascent actin filament, the pathway linking Arc to pCofilin has not been identified (Nikolaienko et al., 2017). Arc does interact with debrin A, another actin-binding protein, which helps to stabilize the actin cytoskeleton by bundling F-actin to the PSD (Nikolaienko et al., 2017).

The Clustered Plasticity Model

This is a good place to return to why there is interest in the events that change the strength of synaptic connections. Briefly, memories are mediated by changes in the synaptic connections among the members of the neuronal ensembles activated by the experience. Retrieving a memory in this scheme depends on the ability of the sending neurons to depolarize the receiving neurons sufficiently to produce action potentials that will propagate the signal within the ensemble. Strengthening of individual synapses should enhance the ability of sending neurons to depolarize receiving neurons, thereby increasing the probability of generating action potentials and thus activating the ensemble.

As discussed earlier, neurobiologists sometimes reduced the problem of changing synaptic strength to the study of single molecules in single spines. However, releasing glutamate onto a single spine has no chance of depolarizing the neuron. So how does synaptic strength influence the likelihood that a neuron will depolarize and propagate the signal? A prevailing view is that the *dendritic branch*, rather than individual spines, is the fundamental storage unit (Branco and Hausser, 2010; Govindarajan et al., 2011). This view can be organized around what is called the **clustered plasticity model** (Govindarajan et al., 2006; Mel, 1992; see van Bommel and Mikhaylava, 2016 for an excellent review). Three ideas are the foundation of this model.

1. Computational models suggest that fewer synaptic inputs are required to initiate an action potential when clusters of synapses are stimulated on a few dendrites than when they are distributed on multiple dendritic branches (Figure 6.11).

2. The dendrite is a functional unit that contains all the machinery required to supply synapses with the proteins needed to ensure enduring change (local protein synthesis).

3. When spines are stimulated they not only attract mRNA and ribosomes for translation, the new protein can be shared among very-close-by spines so that a cluster of modified spines is created.

Although the value of the computational models (Mel, 1992) was appreciated, at the time there was no known biological mechanism that could support strengthening clusters of synapses. This changed as the full implications of local protein synthesis were recognized. Susumu Tonegawa and his colleagues (Govindarajan et al., 2006) proposed that, when considered together with the spatial distribution of synapses along a strip of dendrite, the facts of local protein synthesis favor the strengthening of synapses in clusters. This can happen because (a) synapses are likely activated in clusters which (b) allows them to cooperate to depolarize a local dendritic region to activate NMDA receptors and BDNF release, (c) thereby initiating local protein synthesis in the region of

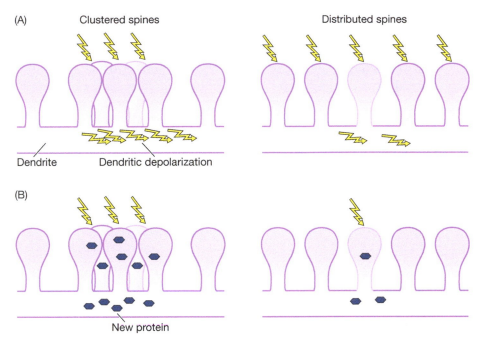

FIGURE 6.11   (A) The activation of spines clustered on a dendrite (left) have a higher probability of depolarizing the local dendritic region than activation of spines that are more spatially distributed (right). (B) Clustered spines can cooperate to initiate local protein synthesis and are positioned to capture and share the new protein (left) compared to more spatially distributed spines (right).

the cluster and (d) allowing members of the cluster to share the new protein at the expense of other spines not belonging to the cluster.

Strong evidence for the clustered plasticity model was provided by Govindarajan et al. (2011). They developed a glutamate uncaging preparation that allowed them to produce either a long-lasting *protein-synthesis-dependent* change or a short-lasting *protein-synthesis-independent* change in the volume of a single spine (Figure 6.12A). In their experiment Spine 1 was stimulated to produce a long-lasting protein-synthesis-dependent enlargement of that spine and Spine 2 was weakly stimulated to produce a normally short-lasting enlargement. The central finding was that proteins created by stimulating Spine 1 *were captured by Spine 2* to create a protein-synthesis-dependent long-lasting LTP (Figure 6.12B). This was because inhibiting protein synthesis normally produced by stimulating Spine 1 prevented Spine 2 enlargement from enduring (Figure 6.12C). However, for Spine 2 to capture protein, the two stimulating events had to occur within about 90 minutes of each other and the two spines had to be spatially clustered on the same dendrite.

(A) Only S1 or S2 stimulated

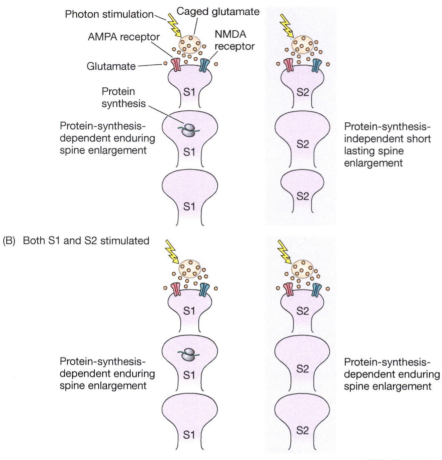

Photon stimulation — Caged glutamate

AMPA receptor — NMDA receptor

Glutamate —

Protein synthesis

Protein-synthesis-dependent enduring spine enlargement

Protein-synthesis-independent short lasting spine enlargement

(B) Both S1 and S2 stimulated

Protein-synthesis-dependent enduring spine enlargement

Protein-synthesis-dependent enduring spine enlargement

(C) Both S1 and S2 stimulated and protein synthesis inhibited

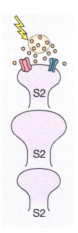

Anisomycin

Spine enlargement short lasting

FIGURE 6.12 (A) Govindarajan and colleagues (2011) developed a preparation that allowed them to create a protein-synthesis-dependent enlarged spine (S1) that would endure and a protein-synthesis-independent enlarged spine (S2) that would shortly return to its baseline size. (B) If both S1 and S2 were stimulated the protein generated by stimulating S1 was captured by S2, with the result that S2 also remained enlarged. (C) Spine enlargement did not endure in either spine if protein synthesis was inhibited by anisomycin. These results provide strong support for the clustered synapse hypothesis. (After A. Govindarajan et al. 2011. *Neuron* 69: 132–146.)

These results support two important conclusions: (1) proteins generated at one spine can be shared with another spine, and (2) the delivery of a weak stimulating event to a spine can temporarily create what is called a **synaptic tag** (Frey and Morris, 1998) that allows it to capture proteins generated elsewhere (further discussed below).

Another potential contributor to spine clustering is the organization of the presynaptic input. For example, Nelson Spruster and his colleagues (Bloss et al., 2018) reported that boutons from a single axon can form synapses onto nearby spines and single boutons also can form synapses onto adjacent spines on distal but not proximal dendrites of CA1 pyramidal cells. Such arrangements would greatly enhance the likelihood that clustered spines would respond to the same excitatory input and cooperate to generate local protein synthesis.

Synaptic Tags and the Regulation of Spine Clusters

The fact that synaptic activity can induce transcription brought with it a problem: *How do mRNAs transcribed in response to synaptic activity find their way from the soma to the correct synapses?* In their influential papers, Julietta Frey and Richard Morris (1997, 1998) proposed the **synaptic tag and capture hypothesis** as the solution.

The basic ideas in their proposal are illustrated in Figure 6.13 and in the following explanation.

1. Synaptic activity that potentiates synapses has two general effects: (1) it can generate a synaptic tag, which will allow the stimulated spine to subsequently capture newly transcribed plasticity molecules such as Arc, and (2) it can engage the translation and transcription machinery to generate new **plasticity products** (**PPs**).

2. Relatively weak stimulation (such as that needed to produce a short-lasting LTP) can create synaptic tags but will not engage the translation and transcription machinery.

3. Relatively strong stimulation will create synaptic tags and also engage the translation and transcription machinery.

4. Newly generated PPs can be captured by any tagged synapses but untagged synapses are not eligible to receive new PPs.

5. Over time, synapses lose their tag and return to their initial state.

6. Over time, the supply of new PPs will deplete.

7. To capture the PPs, the tags and new PPs must overlap in time.

This hypothesis makes an important prediction: weakly stimulated synapses can capture PPs that were generated by strongly stimulating other synapses belonging to the same neuron. This is because the tags generated by weak stimulation make these synapses eligible to capture new PPs, even though these synapses did not participate in generating the new PPs

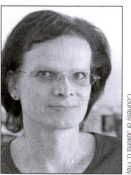

Julietta U. Frey

Courtesy of Julietta U. Frey

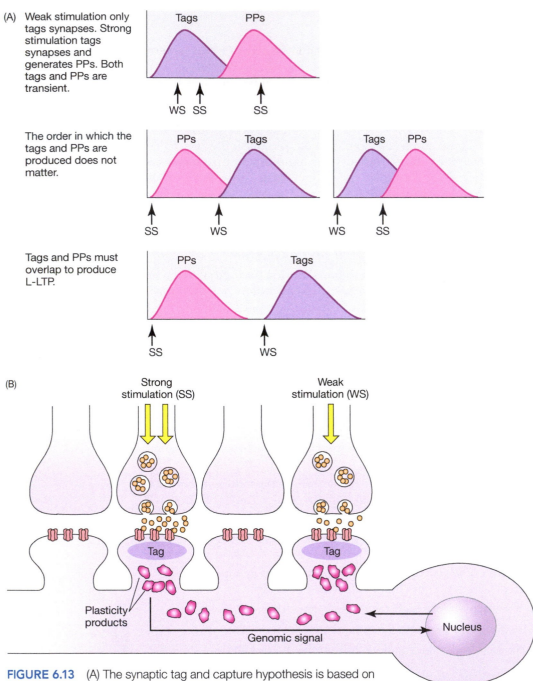

(A) Weak stimulation only tags synapses. Strong stimulation tags synapses and generates PPs. Both tags and PPs are transient.

The order in which the tags and PPs are produced does not matter.

Tags and PPs must overlap to produce L-LTP.

(B)

FIGURE 6.13 (A) The synaptic tag and capture hypothesis is based on three assumptions. (B) A strong stimulus (SS) both tags a synapse and generates a genomic signaling cascade that leads to transcription and translation of proteins (plasticity products or PPs) used to support L-LTP. The function of the tag is to capture the protein. A weak stimulus (WS) will not generate a genomic signaling cascade. However, it can tag synapses and these synapses capture PPs produced by a strong stimulus providing the timing is correct. Note that untagged synapses do not capture PPs. (After U. Frey and R. G. Morris. 1997. *Nature* 385: 533–536.)

(see Frey and Morris, 1998). This important prediction has received experimental support (Figure 6.14).

The development of the clustered plasticity model led to a subtle but important shift in thinking about the synaptic tag and capture hypothesis. Recall

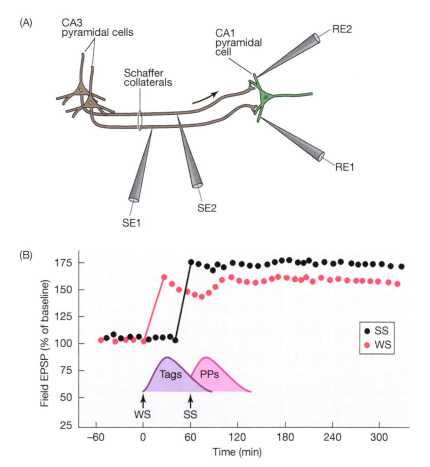

FIGURE 6.14   (A) This schematic illustrates the procedure Frey and Morris (1997, 1998) used to test the synaptic tag and capture hypothesis. It shows that separate sets of Schaffer collateral fibers can synapse on dendrites belonging to the same CA1 neurons. Stimulating electrodes (SE1 and SE2) can generate field EPSPs in the dendritic fields that can be recorded by the extracellular recording electrodes (RE1 and RE2). By controlling the intensity of the stimulation delivered by the stimulating electrodes, it is possible to generate either a short-lasting or long-lasting LTP on synapses belonging to the same neuron. (B) A weak stimulus (WS) that normally would produce a short-lasting LTP will produce a long-lasting LTP if a strong stimulus (SS) is delivered to synapses belonging to the same neuron. Theoretically, this happens because the synaptic tags produced by the weak stimulus will capture plasticity products (PPs) generated by the strong stimulus. (After U. Frey and R. G. Morris. 1997. *Nature* 385: 533–536.)

that there is an abundance of mRNA already available in the dendritic spine region before LTP is induced and stimulating spines will induce its translation. So the issue of how synaptic plasticity products produced in the soma find the correct synapses is largely muted. Yet the idea of a synaptic tag that can capture the protein still applies, but on a much smaller spatial scale (the local dendritic region compared to the entire neuron). Recall that Govindarajan et al. (2011) found that a weakly stimulated (tagged) spine could capture proteins produced by a strongly stimulated spine but the spines need to be within about 50 μm. Moreover, tags only exist for about 50 minutes. So synaptic tag and capture remains an important part of the story, but it is extremely localized.

What Is the Tag?

For a period of time that corresponds roughly to the duration of a short-lasting LTP, a stimulated (tagged) spine can capture protein produced in its local vicinity. *What is the molecular basis of the synaptic tag*? In addressing this question, it is important to keep in mind that tags are rapidly generated but unless reinforced will be temporary. The primary property of a tagged synapse is *almost certainly the enlarged actin cytoskeleton and the interaction with other synaptic proteins it affords* (Redondo and Morris, 2011; Rudy, 2015). Several facts support this assertion.

- There is a large literature indicating that LTP will not persist unless an enlarged actin cytoskeleton is stabilized (see Chapter 4).
- Studies of single spines revealed that interfering with development of the actin cytoskeleton prevents the redistribution of both mRNA and protein into stimulated spines (Bosch et al., 2014; Cajigas et al., 2010).
- The ability of a weakly stimulated but enlarged spine to capture protein generated by a strongly stimulated spine is almost perfectly correlated with its volume at the time the new protein was produced. Spines with large volumes captured the protein but this diminished as spine volume decreased over time (Govindarajan et al., 2011).

As shown earlier in Figure 6.1, mRNA is transported to dendrites by motor proteins that use the microtubule cytoskeleton to reach their initial destination. It is known that microtubule polymerization in the dendritic spine region is also regulated by synaptic activity. The important result is that microtubules polymerize into stimulated spines. Although their stay is relatively short (a few minutes) they can reenter the spine multiple times. Their presence would facilitate the redistribution of mRNAs into the stimulated spines enabling their capture (see Dent, 2017 for a review). Notably, the polymerization of the microtubules into spines requires the presence of debrin, one of the key actin-associated proteins needed to consolidate the enlarged spine (Merriam et al., 2013). This supports the idea that by its interaction with microtubules, the actin cytoskeleton is the basis of the synaptic tag (Figure 6.15).

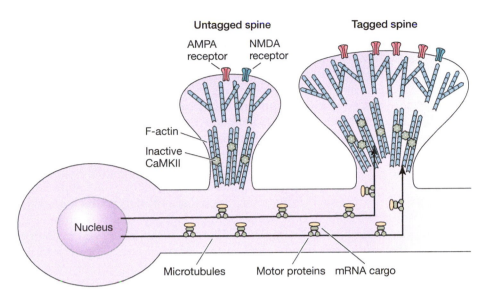

FIGURE 6.15   Tagged spines have an enlarged actin cytoskeleton that induces the invasion of microtubules into the spine where they can deliver cargo containing mRNAs for translation.

Inverse Tags

Clustered synapses tend to be depolarized at the same time and share in resources needed to ensure they are strengthened. *But what happens to other spines on the same dendrite that are not stimulated?* The answer is that their potential contribution to depolarization is reduced. In the aftermath of local protein synthesis produced by synaptic depolarization, over time one of the proteins, Arc, accumulates in the dendrites. Compared to recently activated spines, the nonactive spines contain *inactive* CaMKII. Because there is a strong affinity between Arc and the inactive form of CaMKII, Arc accumulates in the inactive spines where it participates in the removal of AMPA receptors, thereby weakening their contribution to depolarizing the neuron. In this context, CaMKII can be thought of as an **inverse tag** (Okuno et al., 2012, 2018). By capturing late-accumulating Arc, the inverse tag prevents Arc from entering and depotentiating the recently potentiated spines. The net effect is to ensure that the cluster of potentiated spines stabilizes and the contribution of other spines to depolarization is minimized.

A Caveat

It is helpful to note that earlier in this chapter Arc protein was identified as an important contributor to late-stage actin dynamics that stabilized enlarged spines. When this fact is considered together with its role in inverse tagging, it can be correctly inferred that *Arc has multiple functions*. Arc's interaction with other proteins determines what it will do (see Nikolaienko et al., 2017 for a review).

Summary

Local protein synthesis allows for proteins to be produced on demand in the correct spatial location. Messenger RNAs are delivered to dendritic spine regions by motor proteins that carry them via microtubules. Once there, mRNAs periodically move along the dendrite. The release of glutamate results in mRNAs and ribosomal complexes being captured by the stimulated spine where they remain for at least an hour. This results in the synthesis of the relevant proteins.

Local protein synthesis is initiated by the release of BDNF which binds to TrkB receptors to activate mTOR, which then phosphorylates TOP proteins to produce functional ribosomal complexes. This results in enhanced translation capacity in the stimulated spines. None of this occurs if either the NMDA receptors are inhibited or actin polymerization is prevented.

Protein degradation produced by activation of the ubiquitin–proteasome system is critical to protein synthesis. Activation of this system prevents the overexpression of LTP by limiting the translation of TOP proteins. In addition, the UPS degrades both transcription and translation repressor proteins, which is necessary if new protein is to be translated.

Many of the locally translated synaptic proteins are familiar (AMPA receptors, CaMKII, actin). However, the translation of the immediate early gene *Arc* is a novel outcome of the BDNF → TrkB → mTOR → TOP signaling cascade. Preventing *Arc* translation interferes with L-LTP and late-emerging actin polymerization.

The retrieval of a memory requires the activation of the neuronal ensembles that store the experience. It is assumed that this depends on the strengthening of synaptic connections linking neuronal members of the ensemble. Current thinking is organized around the clustered plasticity model. This model assumes that fewer synaptic inputs are required to initiate an action potential when clusters of synapses are stimulated on a few dendrites than when they are distributed on multiple dendritic branches. The facts of local protein synthesis support the clustered plasticity model. Clustered spines can cooperate in depolarizing a local dendritic region and can share in the new protein at the expense of other spines not belonging to the cluster.

The synaptic tag and capture hypothesis was proposed to solve the problem of how plasticity products that are generated in the nucleus find their way to the correct synapses. This hypothesis assumes that stimulated spines are tagged and that tagged synapses capture the new product at the expense of untagged synapses. The development of the clustered plasticity model produced a subtle shift in this view because there is an abundance of mRNA already available in the dendritic spine region. The concept of a synaptic tag that can capture the protein still applies but on a much smaller spatial scale (the local dendritic region compared to the entire neuron). So what is the molecular basis of the synaptic tag? The primary property of a tagged synapse is almost certainly the enlarged actin cytoskeleton and the interaction with other synaptic proteins it affords. In particular the expansion of the actin cytoskeleton is associated with the polymerization of microtubules into the spine so that motor proteins can deliver their cargo of mRNAs to the spine for translation.

Compared to recently activated spines, the nonactive spines contain inactive CaMKII. There is a strong affinity between Arc protein and the inactive form of CaMKII. Thus, Arc accumulates in the inactive spines where it participates in the removal of AMPA receptors, thereby weakening their contribution to depolarizing the neuron. By capturing late-accumulating Arc, the inverse tag prevents Arc from entering and depotentiating the recently potentiated spines. The net effect is to ensure that the cluster of potentiated spines stabilizes and the contribution of other spines to depolarization is minimized.

References

Bingol, B. and Schuman, E. M. (2006). Activity-dependent dynamics and sequestration of proteasomes in dendritic spines. *Nature, 441,* 1144–1148.

Bingol, B., Wang, C. F., Arnott, D., Cheng, D., Peng, J., and Sheng, M. (2010). Autophosphorylated CaMKIIα acts as a scaffold to recruit proteasomes to dendritic spines. *Cell, 140,* 567–578.

Bloss, E. K., Cembrowski, M. S., Karsh, B., Colonell, J., Fetter, R. S., and Spruston, N. (2018). Single excitatory axons form clustered synapses onto CA1 pyramidal cell dendrites. *Nature Neuroscience, 21,* 353–363.

Bosch, M., Castro, J., Saneyoshi, T., Matsuno, H., Sur, M., and Hayashi, Y. (2014). Structural and molecular remodeling of dendritic spine substructures during long-term potentiation. *Neuron, 82,* 444–459.

Bramham, C. R. (2008.) Local protein synthesis, actin dynamics, and LTP consolidation. *Current Opinion in Neurobiology, 18,* 524–531.

Bramham, C. R., Alme, M. N., Bittins, M., Kuipers, S. D., Nair, R. R., Pai, B., Panja, D., Schubert, M., Soule, J., Tiron, A., and Wibrand, K. (2010). The arc of synaptic memory. *Experimental Brain Research, 2,* 125–140.

Bramham, C. and Messaoudi, E. (2005). BDNF function in adult synaptic plasticity: the synaptic consolidation hypothesis. *Progress in Neurobiology, 76,* 99–125.

Branco, T. and Hausser, M. (2010). The single dendritic branch as a fundamental functional unit in the nervous system. *Current Opinion in Neurobiology, 20,* 494–502.

Buxbaum, A. R., Wu, B., and Singer, R. H. (2014). Single β-actin mRNA detection in neurons reveals a mechanism for regulating its translatability. *Science, 343,* 419–422.

Cajigas, I. J., Will, T., and Schuman, E. M. (2010). Protein homeostasis and synaptic plasticity. *The EMBO Journal, 18,* 2746–2752.

Dent, E. W. (2017). Of microtubules and memory: implications for microtubule dynamics in dendrites and spines. *Molecular Biology of the Cell, 28*, 1–8.

Dong, C., Bach, S. V., Haynes, K. A., and Hegde, A. N. (2014). Proteasome modulates positive and negative translational regulators in long-term synaptic plasticity. *Journal of Neuroscience, 34*, 3171–3182.

Dong, C., Upadhya, S. C., Ding, L., Smith, T. K., and Hegde, A. N. (2008). Proteasome inhibition enhances the induction and impairs the maintenance of late-phase long-term potentiation. *Learning and Memory, 15*, 335–347.

Dynes, J. L. and Steward, O. (2012) Arc mRNA docks precisely at the base of individual dendritic spines indicating the existence of a specialized microdomain for synapse-specific mRNA translation. *The Journal of Comparative Neurology, 26*, 433–437.

Ehlers, M. D. (2003). Activity level controls postsynaptic composition and signaling via the ubiquitin-proteasome system. *Nature Neuroscience, 6*, 231–242.

Fonseca, R., Vabulas, R. M., Hartl, F. U., Bonhoeffer, T., and Nagerl, U. V. (2006). A balance of protein synthesis and proteasome-dependent degradation determines the maintenance of LTP. *Neuron, 52*, 239–245.

Frey, U. and Morris, R. G. (1997). Synaptic tagging and long-term potentiation. *Nature, 385*, 533–536.

Frey, U. and Morris, R. G. (1998). Synaptic tagging: implications for late maintenance of hippocampal long-term potentiation. *Trends in Neurosciences, 21*, 181–188.

Govindarajan, A., Israely, I., Huang, S. Y., and Tonegawa, S. (2011). The dendritic branch is the preferred integrative unit for protein synthesis-dependent LTP. *Neuron, 69*, 132–146.

Govindarajan, A., Kelleher, R. J., and Tonegawa, S. (2006). A clustered plasticity model of long-term memory engrams. *Nature Reviews Neuroscience, 7*, 575–583.

Guo, L. and Wang, Y. (2007). Glutamate stimulates glutamate receptor interacting protein 1 degradation by ubiquitin–proteasome system to regulate surface expression of GluR2. *Neuroscience, 145*, 100–109.

Guzowski, J. F., Lyford, G. L., Stevenson, G. D., Houston, F. P., McGaugh, J. L., Worley, P. F., and Barnes, C. A. (2000). Inhibition of activity-dependent arc protein expression in the rat hippocampus impairs the maintenance of long-term potentiation and the consolidation of long-term memory. *Journal of Neuroscience, 20*, 3993–4001.

Hegde, A. N. (2010). The ubiquitin-proteasome pathway and synaptic plasticity. *Learning and Memory, 17*, 314–327.

Hegde, A. N., Goldberg, A. L., and Schwartz, J. H. (1993). Regulatory subunits of cAMP-dependent protein kinases are degraded after conjugation to ubiquitin: a molecular mechanism underlying long-term synaptic plasticity. *Proceedings of the National Academy of Sciences USA, 90*, 7436–7440.

Holt, C. E. and Schuman, E. M. (2013). The central dogma decentralized: new perspectives on RNA function and local translation in neurons. *Neuron, 80*, 648–657.

Huang, E. J. and Reichardt, L. F. (2001). Neurotrophins: roles in neuronal development and function. *Annual Review Neuroscience, 24,* 677–736.

Jia, Y., Gall, C. M., and Lynch, G. (2010). Presynaptic BDNF promotes postsynaptic long-term potentiation in the dorsal striatum. *Journal of Neuroscience, 30,* 14440–14445.

Kang, H. and Schuman, E. M. (1996). A requirement for local protein synthesis in neurotrophin-induced synaptic plasticity. *Science, 273,* 1402–1406.

Karpova, A., Mikhaylova, M., Thomas, U., Knopfel, T., and Behnisch, T. (2006). Involvement of protein synthesis and degradation in long-term potentiation of Schaffer collateral CA1 synapses. *Journal of Neuroscience, 26,* 4949–4955.

Korte, M., Carroll, P., Wolf, E., Brem, G., Thoenen, H., and Bonhoeffe, T. (1995). Hippocampal long-term potentiation is impaired in mice lacking brain-derived neurotrophic factor. *Proceedings of the National Academy of Sciences USA, 92,* 8856–8860.

Korte, M., Kang, H., Bonhoeffer, T., and Schuman, E. (1998). A role for BDNF in the late phase of hippocampal long-term potentiation. *Neuropharmacology, 37,* 553–559.

Lee, S. H., Choi, J. H., Lee, N., Lee, H. R., Kim, J. I., Yu, N. K., Choi, S. L., Lee, S. H., Kim, H., and Kaang, B. K. (2008). Synaptic protein degradation underlies destabilization of retrieved fear memory. *Science, 319,* 1253–1256.

Lessmann, V., Gottmann, K., and Malcangio, M. (2003). Neurotrophin secretion: current facts and future prospects. *Progress in Neurobiology, 69,* 341–374.

Lu, Y., Ji, Y., Ganesan, S., Schloesser, R., Martinowich, K., Sun, M., Mei, F., Chao, M. V., and Lu, B. (2011). TrkB as a potential synaptic and behavioral tag. *Journal of Neuroscience, 31,* 11762–11771.

Mel, B. W. (1992). The clusteron: toward a simple abstraction for a complex neuron. *Advances in Neural Information Processing Systems, 4,* 35–42.

Merriam, E. B., Millette, M., Lumbard, D. C, Saengsawang, W., Fothergill, T., Hu, X., Ferhat, L., and Dent, E. W. (2013). *Neuroscience, 33,* 16471–16482.

Messaoudi, E., Kanhema, T., Soule, J., Tiron, A., Dagyte, G., da Silva, B., and Bramham, C. R. (2007). Sustained Arc/Arg3.1 synthesis controls long-term potentiation consolidation through regulation of local actin polymerization in the dentate gyrus in vivo. *Journal of Neuroscience, 27,* 10445–10455.

Nikolaienko, O., Patil, S., Eriksen, M. S., and Bramham, C. R. (2017). Arc protein: a flexible hub for synaptic plasticity and cognition. *Seminars in Cell & Developmental Biology, 77,* 33–42.

Okuno, H., Akashi, Y., Ishii, N., Yagishita-Kyo, N., Suzuki, K., Nonaka, M., Kawashima, T., Fujii, H., Takemoto-Kimura, S., Abe, M., Natsume, R., Chowdhury, S., Sakimura, K., Worley, P. F., and Bito, H. (2012). Inverse synaptic tagging of inactive synapses via dynamic interaction of Arc/Arg3.1 with CaMKIIβ. *Cell, 149,* 886–898.

Okuno, H., Minatoharo, K., and Bito, H. (2018). Inverse synaptic tagging: an inactive synapse-specific mechanism to capture activity-induced Arc/arg3.1 and to locally regulate spatial distribution of synaptic weights. *Seminars in Cell & Developmental Biology, 77,* 43–50.

Ostroff, L. E., Watson, D. J., Cao, G., Parker, P. H., Smith, H., and Harris, K. M. (2018). Shifting patterns of polyribosome accumulation at synapse over the course of hippocampal long-term potentiation. *Hippocampus, 28,* 416–430.

Panja, D. and Bramham, C. R. (2014). BDNF mechanisms in late LTP formation: a synthesis and breakdown. *Neuropharmacology, 76,* 664–676.

Patrick, G. N., Bingol, B., Weld, H. A., and Schuman, E. M. (2003). Ubiquitin-mediated proteasome activity is required for agonist-induced endocytosis of GluRs. *Current Biology, 13,* 2073–2081.

Redondo, R. L. and Morris, R. G. (2011). Making memories last: the synaptic tagging and capture hypothesis. *Nature Reviews Neuroscience, 12,* 17–30.

Rudy, J. W. (2015). Variation in the persistence of memory: an interplay between actin dynamics and AMPA receptors. *Brain Research, 1621,* 29–37.

Schratt, G. M., Nigh, E. A., Chen, W. G., Hu, L., and Greenberg, M. E. (2004). BDNF regulates the translation of a select group of mRNAs by a mammalian target of rapamycin-phosphatidylinositol 3-kinase-dependent pathway during neuronal development. *Journal of Neuroscience, 24,* 7366–7377.

Tai, H. C. and Schuman, E. M. (2008). Ubiquitin, the proteasome and protein degradation in neuronal function and dysfunction. *Nature Reviews Neuroscience, 9,* 826–838.

Tang, S. J., Reis, G., Kang, H., Gingras, A. C., Sonenberg, N., and Schuman, E. M. (2002). A rapamycin-sensitive signaling pathway contributes to long-term synaptic plasticity in the hippocampus. *Proceedings of the National Academy of Sciences USA, 99,* 467–72.

Tsokas, P., Grace, E. A., Chan, P., Ma, T., Sealfon, S. C., Iyengar, R., Landau, E. M., and Blitzer, R. D. (2005). Local protein synthesis mediates a rapid increase in dendritic elongation factor 1A after induction of late long-term potentiation. *Journal of Neuroscience, 25,* 5833–5843.

Tsokas, P., Ma, T., Iyengar, R., Landau, E. M., and Blitzer, R. D. (2007). Mitogen-activated protein kinase upregulates the dendritic translation machinery in long-term potentiation by controlling the mammalian target of rapamycin pathway. *Journal of Neuroscience, 27,* 5885–5894.

van Bommel, B. and Mikhaylava, M. (2016). Talking to the neighbours: the molecular and physiological mechanisms of clustered synaptic plasticity. *Neuroscience and Biobehavioral Reviews, 71,* 352–361.

Yoon, Y. J., Wu, B., Buxbaum, A. R., Das, S., and Singer, R. H. (2016). Glutamate-induced RNA localization and translation in neurons. *Proceedings of the National Academy of Sciences USA, 113,* E6877–E6886.

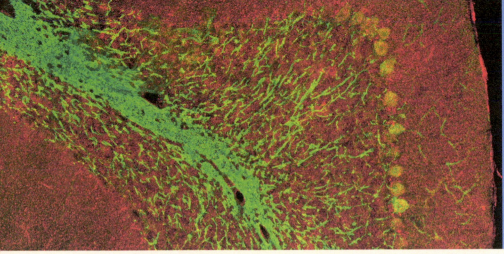

Maintaining Long-Term Potentiation

In a matter of minutes, a series of overlapping core signaling events initiated by the delivery of an LTP-inducing stimulus dramatically increases the ability of dendritic spines to respond to glutamate and depolarize the neuron. These events insert more AMPA receptors into the postsynaptic density, destroy and rebuild the actin cytoskeleton, and synthesize new proteins to reinforce the enlarged spine. Stimulated synapses have been strengthened and consolidated.

As the significance of molecular biology and biochemistry for neurobiology was becoming clear, however, Frances Crick, co-discoverer of the structure DNA, raised a daunting issue—*the molecular turnover problem*. The synaptic molecules that support memory traces are short-lived in comparison to the duration of our memories (Figure 7.1).

Thus, a fundamental question is, *how can the strengthened synapses that support memories outlive the molecules from which they are made?* As Crick (1984, p. 101) put it: "How then is memory stored in the brain so that its trace is relatively immune to molecular turnover?" He also suggested a general answer: "…the molecules in the synapse interact in such a way that they can be replaced with new material, one at a time, without altering the overall state of the structure." Independently, and at about the same time, John Lisman questioned how unstable molecules

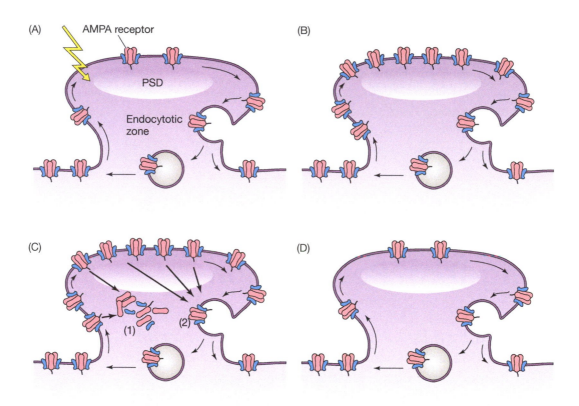

FIGURE 7.1 (A) An unpotentiated synapse is depolarized. (B) As the synapse is potentiated, AMPA receptors are added to the postsynaptic density. (C) Two processes—(1) degradation of AMPA receptors and (2) receptor endocytosis—then pressure the synapse to (D) return to its prepotentiated state.

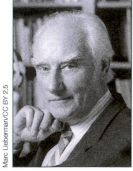

Francis Crick

can store information stably. He suggested that stability in principle could result from "a kinase that is activated by phosphorylation and capable of intermolecular autophosphorylation" (Lisman, 1985, p. 3055).

This chapter describes progress toward providing specific answers to the question, *how in the face of molecular turnover are the consolidated synaptic changes maintained?* In approaching this question, it is important to appreciate that Crick and Lisman put the maintenance burden on synaptic proteins (kinases) with special properties; they can be modified into a persistently active state and have a property of self-perpetuation. These properties would enable the continuously active protein to interact with other synaptic proteins to preserve synaptic strength. Such proteins have been referred to as "memory molecules" and there are a number of them.

However, before considering this idea in some detail, it is useful to frame the memory maintenance question more broadly. For example, Mary Kennedy, whose laboratory discovered CaMKII, remarked: "There is no memory molecule. Synapses are regulated by the mutual interactions of a whole network of proteins" (Bear et al., 2018, p. 8). She also speculated that the need for a synaptic protein whose persistence determines the duration of synaptic strength may be overstated. In line with a suggestion by Richard Morris (2016), she (and Morris) allowed that it is possible that a molecule implicated in memory retention may not need to persist throughout the lifetime of a memory. It might contribute to a structural change in the spine (such as the stability of the actin cytoskeleton or the enhancement of scaffolding proteins such as PSD-95) that give it (the spine) the property of self-perpetuation by altering its ability to capture new replacement proteins. In addition to self-perpetuating protein interactions and structural changes that might support maintenance, part of the solution may be the potential role of genomic factors that ensure the supply of the relevant synaptic proteins. At a minimum, the maintenance problem may require a multifactor solution (Smolen et al., 2019).

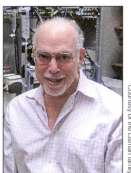

John Lisman

Maintenance Molecules

It should be clear by now that dendritic spines are awash in proteins that contribute to strengthening synapses. So how can one distinguish a "memory molecule" from any of the others that are critically involved in changing synaptic strength? Several criteria have been suggested (see Lisman, 2017). However, only one is the focus of this discussion. Ideally, such a molecule should not be required to generate and initially stabilize/consolidate LTP but should be required for the duration of LTP. This means that interfering with the activity of that molecule at any time following the protein-synthesis-dependent consolidation phase should return the strengthened synapses to their baseline state. In doing so the inhibitor should not alter basic neuronal transmission. This is sometimes referred to as the *erasure* criteria. Some candidate maintenance molecules (such as CaMKII and PKC variants) are discussed in the sections that follow.

CaMKII

> My eureka moment…was that a group of autophosphorylating kinase molecules localized at a synapse could make a stable switch. During LTP induction, these molecules would become phosphorylated, and this would make them active. If a kinase molecule was dephosphorylated or replaced in the course of protein turnover, it could be phosphorylated by other members of the group. The switch could stay on, perhaps indefinitely, and this showed how unstable molecules could produce stable information storage (John Lisman, in Bear et al., 2007, p. 789).

Fortuitously, around the time Lisman proposed that an intramolecular auto-phosphorylation mechanism could provide the basis for a molecular switch that could maintain synaptic strength, Mary Kennedy's laboratory (Bennett et al., 1983; Erondu and Kennedy, 1985; Kennedy et al., 1983) discovered that CaMKII had autophosphorylation properties (see Box 3.1). This led Lisman to propose that the CaMKII holoenzyme could have self-sustaining properties that could maintain synaptic changes (Lisman and Goldring, 1988). Unfortunately, at best, support for this appealing hypothesis has been controversial. For example, inhibition of CaMKII failed to erase LTP in the hippocampus (Otmakhov et al., 1997) and CaMKII activity appears to be short-lived (Lee et al., 2009). In addition, subsequent evidence that inactivating CaMKII erases LTP has been attributed to the inhibitory agent having irreversibly depressed synaptic transmission (Sacktor and Fenton, 2018). Given this state of affairs, a recent review (Smolen et al., 2019) concluded that the literature argues against but does not completely rule out a role for persistently self-sustaining CaMKII activity in maintaining LTP and long-term memory (see also Bear et al., 2018).

PKMζ

In the 1980s, studies of **protein kinase C (PKC)** variants set the stage for the discovery by Todd Sacktor that one variant, called **PKMζ (protein kinase Mζ)** might have properties that qualify it as a maintenance molecule (Sacktor, 2008). PKMζ is a constitutively active form of PKC. Unlike PKC it lacks an **inhibitory domain** that keeps the kinase in an inactive state, so once translated *it is persistently active* and does not require a second messenger to remove the inhibitory domain.

PKMζ mRNA is found in regions of dendritic spines. Like other messengers transported to the dendritic region, translation of PKMζ mRNA is normally suppressed by a translation repressor protein. The translation of PKMζ mRNA occurs locally and initially requires the activity of several kinases—including CaMKII, P13K, MAPK, PKA, and mTOR—to remove the repressing element.

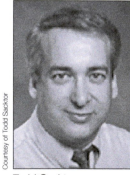

It also requires actin filament. Newly synthesized PKMζ becomes available within about 10 minutes following a strong LTP-inducing stimulus. PKMζ's *self-perpetuating properties* derive from the fact that once translated it too can remove the repressor protein that prevents translation of PKMζ mRNA. Thus, PKMζ participates in a signaling pathway that acts as a positive feedback loop to perpetuate increased translation of PKMζ mRNA (Osten et al., 1996; Sacktor, 2011). As summarized in Figure 7.2, PKMζ has three special properties that qualify it as a potential maintenance molecule.

1. It has no inhibitory domain and thus is constitutively active.
2. It is translated locally.
3. It can self-perpetuate.

Todd Sacktor

Courtesy of Todd Sacktor

(A) PKC

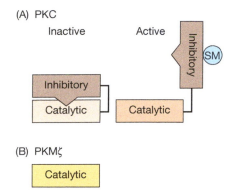

(B) PKMζ

Catalytic

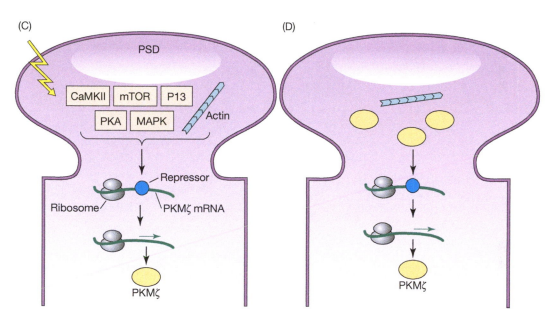

FIGURE 7.2 (A) Kinases like PKC have an inhibitory–regulatory domain and a catalytic domain. Such kinases require a second messenger (SM) to remove the inhibitory domain and expose the catalytic domain. (B) PKMζ has no inhibitory domain so it does not require a second messenger to be catalytic. It is perpetually active. (C) PKMζ mRNA is present in dendritic spine regions and its translation requires synaptic activity to activate several kinases and active filament. (D) Once translated, PKMζ self-perpetuates; it interacts with other proteins to remove the translator repressor and thereby facilitates translation of PKMζ mRNA in dendritic spines where it was initially translated.

INHIBITING PKMζ PREVENTS LTP MAINTENANCE   PKMζ does not have an inhibitory domain; however, it does have a potential binding site for an inhibitory domain. The discovery of the cell-permeable ζ-pseudosubstrate **ZIP (zeta inhibitory peptide)** made it possible to examine the role of PKMζ in LTP. In effect, ZIP can serve as the missing regulatory domain to inactivate PKMζ (Laudanna et al., 1998).

Applying ZIP to inhibit PKMζ prior to the LTP induction stimulus has no effect on the expression of the early form of LTP, but it prevents the late, lasting phase. The critical finding, however, was that application of ZIP reversed the potentiated response even when it was applied 2 or 5 hours after LTP was induced (Serrano et al., 2005), as shown in Figure 7.3. For comparison, other molecules known to be involved in LTP—CaMKII, MAPK, and PKC—are only required for a much shorter time after LTP is induced (Serrano et al., 2005).

PKMζ appears to have a critical role in maintaining potentiated synapses. However, as noted earlier, mutual interactions of a whole network of proteins regulate synapses. Given that this is true, then what other synaptic proteins interact with PKMζ and what does it do?

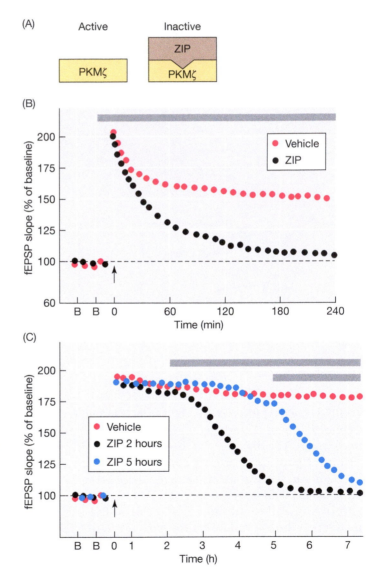

FIGURE 7.3 (A) As noted, PKMζ has no inhibitory domain; however, the peptide ZIP functions as an inhibitory domain and inactivates it. (B) ZIP applied to a hippocampal slice prior to the inducing stimulus does not affect the early induction phase of LTP but does prevent the late phase. (C) ZIP applied 2 or 5 hours following induction reverses late-phase LTP. (After P. Serrano et al. 2005. *J Neurosci* 25: 1979–1984.)

PKMζ RELEASES GLUA2 AMPA RECEPTORS INTO THE SYNAPSE   GluA1 receptors are responsible for the initial potentiation of synapses but are replaced by GluA2 receptors. There is evidence that PKMζ contributes to this outcome. The application of PKMζ to hippocampal slices potentiates synapses (Ling et al., 2002), but inhibiting PKMζ prevents this potentiation (Figure 7.4A). This result implies that PKMζ can traffic AMPA receptors into the PSD, and this implication has been confirmed (Ling et al., 2006).

A pool of GluA2 receptors is maintained outside of the synapse by binding to a complex called PICK1 (protein interacting with C kinase 1). The release of this pool of GluA2s for insertion into the synapse depends in part on a trafficking protein called **NSF** (N-thylmaleimide-sensitive factor). PKMζ forms a complex with NSF and PICK1 and this motif facilitates the disruption of the PICK1–GluA2 complex. This in turn releases the GluA2 receptors into the PSD and potentiates the synapse (Sacktor, 2011; Yao et al., 2008), as shown in Figure 7.4B.

(A)

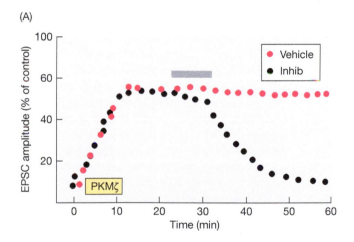

(B)

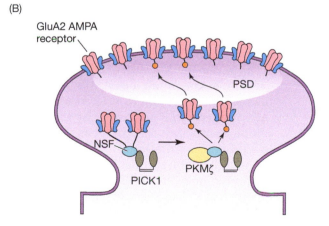

FIGURE 7.4 (A) PKMζ potentiates synapses and a PKMζ inhibitor reverses this effect. Note in this example the data are from intracellular recordings (Excitatory Post Synaptic Current, EPSC). (B) A pool of GluA2 AMPA receptors is trapped outside of the synapse by protein interacting with C kinase 1 (PICK1). Release of this pool depends on a trafficking protein enzyme, NSF. When PKMζ interacts with the NSF–PICK1 complex, the receptors are released for entry into the PSD. (A after D. S. Ling et al. 2006. *Hippocampus* 16: 443–452.)

PKMζ PREVENTS ENDOCYTOSIS OF AMPA RECEPTORS   A major outcome of the generation phase of LTP (see Chapter 3) is the accumulation of AMPA receptors in the postsynaptic density. However, there is continuous pressure to recycle AMPA receptors out of synapses and, left unopposed, the endocytotic cycle will remove additional GluA2 receptors and return the synapse to its basal state (Sacktor, 2011). This is one reason that LTP produced by a weak-inducing stimulus will decay back to its baseline state. For example, Dong et al. (2015) reported that interfering with AMPA-receptor endocytosis with the peptide GluR23γ prevents the decay of LTP normally produced by weak stimulation (see also Migues et al., 2010; Yu et al., 2017).

This result suggests that if LTP is to endure there must exist synaptic protein interactions that protect against the removal of AMPA receptors. PKMζ is one of these proteins. The evidence for this conclusion is that (a) both inhibiting PKMζ function by ZIP and reducing its expression by genetic tools cause normally long-lasting LTP to decay to baseline, and (b) this effect is prevented if GluR23γ is also present. The second result is critical because if interfering with PKMζ function results in the removal AMPA receptors then the addition of another agent that can prevent endocytosis should preserve LTP (Dong et al., 2015). A model proposed by Sacktor (2011) of how PKMζ might interact with other proteins to disrupt the endocytosis of AMPA receptors is presented in Figure 7.5.

PKMζ CLUSTERS PSD-95   PSD-95 is critical for trapping glutamate receptors in the postsynaptic density. The size of PSD-95 clusters determines the number of AMPA receptors that can be maintained. A form of chemically induced LTP generated by the lipid-soluble compound forskolin has been used to study the regulation of PSD-95 clustering in cultured neurons. When applied to tocultured neurons, forskolin increases the presence of PSD-95 clusters in the postsynaptic density but does not change the total

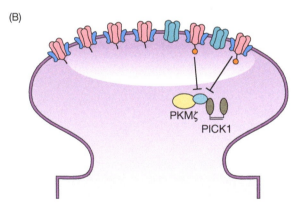

FIGURE 7.5   (A) The activation of tyrosine kinase (Trk) receptors phosphorylates tyrosine sites on GluA2 AMPA receptors. This activity releases the receptors from the PSD into the endocytotic zone where they bond with the NSF–PICK1 complex for recycling. (B) The presence of PKMζ disrupts the normal endocytic cycle—the receptors remain trapped in the PSD and the synapse remains potentiated.

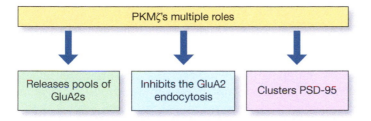

FIGURE 7.6   PKMζ maintains potentiated synapses through multiple parallel and complementary actions. It facilitates the release of nonsynaptic pools of GluA2 receptors to replace GluA1 receptors, interferes with the endocytotic cycle that normally removes GluA2s from the synapse, and it clusters PSD-95 in the postsynaptic density.

amount of PSD-95 in the dendritic spine region. Thus, the forskolin-induced increase in clusters is due to a redistribution of PSD-95 to the postsynaptic density. This redistribution of PSD-95 protein does not occur if PKMζ activity is inhibited (Shao et al., 2012).

MULTIPLE CONTRIBUTIONS OF PKMζ   The important general conclusion from this discussion is that PKMζ maintains potentiated synapses through several parallel and complementary interactions with other proteins (Figure 7.6).

- It facilitates the release of nonsynaptic pools of GluA2 containing AMPA receptors for insertion into the PSD.
- It interferes with the endocytotic cycle that normally removes AMPA receptors from the synapse.
- It mediates the redistribution of PSD-95 clusters to the postsynaptic density.

The combined effects of these processes enable synapses to maintain the complement of AMPA receptors required to support a potentiated synaptic response to glutamate release. Inhibiting the catalytic properties of PKMζ in principle disrupts all of these functions and thus these synapses return to their unpotentiated state.

Redundancy and Compensation

PKMζ is not the only PKC variant that can contribute to LTP maintenance. An enduring LTP can be established even if PKMζ is genetically deleted, as demonstrated in a Volk et al. study (2013) of genetically altered (PKMζ-null) mice. Moreover, in that same study, the application of ZIP erased LTP. These results support three strong conclusions: (1) enduring LTP can be established *independent of the presence of* PKMζ, that is, the maintenance of LTP does not require PKMζ, (2) ZIP is not selective for PKMζ, rather it must also interact with other kinases, and (3) there must be other kinases that can participate in the maintenance of LTP and memories.

These findings were initially interpreted as strong evidence that PKMζ may have no role in memory maintenance. However, this interpretation fails to recognize that *deletion experiments can only reveal what the brain can do in the absence of a particular molecular*. They cannot reveal the normal functions of the molecule. Consistent with this point, Sacktor's laboratory (Tsokas et al., 2016) reported that there is a PKC variant called protein kinase C iota–lambda (PKCι/λ) that can compensate for the absence of PKMζ. However, in wild type mice the expression of PKCι/λ in response to LTP induction is transient. Its full expression only emerges in the PKMζ-null mice.

Although the two kinases (PKMζ and PKCι/λ) share some properties (for example, ZIP can inhibit both), their effects on LTP can be independently altered. As illustrated in Figure 7.7, a PKCι/λ antagonist, ICAP, prevents LTP from enduring in PKMζ-null mice but has no effect on the duration of LTP

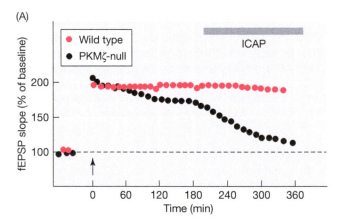

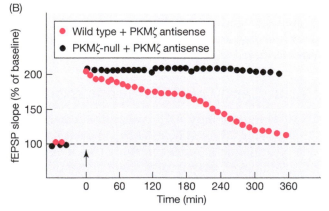

FIGURE 7.7 (A) When the gene for PKMζ is deleted (PKMζ-null mice), LTP can be maintained by another kinase, PKCι/λ. ICAP, which inhibits PKCι/λ, prevents maintenance in PKMζ-null mice but does not prevent maintenance in the wild type mice. (B) Antisense to PKMζ prevents maintenance in the wild type mice but not in the PKMζ-null mice. These results indicate that PKCι/λ can compensate for the absence of PKMζ but it does not contribute to maintenance when PKMζ is present. (After P. Tsokas et al. 2016. *eLife* 2016: 5:e14846. DOI: 10.7554/eLife.14846.)

in wild type mice. Conversely, antisense to PKMζ mRNA prevents LTP from enduring in wild type mice but has no effect on the genetically altered mice. Thus, there are other kinases (PKCι/λ) that can to some extent compensate for the absence of PKMζ. However, under normal circumstances the expression of such kinases may be suppressed, and PKMζ is the primary contributor to enduring LTP.

Genomic Contributions

PKMζ plays a critical role in ensuring the maintenance of synaptic changes that support LTP. Nevertheless, the duration of the synaptic changes needed to support memories that last for weeks will exceed the half-life of PKMζ (Hernandez et al., 2013). For this reason, it is critical that a continuous supply of relevant mRNA, including that for PKMζ, be available long after the initial translation of locally available PKMζ. There is evidence that PKMζ may also be part of an extensive cell-wide positive feedback loop that ensures that levels of PKMζ are available to maintain the potentiated synapses. In response to chemically induced synaptic activity, PKMζ translocates from the cytosol to the nucleus. There it can phosphorylate CREB-binding protein and perhaps increase transcription of PKMζ mRNA and other critical synaptic proteins (Ko et al., 2016). In addition, PKMζ has been localized to the nucleoli, which make ribosomal subunits and ribosomal RNA. These subunits are sent out to the rest of the cell where they combine into complete ribosomes. This outcome could contribute to the continued upregulation of the protein synthesis capacity of potentiated synapses (Tsokas et al., 2005).

Structural Contributions

The strengthening of synapses is highly selective. Only a small fraction of synapses are strengthened by the induction stimulus. In contrast, outflow of newly transcribed mRNA is cell wide. Thus, a critical part of maintenance over the lifetime of a memory is ensuring that only those originally potentiated synapses receive the relevant synaptic products needed for maintenance. The capture of subsequent mRNA proteins, including PKMζ, by unpotentiated synapses could greatly diminish the preciseness of the representation. In effect, the ground work for maintaining selectivity was laid down by structural changes during the stabilization phase; stimulated spines were enlarged by expansion of the actin cytoskeleton which, by their interactions with the microtubules and other synaptic proteins, enabled them to successfully compete for replacement proteins. Thus, the same properties that allowed stimulated spines to capture the available mRNA and polyribosomes at the time of LTP induction would provide a basis for maintaining selectivity over the long haul. One might infer that enlarged spines themselves have self-perpetuating properties because of their ability to capture new proteins needed to replace those that normally degrade, and this is an essential part of maintenance. Without this self-perpetuating property, the mRNA for kinases like PKMζ would get lost on their way from the nucleus.

Summary

Consolidated synapses face the molecular turnover problem. Memories outlive the molecules that support their synaptic basis. Synapses have to be maintained in the face of forces that (a) degrade the molecules that strengthen them and (b) remove the GluA2 receptors from the synapses. "Memory molecules" with self-perpetuating catalytic properties have been proposed as providing a counter to the turnover problem. The most promising is the PKC variant PKMζ. It has several important properties.

- It lacks a regulatory unit and is persistently active.
- PKMζ mRNA is available in dendritic spine regions.
- Once translated it can self-perpetuate.
- It releases pools of GluA2 receptors from the extrasynaptic region.
- It disrupts the endocytotic cycle that normally would remove GluA2 receptors from the synapse.

Another PKC variant, PKCι/λ, also has been identified as a maintenance molecule that can compensate for the absence of PKMζ. Normally, however, the expression of this kinase is suppressed by PKMζ. Maintenance may also be supported by translocation of PKMζ to the nucleus where it can contribute to ensuring a continuing supply of mRNA for synaptic proteins and mRNA needed for their local translation. The success of all these processes depends on the enlarged spines created during the stabilization phase that are able to capture proteins needed to replace those that have been degraded.

References

Bear, M. F., Connors, B. W., and Paradiso, M. A. (2007). *Neuroscience: Exploring the Brain*. 3rd ed. Philadelphia, PA: Lippincott Williams and Wilkins.

Bear, M. F., Cooke, S. F., Giese, K. P., Kaang, B. K., Kennedy, M. B., Kim, J. I., Morris, R. G. M., and Park, P. (2018). In memoriam: John Lisman—commentaries on CaMKII as a memory molecule. *Molecular Brain, 11,* 76.

Bennett, M. K., Erondu, N. E., and Kennedy, M. B. (1983). Purification and characterization of a calmodulin-dependent protein kinase that is highly concentrated in brain. *Journal of Biological Chemistry, 258,* 12735–12744.

Crick, F. (1984). Memory and molecular turnover. *Nature, 312,* 101.

Dong, Z., Han, H., Li, H., Bai, Y., Wang, W., Tu, M., Peng, Y., Zhou, L., He, W., Wu, X., Tan, T., Liu, M., Wu, X., Zhou, W., Jin, W., Zhang, S., Sacktor, T. C., Li, T., Song,

W., and Wang, Y. T. (2015). Long-term potentiation decay and memory loss are mediated by AMPAR endocytosis. *The Journal of Clinical Investigation, 125,* 234–247.

Erondu, N. E. and Kennedy, M. B. (1985). Regional distribution of type II Ca^{2+}/calmodulin-dependent protein kinase in rat brain. *Journal of Neuroscience, 5,* 3270–3277.

Hernandez, A. I., Oxberry, W. C., Crary, J. F., Mirra, S. S., and Sacktor, T. C. (2013). Cellular and subcellular localization of PKMζ. *Philosophical Transactions of the Royal Society of London. Series B, Biological sciences, 369* (1633), 20130140.

Kennedy, M. B., Bennett, M. K., and Erondu, N. E. (1983). Biochemical and immunochemical evidence that the "major postsynaptic density protein" is a subunit of a calmodulin-dependent protein kinase. *Proceedings of the National Academy of Sciences USA, 80,* 7357–7361.

Ko, H. G., Kim, J. I., Sim, S. E., Kim, T., Yoo, J., Choi, S. L., Baek, S. H., Yu, W. J., Yoon, J. B., Sacktor, T. C., and Kaang, B. K. (2016). The role of nuclear PKMζ in memory maintenance. *Neurobiology of Learning and Memory, 135,* 50–56.

Laudanna, C., Mochly-Rosen, D., Liron, T., Constantin, G., and Butcher, E. C. (1998). Evidence of zeta protein kinase C involvement in polymorphonuclear neutrophil integrin-dependent adhesion and chemotaxis. *Journal of Biological Chemistry, 273,* 30306–30315.

Lee, S-J. R., Escobedo-Lozoya, Y., Szatmari, E. M., and Yasuda, R. (2009). Activation of CaMKII in single dendritic spines during long-term potentiation. *Nature, 458,* 299–306.

Ling, D. S., Benardo, L. S., and Sacktor, T. C. (2006). Protein kinase Mζ enhances excitatory synaptic transmission by increasing the number of active postsynaptic AMPA receptors. *Hippocampus, 16,* 443–452.

Ling, D. S., Benardo, L. S., Serrano, P. A., Blace, N., Kelly, M. T., Crary, J. F., and Sacktor, T. C. (2002). Protein kinase Mζ is necessary and sufficient for LTP maintenance. *Nature Neuroscience, 5,* 295–296.

Lisman, J. E. (1985). A mechanism for memory storage insensitive to molecular turnover: a bistable autophosphorylating kinase. *Proceedings of the National Academy of Sciences USA, 82,* 3055–3057.

Lisman, J. E. (2017). Criteria for identifying the molecular basis of the engram (CaMKII, PKMζ). *Molecular Brain, 10,* 55.

Lisman, J. E. and Goldring, M. A. (1988). Feasibility of long-term storage of graded information by the Ca^{2+}/calmodulin-dependent protein kinase molecules of the postsynaptic density. *Proceedings of the National Academy of Sciences USA, 85,* 5320–5324.

Migues, P. V., Hardt, O., Wu, D. C., Gamache, K., Sacktor, T. C., Wang, Y. T., and Nader, K. (2010). PKMζ maintains memories by regulating GluR2-dependent AMPA receptor trafficking. *Nature Neuroscience, 13,* 630–634.

Morris, R. G. M. (2016). Memory: forget me not. *eLife* 2016: 5:e16597. DOI: 10.7554/eLife.16597

Osten, P., Valsamis, L., Harris, A., and Sacktor, T. C. (1996). Protein synthesis-dependent formation of protein kinase Mζ in LTP. *Journal of Neuroscience, 16,* 2444–2451.

Otmakhov, N., Griffith, L. C., and Lisman, J. E. (1997). Postsynaptic inhibitors of calcium/calmodulin-dependent protein kinase type II block induction but not maintenance of pairing-induced long-term potentiation. *Journal of Neuroscience, 17,* 5357–5365.

Sacktor, T. C. (2008). PKMζ, LTP maintenance, and the dynamic molecular biology of memory storage. *Progress in Brain Research, 169,* 27–40.

Sacktor, T. C. (2011). How does PKMζ maintain long-term memory? *Nature Reviews Neuroscience, 12,* 9–15.

Sacktor, T. C. and Fenton, A. A. (2018). What does LTP tell us about the roles of CaMKII and PKMζ in memory? *Molecular Brain, 11,* 77.

Serrano, P., Yao, Y., and Sacktor, T. C. (2005). Persistent phosphorylation by protein kinase Mζ maintains late-phase long-term potentiation. *Journal of Neuroscience, 25,* 1979–1984.

Shao, C. Y., Sondhi, R., van de Nes, P. S., and Sacktor, T. C. (2012). PKMζ is necessary and sufficient for synaptic clustering of PSD-95. *Hippocampus, 22,* 1501–1507.

Smolen, P., Baxter, D. A., and Byrne, J. H. (2019). How can memories last for days, years, or a lifetime? Proposed mechanisms for maintaining synaptic potentiation and memory. *Learning and Memory, 26,* 133–150.

Tsokas, P., Grace, E. A., Chan, P., Ma, T., Sealfon, S. C., Iyengar, R., Landau, E. M., and Blitzer, R. D. (2005). Local protein synthesis mediates a rapid increase in dendritic elongation factor 1A after induction of late long-term potentiation. *Journal of Neuroscience, 25,* 5833–5843.

Tsokas, P., Hsieh, C., Yao, Y., Lesburguères, E., Wallace, E. J. C., Tcherepanov, A., Jothianandan, D., Hartley, B. R., Pan, L., Rivard, B., Farese, R. V., Sajan, M. P., Bergold, P. J., Hernández, A. I., Cottrell, J. E., Shouval, H. Z., Fenton, A. A., and Sacktor, T. C. (2016). Compensation for PKMζ in long-term potentiation and spatial long-term memory in mutant mice. *eLife* 2016: 5:e14846. DOI: 10.7554/eLife.14846.

Volk, L. J., Bachman, J. L., Johnson, R., Yu, Y., and Huganir, R. L. (2013). PKMζ is not required for hippocampal synaptic plasticity, learning and memory. *Nature, 493,* 420–423.

Yao, Y., Kelly, M. T., Sajikumar, S., Serrano, P., Tian, D., Bergold, P. J., Frey, J. U., and Sacktor, T. C. (2008). PKMζ maintains late long-term potentiation by N-ethylmaleimide-sensitive factor/GluR2-dependent trafficking of postsynaptic AMPA receptors. *Journal of Neuroscience, 28,* 7820–7827.

Yu, N. K., Uhm, H., Shim, J., Choi, J. H., Bae, S., Sacktor, T. C., Hohng, S., and Kaang, B. K. (2017). Increased PKMζ activity impedes lateral movement of GluA2-containing AMPA receptors. *Molecular Brain, 10,* 56.

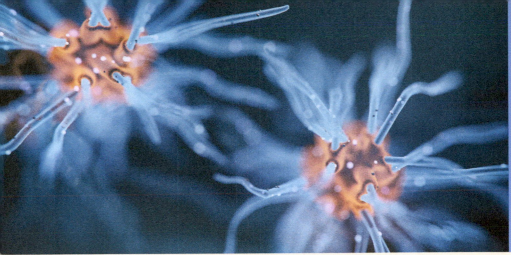

8

Bringing It All Together

Synapses are the fundamental units connecting members of neuronal ensembles that support memory. They are remarkably plastic so that the strength of existing connections can be modified by their activity. Whether the changes in synaptic strength endure depends on the totality of cellular molecular processes engaged by the stimulation that induces LTP. Since the discovery of LTP, neurobiologists have made significant progress toward identifying many of the molecules and their interactions that contribute to altering the strength of synaptic connections. To understand some of the core processes involved in altering synaptic strength, the field was organized into a framework that assumes that changes in synaptic strength evolve over four distinct temporally ordered but overlapping stages: generation, stabilization, consolidation, and maintenance. These stages can be distinguished by the different molecular events that are engaged. The general points summarized in this chapter are presented in Figure 8.1 and amplified in the sections that follow.

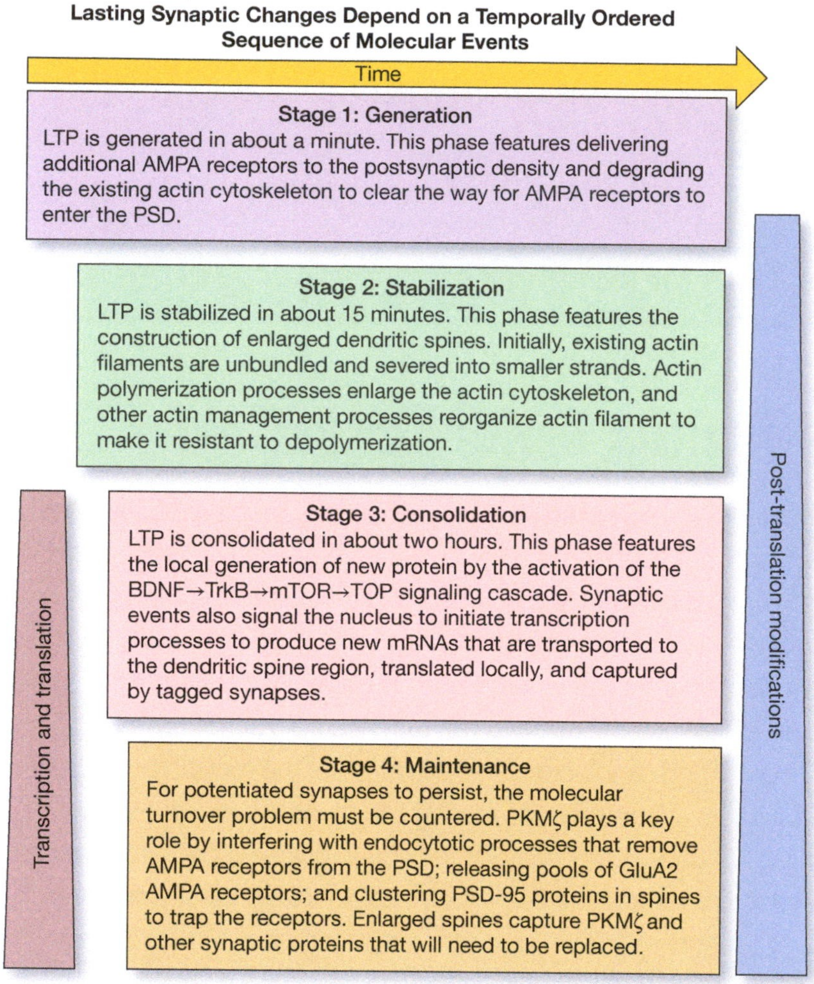

Lasting Synaptic Changes Depend on a Temporally Ordered Sequence of Molecular Events

Time →

Stage 1: Generation
LTP is generated in about a minute. This phase features delivering additional AMPA receptors to the postsynaptic density and degrading the existing actin cytoskeleton to clear the way for AMPA receptors to enter the PSD.

Stage 2: Stabilization
LTP is stabilized in about 15 minutes. This phase features the construction of enlarged dendritic spines. Initially, existing actin filaments are unbundled and severed into smaller strands. Actin polymerization processes enlarge the actin cytoskeleton, and other actin management processes reorganize actin filament to make it resistant to depolymerization.

Stage 3: Consolidation
LTP is consolidated in about two hours. This phase features the local generation of new protein by the activation of the BDNF→TrkB→mTOR→TOP signaling cascade. Synaptic events also signal the nucleus to initiate transcription processes to produce new mRNAs that are transported to the dendritic spine region, translated locally, and captured by tagged synapses.

Stage 4: Maintenance
For potentiated synapses to persist, the molecular turnover problem must be countered. PKMζ plays a key role by interfering with endocytotic processes that remove AMPA receptors from the PSD; releasing pools of GluA2 AMPA receptors; and clustering PSD-95 proteins in spines to trap the receptors. Enlarged spines capture PKMζ and other synaptic proteins that will need to be replaced.

Transcription and translation

Post-translation modifications

FIGURE 8.1 Synapses are strengthened in four overlapping stages. This figure illustrates the relative duration of each stage and important events that occur during each stage. Note that all stages depend on the activation of post-translation processes that modify and rearrange existing proteins. Translation and transcription processes are initiated within minutes of strong synaptic activity. The consolidation phase uniquely depends on signaling cascades that initiate local translation and transcription.

Generation

Under basal conditions, primarily by diffusion, AMPA receptors are trafficked around the dendritic spine into the postsynaptic density (PSD) where they are briefly trapped. The delivery of the LTP-inducing stimulus alters the dynamics of this trafficking to insert more AMPA receptors into the PSD. This result requires the rapid increase in calcium levels in the spine compartment. This occurs when glutamate binds to AMPA and NMDA receptors and the resulting synaptic depolarization removes the Mg^+ from NMDA receptors. A small influx of calcium via NMDA receptors is amplified by calcium released from the endoplasmic reticulum when calcium binds to ryanodine receptors. This increase in calcium modifies calmodulin so that it can then place CaMKII into a persistently active state. One important consequence is that CaMKII phosphorylates the TARP stargazin, associated with GluA1 AMPA subunits. This modification releases stargazin from the plasma membrane so that it can bind to PSD-95 proteins and trap these GluA1 receptors in the postsynaptic density. A consequence is that the AMPA receptors that normally diffuse through the postsynaptic density stay longer. These events are followed shortly by recycling endosomes that deliver additional intracellular pools of receptors to the PSD.

In parallel with this activity, the increase in calcium levels activates calpain proteins that degrade spectrins that crosslink actin filaments. Additionally, the depolymerization properties of cofilin are temporarily enhanced. Together, these processes clear a path for the rapid insertion of GluA1 AMPA receptors into the PSD. All of this takes place in about a minute and is not accompanied by an increase in spine size. These initial changes result in a potentiated synapse, but they are transient and subject to reversal by low-frequency stimulation.

This generation stage does not depend on either the transcription of new mRNA or the translation of new proteins and is carried by the modification and rearrangement of existing synaptic proteins. However, in response to calcium signaling produced by glutamate, to limit the extent to which synapses are potentiated the ubiquitin–proteasome system (UPS) initially degrades proteins that are part of the local translation machinery.

It is relatively easy to potentiate a synapse. All that is required is enough glutamate to depolarize the synapse, cause a brief increase in the calcium content in a spine, and momentarily trap additional AMPA receptors in the PSD. That being so, one can imagine that intrinsic neural activity as well as neural activity generated by sensory input are constantly potentiating the synapses they activate. However, there are endogenous mechanisms in play that are designed to remove these receptors and return the synapses to their prepotentiated state. Thus, these synapses are only temporarily potentiated.

Stabilization

If potentiated synapses are to endure, additional processes must be recruited that enlarge and stabilize the actin cytoskeleton. Stabilization can be divided into three phases. The first begins with the activation of a number of processes whose goal is to unbundle existing actin filaments and sever them into multiple small strands. These strands provide seeds for the next phase—rebuilding and enlarging the actin cytoskeleton—that is controlled by GTPase signaling to phosphorylate cofilin and temporarily turn off its severing activity to create a large stable pool of F-actin. During the third phase, actin stabilizing proteins return to rebundle actin filaments, crosslink them, and bind them to the plasma membrane. These activities are further reinforced by (a) integrin receptors that respond to molecules in the extracellular matrix and contribute to crosslinking actin filaments and to deactivating cofilin, and (b) a reorganization of N-cadherins to tightly couple the pre and postsynaptic components and position the glutamate receptors to receive glutamate released from their presynaptic terminals. Stabilization requires about 15 to 20 minutes to complete. If any of these pathways are inhibited during this time period, potentiated synapses will return to their initial baseline state. Although the consolidation phase, discussed next, requires new protein, one could argue that the consolidating event actually occurs in the stabilization phase during which enlarged stable spines are constructed.

Consolidation

The generation and stabilization of LTP are the product of post-translation processes that modify and rearrange existing proteins. No new protein is required. In contrast, the transcription and translation processes dominate the consolidation stage. If the LTP-inducing stimulus is strong, it will activate signaling cascades (synapse to nucleus and soma to nucleus) that then activate transcription factors in the nucleus. These transcription factors target genes for synaptic proteins that can be transported to the dendritic spine region for translation. The translation of synaptic proteins, however, is a local event.

Local protein synthesis enables new proteins to be produced on demand and in the correct synaptic locations. Thus, protein synthesis occurs after mRNAs have been transported via microtubules to the dendritic spine region. Under nonstimulated conditions, mRNAs in the dendritic spine region change their locations periodically. When glutamate stimulates NMDA receptors they redistribute to the stimulated spines where they are captured and maintained for an hour or more. At about the same time the ribosomal machinery responsible for translation also is captured by stimulated spines. The distribution of neither mRNAs nor ribosomes occurs if actin polymerization is inhibited. Thus, the construction of an enlarged spine is a critical prerequisite for this redistribution.

Local protein synthesis is under the control of signaling events that increase the number of functional ribosomal complexes in the region of stimulated spines. This requires the coordinated translation of mRNAs called TOPs (also known as translation factors). This results in a rapid increase of translation capacity of enlarged spines. Two major signaling pathways contribute to the synthesis of these translation factors. One pathway is initiated primarily by glutamate receptors (NMDA and mGluR) and goes through the mitogen-activated protein kinase (MAPK). The second pathway is activated by glutamate receptors and BDNF binding to TrkB and goes through mTOR. A common target of both pathways is the phosphorylation of the TOP protein 4E-BP, which otherwise would interfere with the assembly of the other translation factors (initiation and elongation factors) with small ribosomal complexes.

The ubiquitin–proteosome system also plays a critical role during the consolidation stage. It initially operates to regulate the level of protein translated locally to ensure that synapses are not overly potentiated. This system is also engaged (a) in the nucleus where it degrades proteins that normally prevent transcription of mRNAs that are needed for enduring LTP and (b) in the dendritic spine region where it degrades translation inhibitors.

Many of the proteins synthesized locally existed prior to LTP induction (for example, AMPA receptors, CaMKII, actin); however, the case can be made that the translation of the *Arc* gene represents a new contribution to the mix. Translated Arc contributes to the stabilization of the actin cytoskeleton. However, the precise pathways through which Arc exerts its impact are unknown.

When LTP is induced, small clusters of spines are potentiated. Members of the cluster can share in the protein resources needed to sustain potentiation and the stimulation of spine clusters is more likely to depolarize the neuron than would the stimulation of spines distributed along a dendritic branch. The sharing of resources among spines is possible because stimulated or tagged spines are thought to have properties that enable them to capture mRNAs and proteins in their vicinity. The concept of a synaptic tag represents this property. A principal feature of tagged synapses is an enlarged actin cytoskeleton that interacts with microtubules to facilitate the capture of proteins.

In a couple hours following the initial induction of LTP, the need for new protein generated by the LTP-inducing event has ended. Functionally, this means that briefly inhibiting transcription and translation processes will no longer return potentiated synapses to their baseline state.

Maintenance

The processes just described are important for establishing an enlarged, well-formed spine that contains enough new AMPA receptors in the PSD to support an enhanced synaptic response to a subsequent encounter with glutamate. However, for the potentiated synapse to persist for days the molecular turnover problem must be overcome. This requires the initiation of processes that will perpetuate the established synaptic changes. Kinases with self-perpetuating properties have been proposed to provide a molecular basis for maintaining potentiated synapses. PKMζ has emerged as a key maintenance molecule. It can self-perpetuate and interact with other proteins to release additional GluA2 AMPA receptors into the PSD and prevent their endocytosis. PKMζ also mediates the redistribution of clusters of PSD-95 into the PSD to facilitate the trapping of AMPA receptors. Another kinase, PKCι/λ, can compensate to some extent for the absence of PKMζ. However, the full expression of this protein is suppressed in normal animals, which implies that under normal conditions, PKMζ is the primary maintenance molecule.

Although PKMζ's presence in synapses is critical, memories can endure for longer than PKMζ. Thus, PKMζ mRNA must be continuously transcribed and transported to dendritic spine regions. PKMζ may also contribute to this outcome because it translocates from the dendritic spine region to the nucleus and phosphorylates the transcription factor CREB-binding protein to target genes for synaptic proteins, including PKMζ mRNA.

Successful maintenance requires the *selective delivery* of PKMζ mRNA transcribed days after LTP is initially consolidated to spines that were originally potentiated. This is made possible because potentiated spines have an enlarged actin cytoskeleton which enables them to capture PKMζ and other replacement proteins.

And So It Is

Although the story is not complete, a general picture has emerged. The multiple intracellular events that change the strength of synaptic connections conspire to produce two major outcomes.

1. They increase the representation of AMPA receptors in the PSD by reconfiguring constitutive trafficking processes and increasing the presence of scaffolding proteins such as PSD-95 that provide anchors for these receptors.
2. They enlarge and stabilize dendritic spines through processes that regulate actin dynamics. Enlarged spines are able to capture synaptic proteins to replace those (including PKMζ) that over time will degrade and thereby self-maintain.

At the end of the day this is a whole-cell operation that involves local interactions among synaptic proteins, genomic signaling, and mRNA transport to provide a continuous supply of the relevant mRNAs to the enlarged spines. It's a miracle!

PART 2
Molecules and Memory

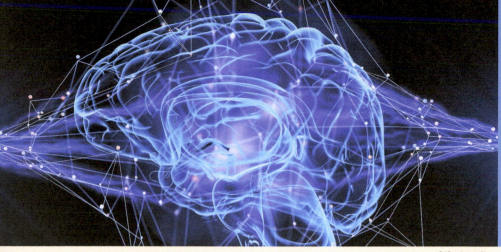

Making Memories: Conceptual Issues and Methodologies

A fundamental question for many students of memory is, *how is information contained in a behavioral experience stored in the brain?* Many researchers believe that the synapse is the basic information storage unit, and previous chapters describe some of the essential findings and ideas about how synapses can be modified. This chapter uses this foundation to explore how memories might be made.

In studies of synaptic plasticity, the stimulus that modified synapses was high-frequency electrical stimulation. Memories, however, are established as a result of a **behavioral experience**, that is, a behaving organism interacting with its environment. This experience is assumed to produce changes in synaptic strength in regions of the brain that store the experience. Memory researchers are thus in the difficult position of connecting the mechanisms of synaptic plasticity to behavioral experience. To do this, the researcher has to navigate a number of difficult conceptual and interpretive issues, and the research requires behavioral and brain methodologies that have not yet been discussed. Thus, the goal of this chapter is to provide an understanding of some of these issues and methodologies.

LTP and Memory

If the synapse is the fundamental storage unit in the brain, and if studies of LTP have produced a complete understanding of how synapses are modified (which they have not), then one might argue that we already know how memories are made. The problem with this argument is that the information acquired by studying LTP comes from a highly artificial preparation.

First, the experience used to induce LTP is a low-intensity, high-frequency electrical event that bypasses all the sensory inputs that normally bring environmental information into the brain. No one has any firm idea about exactly how the pattern of electrical stimulation used to produce LTP corresponds to the pattern of neural activity generated by normal sensory stimulation that initiates the formation of a memory trace in a behaving organism. It should be appreciated that a slightly more intense inducing stimulus would generate seizure activity in a normal brain.

Second, the modified synapses typically are in slices of brain tissue that are maintained in a chemical cocktail to keep them functional. There are consequences associated with the removal of the tissue, which requires a number of preparatory steps just to get a functional preparation. In short, to produce LTP an unnatural stimulus is often delivered to an abnormal neural preparation. So in principle all the results and ideas that have been discussed thus far might have no relevance to how a normal brain stores the information contained in natural experiences.

Fortunately, even though there are enormous differences between the sensory consequences of a behavioral experience arriving into an intact brain and the electrical stimulation arriving into a population of neurons, studies of LTP have yielded important ideas about how memories are formed. Thus, although the synaptic changes that are recorded as LTP do not constitute a memory, studies of synaptic plasticity are the fundamental source of hypotheses about how the brain makes memories. So much of what has already been presented will help in understanding the molecules that make memories.

Behavior and Memory

As previously stated, memories are the product of behaving organisms interacting with their environments. Chapter 1 makes the point that memory is a concept offered to explain why behavioral experiences can influence subsequent behavioral responses to the environment. No one has ever directly observed a memory. This state of affairs has important implications for trying to understand the biological basis of memory. In reality, the effort requires trying to link some physical properties of the brain to an abstract, unobservable concept. To approach this endeavor requires some discussion about the relationship between memory and behavior.

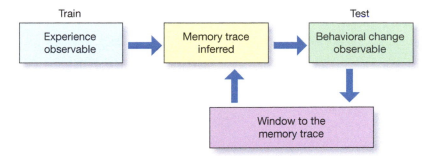

FIGURE 9.1 All experimental investigations of memory require a training phase to establish a memory and a test phase to detect the memory. The existence of a memory trace is inferred when the training experience influences behavior. Thus, test behavior can be thought of as the window to the memory trace.

To start the discussion, consider the basic paradigm used in all studies of learning and memory (Figure 9.1). The inference that a memory has been established requires that the subject in the experiment have a particular experience and then be tested with some component of that experience. If the experience influences the behavioral test, then one might infer that a memory has been established. Recall, for example, that Ebbinghaus trained himself on lists of nonsense syllables and then tested himself to see if he remembered them (see Chapter 1).

Test Behavior: The Window to the Memory Trace

Given that Ebbinghaus recalled the nonsense syllables, one might infer that a memory was established. However, this was because his past behavioral experience influenced his test behavior. The memory was not observed. What was observed was that studying the lists influenced his recall of the nonsense syllables. Note that without a measurable behavioral test response, there would be no evidence that his studying produced a memory trace. Thus, one might conclude that test behavior is the window to the memory trace. Unless the researcher can demonstrate that experience alters test behavior, there is no basis to say it established a memory.

If memory were the only thing that influenced behavior, the study of the biological basis of learning and memory would still be difficult, but far simpler. Unfortunately, this is not the case; a measurable behavior is the final product of many different component processes (Figure 9.2). To list just a few, there are:

- sensory, attentional, and perceptual processes that determine what the subject experiences at the time of training and testing;
- motivational processes that determine the subject's willingness to initiate a response;

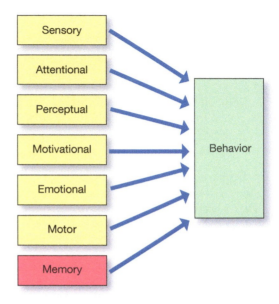

FIGURE 9.2 An organism's behavioral response is determined by the interaction of many different component processes. Thus, before one can conclude that some biological manipulation influenced some aspect of memory, one has to be sure that it did not influence some other component that influences behavior.

- emotional processes that can interfere with the subject's ability to access stored information;
- motor systems that provide the basis for the behavioral response to be expressed; and
- a memory system that stores the experience.

What are the implications of this state of affairs? In studying the biological basis of memory, neurobiologists use a variety of methods to influence brain function. They include:

- experimentally damaging a particular region of the brain;
- injecting drugs into the brain that are designed to influence some aspect of neural function; and
- genetic engineering to increase or decrease the expression of some potential memory molecule.

These methods are discussed in greater detail later in this chapter. To interpret the results produced by any of these methods, the researcher has to confront the possibility that the treatment influenced behavior by its effect on one or more of the component processes listed above.

To illustrate this point, consider the hypothesis that a specific region of the brain stores the memory for some particular experience. To test this hypothesis the experimenter damages this region and then provides the subjects with a learning experience. The results are stunningly clear: compared to control subjects that had no brain damage, subjects with brain damage display no behavioral evidence that they ever had the training experience. They behave as if they have no memory for the experience. What can be concluded from this outcome?

The proper conclusion would be simply that the data are consistent with the hypothesis. Unfortunately, the results are also consistent with other explanations. Before anyone would believe that the damaged region was critical to memory formation, additional experiments would need to be performed to rule out alternative explanations. The lesion might have impaired (1) sensory, attentional, or perceptual processes, (2) motivational or emotional processes, or (3) motor processes. Thus, the experimenter's work has just begun. This caveat applies to the interpretation of any manipulation of brain processes that alters the behavioral measure of memory.

The Learning–Performance Distinction

Successful inroads into understanding the biological basis of memory depend on researchers establishing a strong basis for their conclusions. They must be able to show that the brain manipulation in their experiment influenced behavior by selectively influencing the unobservable memory component and not by affecting some other component process. Psychologists call this problem the **learning–performance distinction**. It recognizes that the researcher has be sure that the treatment exerted its effect by its influence on the memory component and not on some other component process that could also influence performance. To rule out the possibility that the brain manipulation did not influence other component processes is a daunting task. In spite of these complexities, however, memory researchers have made significant advances in this area.

Dimensions of Memory Traces

At least since William James's treatise on psychology, some memory researchers have believed that behavioral experience produces a succession of memory traces in the brain. How many traces are created is a matter of debate that does not need to be considered here. However, most researchers who study the biological basis of memory agree that experience initiates at least two memory traces: a **short-term memory (STM) trace** that decays relatively quickly and a more stable, **long-term memory (LTM) trace** that has a much slower decay rate (Figure 9.3). Because this distinction is so important to neurobiological memory research, it is important to discuss it more fully.

The idea that short-term and long-term memory traces have different decay rates is important. This duration distinction also is tied to two other dimensions: the state of the memory trace (active versus inactive) and its vulnerability to disruption. For example, a football player who receives a blow to the head may not recall any events he experienced several minutes prior to the blow but he may have full recall of everything that happened in the

Dimensions of memory traces

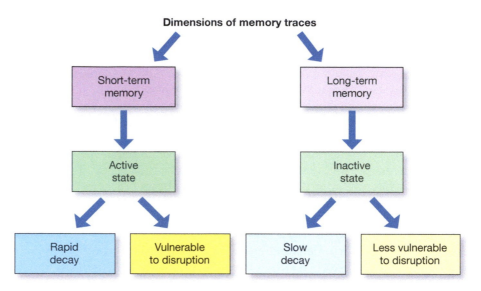

FIGURE 9.3 Memory traces can differ on at least three dimensions: duration, state, and vulnerability to disruption.

locker room before the game started. The blow to the head produced a very time-limited **retrograde amnesia** (a failure to remember an experience that happened prior to the occurrence of the disrupting event). Not all memories were lost; the amnesia was limited only to events that occurred just before the causal event, that is, the blow to the head. One explanation for the limited retrograde amnesia is that the blow affected only the memory traces in the active state. Memories that had achieved long-term memory status and were not in the active state at the time of the trauma were not lost. This point is illustrated in Figure 9.4.

FIGURE 9.4 A football player has two sets of experiences. E1 represents the locker room experiences prior to the game. E2 represents experiences just prior to the head trauma. Thus, the E1 memories are older than the E2 memories. The trauma produces amnesia for only the newer E2 memories because they are still in an active state at the time the trauma occurs. The E1 memories are not affected because they had achieved the inactive, long-term memory state. Key: STM = short-term memory; LTM = long-term memory; A = active state; IA = inactive state; E1 = experience 1; E2 = experience 2.

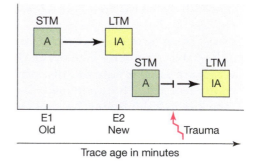

The Concept of Memory Consolidation

Following a learning experience, the memory trace is vulnerable to disruption. With the passage of time, the trace becomes more stable and resistant to memory disruption. This outcome is attributed to a process called **memory consolidation**, a concept introduced over 100 years ago by Müller and Pilzecker (1900). This concept is illustrated in Figure 9.5.

Electroconvulsive Shock and Memory Disruption

Experimental investigations of memory disruption associated with brain trauma did not emerge until nearly half a century after Müller and Pilzecker's research (see McGaugh, 2003 for a review of the history of this development). In the late 1930s, two Italian physicians, Ugo Cerletti and Lucio Bini, began to use **electroconvulsive shock** (**ECS**) to treat psychiatric disorders (Cerletti and Bini, 1938). Clinical observations indicated that patients treated with ECS often did not recall their experiences in the time period leading up to the treatment. A decade later, Carl Duncan (1949) recognized that ECS might be a useful tool for experimentally producing amnesia in animals. He trained rats and administered ECS within a minute or so of training, or an hour later. Rats that received ECS shortly after training displayed a memory impairment. Dozens of experiments were subsequently conducted that used the ECS methodology. Unfortunately, however, this research did not answer any fundamental questions about memory consolidation (McGaugh, 2003). In essence, based on clinical examples, it was already known that brain trauma can disrupt recently established memories and the ECS methodology did not advance understanding beyond this point.

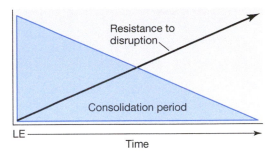

FIGURE 9.5   This figure illustrates the concept of memory consolidation. Following a learning experience (LE), a memory trace is vulnerable to disruption. With the passage of time, resistance to memory disruption increases and the trace becomes more stable. The term memory consolidation is used to describe this change from vulnerable to less vulnerable. The consolidation period is the time it takes to achieve this outcome.

Memory Disruption: A Storage or Retrieval Failure?

In the preceding discussion, the term memory disruption is used to describe the vulnerability of newly established memory traces. Sergei Korsakoff (1897) recognized that memory can be disrupted for two reasons (see Chapter 1).

1. The impairment is a **storage failure**. According to this hypothesis, the agent that produces amnesia, for example a blow to the head, interferes with the processes responsible for storing the memory. The implication of this idea is that events experienced prior to the trauma will never be remembered. A memory not stored can never be recovered.

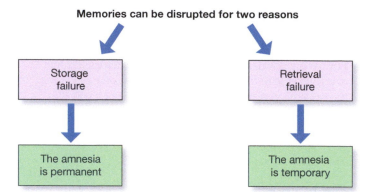

FIGURE 9.6 A disrupting event can interfere with the storage of the memory trace or it can interfere with processes involved in retrieval.

2. The impairment is a **retrieval failure**. According to this hypothesis the memory is stored but cannot be accessed. The agent that produces amnesia in some way disrupts the neural pathways that enable the memory to be retrieved. The implication of this idea is that the memory loss is temporary. Even without trauma, we often have retrieval failures. For example, it is common to forget the location of a book or a coffee cup, only later to remember it. In this case the information had been stored but for some reason could not be accessed or retrieved (Figure 9.6).

The ECS methodology contributed very little to the understanding of how memories are formed. However, it sensitized researchers to the idea that memory failures produced by brain trauma can be either a storage failure or retrieval failure. For a time, research on memory consolidation stalled because researchers using this methodology could not resolve the question of whether or not an event that produced a memory impairment interfered with storage or retrieval. The possibility that a memory impairment can be due to retrieval failures must always be considered when someone claims that their brain manipulation interferes with the consolidation processes that store the memory. The retrieval hypothesis is diabolical because it is impossible to completely disprove. It can never be proved that a memory will not recover with time. The question is, *how much time must be allowed before concluding that the impairment is due to a storage failure: a day, a week, a month?* There is no good answer to this question except that longer is better.

Some Behavioral Test Methods for Studying Memory

Memory researchers use a wide variety of behavioral test methods to study the biological basis of memory. It would be impossible to cover even a small fraction of what is known in this area, so choices have to be made. Much of what we know about the biological basis of memory can be illustrated by initially focusing on results and ideas that have emerged from four extensively used methods: (1) inhibitory avoidance conditioning, (2) fear conditioning, (3) spatial learning in a water-escape task, and (4) recognition memory task. This section describes these methods and some of the advantages they have for memory research. Other methods are described in subsequent sections.

Inhibitory Avoidance Conditioning

An illustration of the apparatus used to study **inhibitory avoidance conditioning** is shown in Figure 9.7. The basic procedure is simple. A rodent (rat or mouse) is placed in the bright side of the apparatus. Rodents generally prefer to be in dimmer environments, so within 10 seconds or so it will cross over to the dark side. When this occurs, a brief electrical shock is applied to its feet and the subject is removed. Some time later the rodent is again placed in the bright side of the apparatus, and the experimenter measures the time it takes the rodent to enter the dark side of the compartment. The expectation is that if the rodent remembers that it was shocked in the dark side, it will be reluctant

(A)

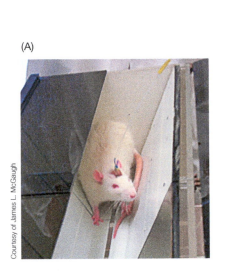

Courtesy of James L. McGaugh

(B)

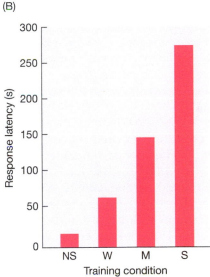

FIGURE 9.7 (A) A photograph of an apparatus used to study inhibitory avoidance learning. The rat is placed in the bright end of the apparatus. When it crosses to the dark side, it receives an electric shock across its feet. To assess the memory for this experience, the rat is placed again in the bright end and the time it takes to cross to the dark side (crossover latency) is measured. (B) The graph illustrates the effect of increasing shock intensity on response latency. Note that as shock intensity increases, so does response latency. Key: NS = no shock; W = weak shock; M = moderate shock; S = strong shock.

to cross over. So the latency to cross over to the dark side should increase. This methodology is called inhibitory avoidance because the rodent has to inhibit its tendency to cross over and thus avoid the place where it was shocked. Note that in using this task, the researcher assumes that the strength of the memory trace is reflected in the response latency, that is, longer latencies reflect a stronger memory trace.

Inhibitory avoidance conditioning has two important attributes. First, only one training trial is required to produce a memory for the experience, although more trials can be given. Second, the rodent's crossover latency is quite sensitive to the intensity of the shock. As shock intensity is increased, the latency to cross over also increases.

Experimental treatments may be hypothesized to either increase or decrease the strength of the memory. So when investigating a drug or some other manipulation that is hypothesized to strengthen a memory trace, a low-intensity shock should be used. This is because if a strong shock is used, the rodent's crossover latency would be so long that it might obscure the possibility of seeing the enhanced latency predicted by the hypothesis. This outcome is called a **ceiling effect** because if the response measure is at the maximum (ceiling), there is no way to see the influence of some other manipulation.

In contrast, if the treatment is hypothesized to impair the memory processes that produce avoidance behavior, then a somewhat higher level of shock that produces a long latency would be used. If a weak shock that produces a short crossover latency is used, it may not be possible to observe the predicted decrease in performance. This outcome is called a **floor effect** because the performance measure is too low to be further reduced by the drug.

Fear Conditioning

Fear conditioning methods are widely used to study the biological basis of memory. The basic methodology, illustrated in Figure 9.8, is a version of Pavlovian conditioning described in Chapter 1. There are two types of tasks based on fear conditioning. One type is called **auditory-cue fear conditioning**. In this case, sometime after a rodent is placed into what is called a conditioning chamber, an auditory stimulus (the conditioned stimulus, CS) is presented. About 10–15 seconds after the onset of the auditory stimulus, electrical shock (the unconditioned stimulus, US) is delivered to the rodent's feet. One can administer one or several training trials. To test for conditioning the rodent is returned to a different chamber and about 2 minutes later the auditory cue is presented for several minutes. The conditioned response (CR), an innate defensive response called **freezing** (see Chapter 20), is often used because in the presence of a danger signal, such as the sight or sounds of a predator, rodents instinctively become still or immobile. This behavior has survival advantages because a moving animal is more likely to be detected by a predator.

The second type of task is called **contextual fear conditioning**. In this case the animal is placed into the conditioning chamber—also called the conditioning

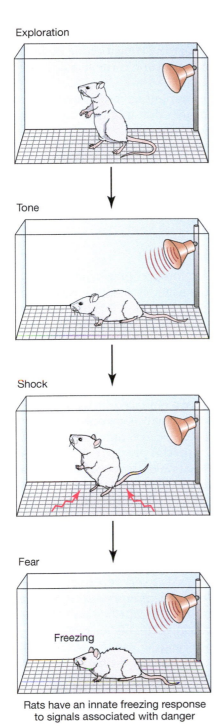

Exploration

Tone

Shock

Fear

Freezing

Rats have an innate freezing response
to signals associated with danger

FIGURE 9.8   In fear conditioning, after
the rat has explored the conditioning
context, an auditory cue (tone) is presented for about 15 seconds. Shock
is delivered when the tone terminates.
Rats are then tested for their fear of the
context–place where shock occurred
and later for their fear of the tone.
Shocked rats display more freezing than
rats that were not shocked.

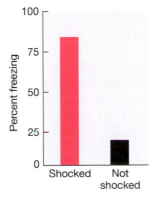

context—and after about 2 minutes the electrical foot shock is presented one or more times. The rodent is then removed from the conditioning context. Sometime later the rodent is returned to the conditioning context and the experimenter measures the time it spends freezing.

The fear conditioning procedure also has important advantages. It allows the experimenter very precise control over factors that might influence the strength of a memory such as (1) the intensity of the CS and US, (2) the time separating the CS and US, and (3) the number of training trials. The innate freezing response that is the CR is easy to measure. Usually the experimenter will observe the rodent and determine the time it spends freezing. However, there are automated methods available to measure this behavior. The basic assumption is that the duration of the freezing response is an indicator of the strength of the memory.

Spatial Learning in a Water-Escape Task

Spatial learning in a water-escape task is a far more complex behavioral test method than the other two described above. The water-escape task was developed by Richard Morris (1981) to allow researchers a method for studying how animals acquire maplike representations of their environments. Essentially, a small platform is located in a large, circular pool of water into which rodents are placed and then tested on finding the location of the platform (Figure 9.9). There are two versions of the water-escape task: the place-learning task and the visible-platform task.

To create the **place-learning task**, the platform is placed in the pool just below the surface of the water but invisible to the rodent. The rodent is placed in the water at the edge of the pool and is released. It can escape from the pool by finding the invisible platform. Note that a special property of this basic task is that the platform remains in the same location of the pool over a block of training trials. The location is specified in relationship to the features of the room in which the pool is located. Typically, the rodent is started randomly from one of several locations inside the side of the pool. This ensures that it has to learn the location of the platform and does not learn just to swim in a particular direction in relationship to some single feature in the room. Rodents are excellent swimmers and, even though the platform is invisible, once the rodent habituates to the surprise of being in the water, it takes very few trials for it to learn to swim quickly and directly to the platform. Successful performance on this task is measured in several ways. During training, **escape latency** (the time it takes to find the platform) decreases dramatically. The distance the rodent swims before it finds the platform, called **path length**, also improves. With practice the rodents swim directly to the platform. Usually escape latency and path length are highly connected because, other things being equal, on a trial when the rodent swims a short distance to find the platform the escape latency will be shorter than when it swims a long distance before locating the platform.

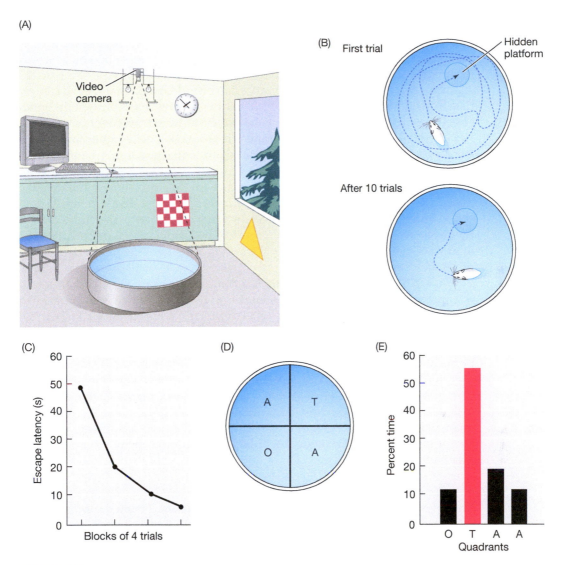

FIGURE 9.9   An illustration of place learning in the Morris water-escape task. (A) A circular swimming pool in the laboratory. (B) On the first trial, the rodent swims a long distance before it locates the platform. After several trials, it learns to swim directly to the platform. (C) Escape latency, the time it takes the rat to find the hidden platform, decreases as a function of training trials. (D) A schematic of the swimming pool that divides it into four quadrants: T, the training quadrant; A, the two adjacent quadrants; O, the quadrant opposite the training quadrant. (E) The results of a probe trial with the platform removed from the pool. Note that the rats spend more time swimming in the training quadrant than in the other quadrants.

Researchers use what is called a **probe trial** to further assess the rodent's memory for the location of the platform. On a probe trial, the platform is removed from the pool and the rodent is placed in the pool and allowed to search for it. The duration of the search can vary (20 to 60 seconds), depending on the experimenter. The rodent's performance can be videotaped or a special camera that feeds data into a computer for further processing can capture it. In either case the experimenter collects information about where the rodent swims.

One standard measure of performance in this task is called **quadrant search time**. The pool is divided conceptually into four equal quadrants. During training the platform is in one quadrant. A rodent that has stored a memory of the location of the platform will spend more of its search time in the training quadrant than it will in the other quadrants. Another performance measure is called **annulus crossings**. In this case, the measure is how many times during the probe trial the animal actually crosses the exact place where the platform is located compared to how many times it crosses the equivalent area in the other quadrants.

The **visible-platform task** is often used as a control task to evaluate alternative interpretations of the effect of some brain manipulation on performance in the place-learning task. In this task the platform sits above the water surface and usually is painted to make it contrast with the water. The platform location usually varies on each trial. If some drug, genetic manipulation, or lesion disrupts performance on the place-learning version of the task, one would want to know that this treatment did not disrupt sensory, motivational, emotional, or motor systems. If the treatment has no effect on performance on the visible-platform task, then one would be more confident about concluding that the treatment influenced some aspect of memory. If, however, the same treatment disrupted performance on this task, then it would be difficult to conclude that the treatment affected memory.

Recognition Memory Tasks

Three versions of tasks based on **recognition memory** are illustrated in Figure 9.10. In all versions the rodent is first allowed to habituate to a large arena. In the **object-recognition task**, the rodent is allowed to explore two identical objects. To test recognition memory for the experienced object, in the test session the animal is returned to the area that contains one of the training experience objects and a new object. The rodent demonstrates that it remembers (recognizes) the old object if it spends more time exploring the new object. In the **object-place-location task**, the animal is allowed to explore two different objects. In the test, one object is moved to a new location. The rodent demonstrates that it remembers the location of the objects if it spends more time exploring the object that is now in a new location. In the **object-in-context task** the animal explores two identical objects in context A and two other but identical objects in context B. In the test, one object from each experienced context is presented in a different context. The rodent demonstrates that it remembers where it experienced the

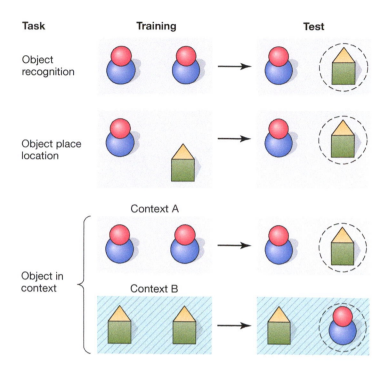

Task	Training	Test
Object recognition		
Object place location		
Object in context		

Context A

Context B

FIGURE 9.10   Three tasks based on recognition memory. In each task the rodent demonstrates that it remembers the training experience by exploring the circled object more than the other objects. See text for a complete description.

object by spending more time exploring the object that is now in a different context. These tasks make different demands on the rodent's memory systems and have the advantage of being the product of the rodent's natural tendency to explore the environment.

Methods for Manipulating Brain Function

Our understanding of how memories are made in the brain requires that the researcher be able to manipulate the brain to determine if a particular region or molecule is critical to creating a memory. This section addresses two general ways this is accomplished. One method, based on damaging or chemically altering neurons in a specific region of the brain, depends on **stereotaxic surgery**. The other method utilizes **genetic engineering** techniques to target specific genes.

Stereotaxic Surgery

Stereotaxic surgery uses a coordinate system to locate specific targets inside the brain to enable some procedure to be carried out on them (for example, a lesion, injection, or implantation). As illustrated in Figure 9.11, a stereotaxic surgery device allows the researcher to lower a fine wire, called an **electrode**, into a precise region of the brain. By passing electric current through the tip of

(A)

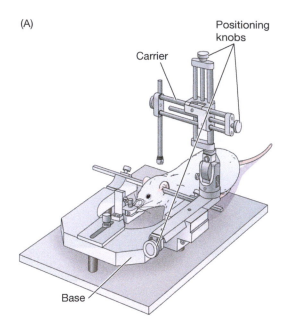

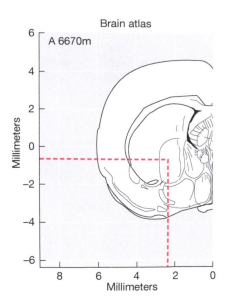

(B)

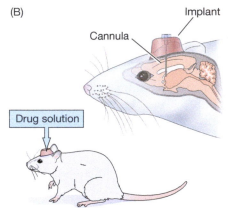

FIGURE 9.11 (A) A stereotaxic device is used during surgery for precise placement of a fine wire (electrode) or a small injection needle (cannula) for targeting electrical current or a chemical solution into a specific region of the brain. The base holds the anesthetized animal's head and neck in a stationary position. The carrier portion places the electrode or cannula in a precise location based on the coordinates of the target area identified with a brain atlas. (B) A cannula guide is implanted deep into the rat's brain. Drugs can then be delivered to specific regions of the brain of an awake and moving rat by inserting a cannula into the guide.

this wire, the researcher can damage neurons in the region of the electrode tip. The device can also be used to position a small injection needle (often referred to as a **cannula**) into a precise brain region so that the researcher can inject into that region a chemical solution that can also damage neurons. Both of these methods are used to damage a particular brain region.

Genetic Engineering

Pharmacological agents have been used with much success in elucidating some of the major molecules that contribute to memory. However, drugs are often "dirty," meaning they are not highly selective to the intended target. This state of affairs can have unintended consequences that can make it difficult to

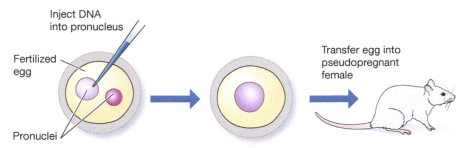

FIGURE 9.12   DNA is injected into a pronucleus from a fertilized egg. This DNA can be designed to replace or knock out a particular gene or it can substitute for another gene.

interpret results. Moreover, controlling the spread of the drug to other regions is also difficult and presents other interpretative problems.

Genetic engineering methods permit much more precise targeting of specific molecules that might play a role in making memories. By using biotechnology to directly influence the genome, it is possible to modify or delete the gene for a particular protein or to transfer new genes into the genome. These methods have made it possible to alter the DNA in a fertilized egg and thereby alter specific genes. Moreover, because this occurs in the fertilized egg, which is then implanted back into the pseudo pregnant animal, this experimentally induced mutation will be carried by the offspring. In general, a particular gene can be removed or "knocked out" or a transgenic animal can be produced, in which case a replacement gene is substituted for the original gene (Figure 9.12).

Researchers often apply genetic engineering methods to mice to study learning and memory. In the first generation of genetically engineered mice, the offspring develop with the mutation and, since a given gene can play an important role in many different functions of the organism, even if the animal survives it might be abnormal in many ways that make it quite difficult to determine the importance of the gene for learning and memory.

However, genetic engineering methods have become much more sophisticated. So there now exists what is called a **conditional knockout methodology**. Under the right conditions, this methodology allows the experimenter to knock out a particular gene in a very well specified region of the brain, such as the CA1 region of the hippocampus, and to do this at different times in development. Moreover, the results of these new techniques can be reversed. Thus, a given gene might be turned off for some period of time and then turned back on, so one can study the same animal with a particular gene knocked out or with that gene functioning.

VIRAL VECTORS   Regional and temporal specificity also have been improved by the use of a **viral vector** methodology—the use of viruses to deliver new genetic material into specific cells (Waehler et al., 2007). Viruses contain genetic material that provides the basic instructions for self-replication. However, they

FIGURE 9.13 This figure illustrates a viral vector methodology used to deliver new genes to the brain where they will be expressed in neurons infected by the viruses. (A) A genetic construct is made that contains the relevant new genetic material and genes for a promotor that drives expression of the gene-infected neurons. (B) This genetic construct is then packaged into the virus and (C) injected into targeted neurons.

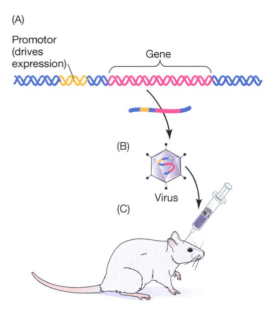

do not have the machinery and metabolism to replicate. Thus, to replicate they must invade a host and hijack the host machinery for this purpose. Viruses can be modified to deliver desired genes into host cells. This is accomplished by deleting some or all of the coding regions of the viral genome and replacing them with a genetic construct that contains the desired new genetic material—the vector genome—and additional genetic elements that control the expression of the gene. This is called a promotor sequence. When the virus is injected into target neurons, the vector genome will then be expressed (Figure 9.13). It is also possible to associate the vector genome with a green fluorescent protein (GFP), a protein that displays bright green fluorescence when exposed to light in the blue-to-ultraviolet ranges. This enables the researcher to identify cells that have been infected by the virus.

OPTOGENETICS   As the name **optogenetics** implies, this methodology combines genetic engineering with optics, the branch of physics that studies the properties of light, to provide a way to control the activity of individual neurons (Deisseroth, 2011; Fenno et al., 2011). Although signaling cascades that regulate neuroplasticity involve interactions among molecules in single neurons, brain functions (vision, motor behaviors, emotional behaviors, and memories) are ultimately the product of neurons communicating with each other. Thus, a fundamental challenge to brain science is to identify the specific neurons and their contribution to the basic brain functions. To do this requires a method that allows scientists to control one type of cell without altering other types.

Existing techniques, based on electrical or chemical stimulation, do not allow this type of control. Francis Crick (1979) suggested that light might be able to control neurons with the temporal and regional specificity needed to map out complex functional circuits of the brain. The development of optogenetics has proven Crick correct.

The discovery that some microorganisms produce proteins that in response to light can regulate the flow of ions across the membrane was fundamental to this development. The genes that code for these proteins are called **opsins**. In 2005, Karl Deisseroth and his colleagues reported that by using the viral vector methodology genes that code for a class of opsins, called channelrhodopsins, could be targeted to hippocampal neurons and would be expressed (Boyden et al., 2005). When activated by blue light, these channel proteins could be stimulated to open and close with millisecond precision and conduct positive ions with the result being depolarization of the neuron. To provide the light source (either with laser light or with light-emitting diodes) optical fibers are implanted into the brain region thought to express the protein, and light will activate only those neurons expressing channelrhodopsin. Another class of opsins, called halorhodopsins, has the opposite effect—when stimulated with green light they conduct negatively charged chloride ions and thereby hyperpolarize the neuron (Figure 9.14). With these tools, the experimenter can excite or inhibit the firing of specific neurons.

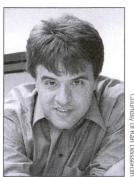

Karl Deisseroth

(B)

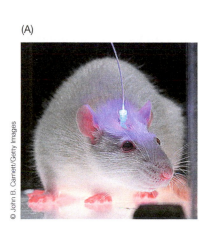

(A)

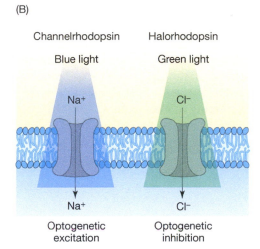

FIGURE 9.14   After rhodopsin genes have been expressed on membranes, they can be activated by light to excite neurons (channelrhodopsin) or to inhibit neurons (halorhodopsin). Channelrhodopsin is activated by blue light and halorhodopsin is activated by green light.

DREADD   DREADD stands for *designer receptor exclusively activated by designer drugs*. This methodology provides another way to regulate neurons. The researcher uses a viral vector to introduce a novel receptor into neurons of interest. It requires about two weeks for the target neurons to express the receptors. These receptors are designed so that they will not respond to any natural ligand. Instead, a synthetic agent such as clozapine N-oxide (CNO) is injected to activate the receptor. A major difference between the optogenetic and DREADD technologies is the time scale. Optogenetics operate on a subsecond time scale to immediately activate the target receptors, whereas the time scale for the synthetic ligand (CNO) to activate the receptors is gradual, taking as much as an hour to exert its effect. DREADD receptors can be engineered to target excitatory or inhibitory neurons and to activate or inhibit them (Roth, 2016).

Summary

Memory researchers must confront a number of conceptual and interpretative issues. Memories cannot be directly observed, so behavior has to be tested in order to infer that a memory has been established. However, behavior is the final product of many different processes. This problem is recognized as the learning–performance distinction. Alternative explanations of the results have to be eliminated before it can be concluded that some brain manipulation influenced memory processes and not some other components that influence behavior. Two ideas are fundamental to confronting these issues: (1) experience can produce memory traces with different properties and (2) memory traces need to consolidate. Interpreting memory impairments is difficult because the experimental treatment can impair processes that store the memory trace (storage failure) or processes that retrieve the memory trace (retrieval failure). Memory researchers depend upon behavioral procedures such as inhibitory avoidance, fear conditioning, and place learning to measure memory, and they depend on methods such as stereotaxic surgery, pharmacology, and genetic engineering to manipulate the brain.

References

Boyden, E. S., Zhang, F., Bamberg, E., Nagel, G., and Deisseroth, K. (2005). Millisecond-timescale, genetically targeted optical control of neural activity. *Nature Neuroscience, 8*, 1263–1268.

Cerletti, U. and Bini, L. (1938). Electric shock treatment. *Bollettino Accademia Medico Roma, 64*, 136–138.

Crick, F. H. (1979). Thinking about the brain. *Scientific American, 241*, 219–232.

Deisseroth, K. (2011). Optogenetics. *Nature Methods, 8*, 26–29.

Duncan, C. P. (1949). The retroactive effect of electroshock on learning. *Journal of Comparative and Physiological Psychology, 42*, 332–344.

Fenno, L., Yizhar, O., and Deisseroth, K. (2011). The development and application of optogenetics. *Annual Review of Neuroscience, 34,* 389–412.

Korsakoff, S. S. (1897). Disturbance of psychic function in alcoholic paralysis and its relation to the disturbance of the psychic sphere in multiple neuritis of nonalcoholic origins. *Vesin. Psychiatrii 4:* fascicle 2.

McGaugh, J. L. (2003). *Memory and Emotion.* New York: Columbia University Press.

Morris, R. G. M. (1981). Spatial localization does not depend on the presence of local cues. *Learning and Motivation, 12,* 239–260.

Müller, G. E. and Pilzecker, A. (1900). Experimentalle beitrage zur lehre vom gedachtinis. *Zeitschrift für Psychologie und Physiologie der Sinnesorgane, I,* 1–288.

Roth, B. L. (2016). DREADDs for neuroscientists. *Neuron, 89,* 683–694.

Waehler, R., Russell, S. J., and Curiel, D. T. (2007). Engineering targeted viral vectors for gene therapy. *Nature Reviews Genetics, 8,* 573–587.

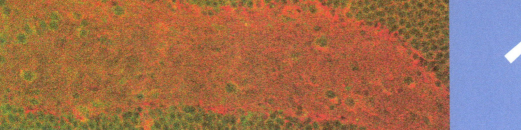

Memory Formation: Early Stages

Memories are produced by experience. The goal of this and the next three chapters is to discuss some of the important cellular–molecular processes that translate experience into memories. These chapters are organized around three basic ideas already presented in the previous chapters on LTP (synaptic plasticity): (1) synaptic changes supporting LTP depend on the binding of glutamate to NMDA and AMPA receptors, (2) post-translation processes can support short-lasting LTP, (3) but long-lasting LTP requires new protein that results from transcription and translation processes. From the perspective of how memories are made, these ideas suggest that post-translation processes can establish a short-term memory trace but experience has to engage transcription and translation processes if the memory is to endure.

It is generally assumed that the formation of a memory trace begins when a behavioral experience activates an ensemble of neurons that might potentially represent the content of the experience. Activated neurons then release glutamate onto the postsynaptic sites and initiate the cascade of cellular–molecular events that strengthen synaptic connections among this set of neurons (Figure 10.1). The signaling cascades that lead to memory formation begin with the release of the first

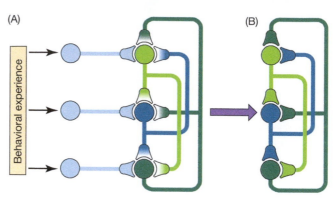

(A)

(B)

Behavioral experience

FIGURE 10.1 (A) The formation of a memory trace begins when a behavioral experience activates a set of weakly connected neurons. (B) The cellular–molecular processes activated in these neurons strengthen their synaptic connections, thereby creating a neural representation of the behavioral experience, called a memory trace.

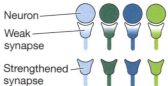

Neuron

Weak synapse

Strengthened synapse

messenger glutamate and the activation of glutamate receptors—a good place to begin the discussion of the early stages of memory formation.

This chapter first addresses the contribution of glutamate receptors (NMDA and AMPA) to memory formation, acquisition, and retrieval; then examines the roles of CaMKII and actin regulation in memory formation; and concludes with a discussion of the dependence of working and reference memory on glutamate receptors.

NMDA Receptors and Memory Formation

Given the critical contribution NMDA receptors make in the initiation of processes that strengthen synapses, one would expect that these receptors are also important for the initiation of memories for behavioral experience. Researchers have used both pharmacological and genetic engineering methodologies to test this hypothesis.

Pharmacological Alteration

Richard Morris (Morris et al., 1986) was the first researcher to experimentally test the hypothesis that the initial formation of a memory trace depends on the activation of NMDA receptors. To do this he implanted a cannula to deliver the NMDA receptor antagonist APV into the ventricular system of a rat's brain where it would enter the **cerebral spinal fluid**. Cerebral spinal fluid is the substance that covers the brain and spinal cord and cushions them against impact. It also provides them with oxygen and nutrients and removes waste products (Figure 10.2).

Morris reasoned that APV injected into this fluid would widely diffuse and occupy NMDA receptors throughout the brain. If NMDA receptors are involved in creating memories for behavioral experiences, then blocking glutamate's access to these receptors at the time of the learning experience

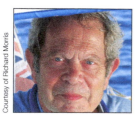

Richard Morris

(A)

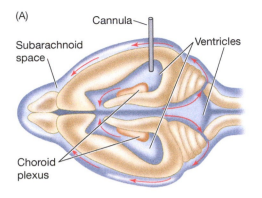

Cannula

Subarachnoid space

Ventricles

Choroid plexus

(B) Computer for image analysis   Video camera

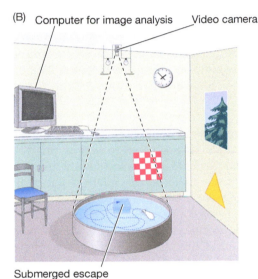

Submerged escape platform

(C) LTP in dentate gyrus

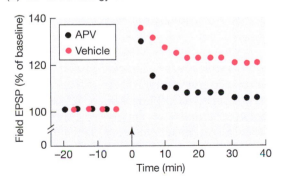

(D)

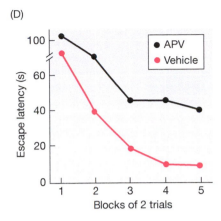

(E)

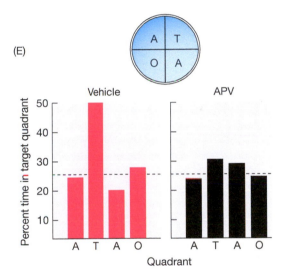

FIGURE 10.2 This figure illustrates the components of the classic Morris experiment. (A) A cannula was implanted into the ventricles of the rat's brain and attached to a time-release pellet that contained the NMDA receptor antagonist APV. (B) Rats were trained on the place-learning version of the water-escape task. (C) Rats infused with APV could not sustain LTP in the dentate gyrus. (D) Rats infused with APV were impaired in learning the location of the hidden platform. (E) Control rats selectively searched the quadrant that contained the platform during training, but rats infused with APV did not. Key: T = training quadrant; A = adjacent quadrant; O = opposite quadrant. (C after R. G. Morris et al. 1990. *Philos Trans R Soc Lond B Biol Sci* 329: 187–204; D, E after R. G. Morris et al. 1986. *Nature* 319: 774–776.)

NMDA receptor subtypes

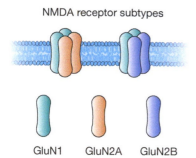

GluN1   GluN2A   GluN2B

FIGURE 10.3 NMDA receptors are composed of four subunits. All functional NMDA receptors contain GluN1 subunits. There are a variety of GluN2 subunits. This figure illustrates NMDA receptor complexes composed of GluN1–GluN2A and GluN1–GluN2B subunits.

should impair memory formation. Morris infused APV dissolved in a vehicle solution into the brain for several days in order to ensure that it occupied NMDA receptors. Control rats were infused with just the vehicle solution. He then trained these rats in the place-learning version of the water-escape task (see Chapter 9).

Morris's experiments revealed that APV prevented the induction of LTP in the dentate gyrus of the hippocampus and, more importantly, dramatically impaired the rat's ability to learn the location of the hidden platform. Morris thus provided the first evidence that NMDA receptors, which are critical to the induction of LTP, may also participate in the initiation of a memory trace. Since the original publication of Morris et al. (1986), there have been many studies using APV to successfully implicate a role for NMDA receptors in memory formation (for example, Campeau et al., 1992; Fanselow and Kim, 1994; Matus-Amat et al., 2007; Morris et al., 1990; Stote and Fanselow, 2004).

Genetic Engineering

Results provided by the genetic engineering approach (see Chapter 9) have strengthened and extended conclusions based on pharmacology. By using these techniques, researchers are able to selectively delete or selectively overexpress the gene for a particular molecule that might be important for making memories. Before considering some of the key findings, however, the composition of the NMDA receptor needs to be more fully described.

The NMDA receptor is composed of four subunits (Figure 10.3). The subunits can be divided into two classes: GluN1 and GluN2. There are several subtypes of GluN2 receptors, designated GluN2A, GluN2B, GluN2C, and GluN2D. All NMDA receptor complexes contain the GluN1 subunit, but a combination of both GluN1and GluN2 subunits is required to form a functional channel that can open to allow Ca^{2+} into the neuron. Researchers interested in the contribution of NMDA receptors to memory have taken advantage of their structure and used genetic engineering methods to selectively delete or overexpress one of these subunits in mice.

DELETION Susumu Tonegawa and his colleagues (Tsien et al., 1996) were able to selectively delete the GluN1 subunit in pyramidal cells in the CA1 field of the mouse hippocampus. This mouse is called a CA1 knockout (CA1KO). These researchers then stimulated the Schaffer collateral fibers and recorded field potentials in slices taken from the CA1KO mice. As one would expect, since the GluN1 subunit is needed to form a functional NMDA receptor, LTP could not be induced in the CA1 field. Note, however, that GluN1 subunits were expressed in neurons in the dentate gyrus (the location where LTP was discovered by Bliss and Lømo; see Chapter 2). Thus, NMDA receptors in this region should be functional, and it was possible to induce LTP in CA1KO mice by stimulating the perforant path and recording field potentials in the dentate gyrus (Figure 10.4).

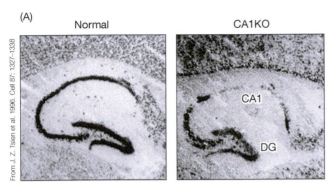

FIGURE 10.4   (A) This photomicrograph shows a section of a normal hippocampus that has been stained to reveal the presence of the GluN1 subunit. Note that the GluN1 subunit is absent in the CA1 region of the section taken from the genetically engineered mouse, called a CA1 knockout or CA1KO, but is present in the dentate gyrus (DG). (B) LTP cannot be induced in CA1 in slices taken from mice lacking the GluN1 subunit. (C) LTP can be induced in the dentate gyrus in slices taken from the genetically engineered mice because the GluN1 subunit is still present. (D) The CA1KO mice are impaired on the place-learning version of the Morris water-escape task. (E) These mice also do not selectively search the training quadrant on the probe trial. (B–E after J. Z. Tsien et al. 1996. *Cell* 87: 1327–1338.)

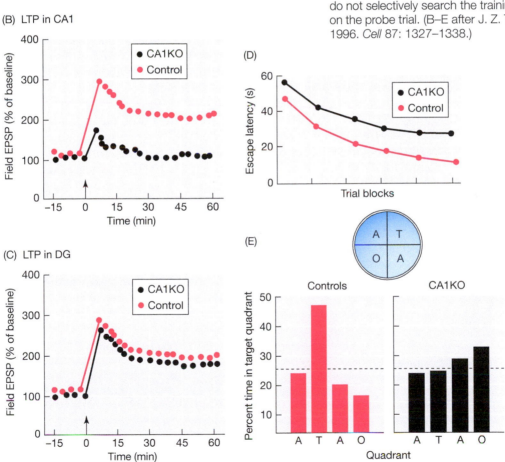

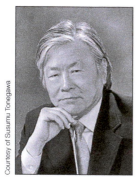

Susumu Tonegawa

The most important results, however, were those that demonstrated that the NMDA receptors in the CA1 field were critical for memory. The researchers tested the CA1KO mice in both the place-learning and visible-platform versions of the Morris water-escape task. These mice were very impaired in acquiring the memory for the location of the hidden platform but were able to learn to swim directly to the visible platform.

Tonegawa and his colleagues (Nakazawa et al., 2003) have also deleted the GluN1 receptor from the CA3 region of the hippocampus. Mice with this deletion were not impaired on the standard place-learning task. However, these researchers also employed a modified version of this task that required mice to learn the location of the platform in one trial. In this study, the mice received four training trials daily, but the platform was moved to a new location each day. Normal mice showed that they acquired the memory for the platform in one trial because their escape latency decreased dramatically between Trial 1 and Trial 2. The escape latency of mice with the GluN1 subunit deleted in CA3, however, did not show a change between the two trials. Thus, this experiment implied that the GluN1 subunit in the CA3 region is necessary for one-trial place learning but not for learning the location of the platform when it remained in the same location every trial.

OVEREXPRESSION   Results of studies discussed thus far indicate that if NMDA receptor function is compromised either by a pharmacological blockade or a genetic deletion of one of its subunits, memory formation can be impaired. Joe Tsien and his colleagues (Tang et al., 1999), however, asked a different question: *can memory formation be improved by enhancing NMDA function?*

During the development of the nervous system, the composition of the NMDA subunits changes. Early in development when the nervous system is being assembled, the GluN2B subunits are dominant, but later these subunits tend to be replaced by GluN2A subunits (Figure 10.5). This shift in the ratio of NMDA receptors containing GluN2B and GluN2A subunits is also associated with different channel opening properties. NMDA receptor complexes that contain

FIGURE 10.5 This figure illustrates the shift in the ratio of GluN1–GluN2A and GluN1–GluN2B NMDA receptors that takes place as the brain develops. (A) During the early postnatal period there are relatively more GluN1–GluN2B receptor complexes. (B) With maturation there is a shift in the balance so that there are more GluN1–GluN2A receptor complexes.

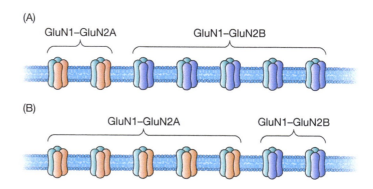

GluN2B subunits remain open longer than those that contain GluN2A subunits and presumably permit more Ca^{2+} to enter the spine. When the GluN2B subunits dominate, it is easier to induce LTP than when GluN2A subunits dominate.

Based on these findings, Tsien reasoned that if one could genetically modify mice to overexpress the GluN2B subunits, it might be possible to improve memory formation. Tsien was successful in engineering this specific overexpression in the cortex and hippocampus of mice in his study. As expected, these mice showed enhanced LTP compared to control mice. The exciting result, however, was that, in addition to enhanced LTP, these mice also demonstrated enhanced memory formation. Their performance in the place-learning version of the water maze was superior to the control mice. They displayed enhanced place learning as well as stronger contextual and auditory-cue fear conditioning, and their object-recognition memory was improved. Tsien called the smart mice Doogie mice after an intellectually precocious teenage character in a once popular television show (Figure 10.6).

Cautions and Caveats

Pharmacological and genetic alteration of the NMDA receptor complex provide evidence that the NMDA receptor can make an important contribution to memory function and thus can play an important role in memory formation. However, it is also important to note that: (a) the interpretation of some of these results has been challenged, and (b) there have been reports that memories can be formed even in the face of a strong pharmacological blockade of NMDA receptors (for example, Cain et al., 1997; Niewoehner et al., 2007; Saucier and

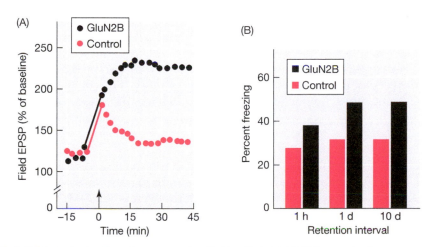

FIGURE 10.6 In the Doogie mouse, the GluN1–GluN2B NMDA complex is overexpressed in several regions of the brain, including the cortex, hippocampus, and amygdala. (A) Slices from the Doogie mouse show enhanced LTP. (B) The Doogie mouse shows a stable and enhanced memory for a contextual-fear-conditioning experience. (After Y. P. Tang et al. 1999. *Nature* 401: 63–69.)

Cain, 1995). The classic Morris et al. (1986) paper—reporting that blocking the NMDA receptor with APV impaired the rat's performance on the place-learning task—can serve to illustrate this issue. This result is, of course, consistent with the idea that NMDA receptors are important in memory formation.

It is often the case that when important new results are reported, the scientific community greets them with caution and skepticism. A number of researchers initially challenged the conclusion that APV impaired performance on this task because it interfered with a process critical to memory formation. As stated previously, any brain manipulation that alters performance can do so for many reasons. Some researchers believe that APV impaired the processes that support the sensory and motor requirements of the task (Bannerman et al., 2006; Cain, 1997; Keith and Rudy, 1990).

In fact Saucier and Cain (1995) reported that if rats are provided with the experience of swimming in a pool before training on the place-learning task, blocking NMDA receptors and LTP in the dentate gyrus has no effect on performance. Bannerman and his colleagues (2006) have discussed many other examples.

Moreover, Brian Wiltgen and his colleagues have reported that mice can learn to fear a new context paired with shock even when NMDA receptors in the hippocampus are pharmacologically inhibited by APV. However, this happens only if the mice were recently conditioned to another similar context. These findings imply that experience can modify the dependency of learning on NMDA receptors and enhance the ability of calcium from other sources to compensate for calcium influxed through NMDA receptors (Taylor et al., 2011; Wiltgen et al., 2010).

There are several lessons to be taken from this discussion.

- Drugs and genetic manipulations can modify behavior without affecting learning and memory.
- These agents can have multiple effects. Even if the targeted molecule or receptor does make a contribution to memory, it might be involved in some other component system that influences behavior.
- Memory formation may take place without the contribution of NMDA receptors.

There is also a more general point that is worth making. As noted, Saucier and Cain (1995) reported that once sensory–motor impairments were reduced, rats easily learned to find the hidden platform even when NMDA receptors were blocked. What should one conclude from this finding? It is tempting to conclude that NMDA receptors do not participate in establishing a memory for the location of the platform. But that would be wrong. Saucier and Cain's observation may mean that there are other mechanisms that can produce memories when NMDA receptors are not functional. They do not, however, exclude the possibility that NMDA receptors normally contribute to creating place memories.

The general point is that when a component of the brain is removed and this has no effect on memory formation, one cannot say the component (for example, brain region, cell, or molecule) is not involved in memory formation when it is normally present. The brain has redundant mechanisms that might substitute for each other. So the absence of an effect primarily reveals what the brain can do without the component. It does not reveal what that component does in the normal brain.

AMPA Receptors and Memory Formation

AMPA receptors play a major role in strengthening synapses. By participating in depolarizing the neuron, they contribute to opening the NMDA calcium channel and thus to initiating intracellular events that strengthen synapses. Moreover, the end product of the biochemical changes that produce LTP is an increase in AMPA receptor function. Existing receptors may stay open longer and more of them are present in the PSD.

Based on these facts one should expect to find evidence that AMPA receptors are involved in both the formation and retrieval of a memory. Indeed, there is evidence that supports this prediction. For example, it is known that object-recognition memory critically depends on a cortical region adjacent to the hippocampus called **perirhinal cortex**. Winters and Bussey (2005) infused the AMPA receptor antagonist 6-cyano-7-nitroquinoxaline (CNQX) into the perirhinal cortex of rats to temporarily reduce AMPA receptor function. Infusing this drug before training prevented the rats from forming a memory of the object, while injecting the drug before testing prevented them from retrieving the memory.

Fear Conditioning Drives GluA1 AMPA Receptors into Spines

It is generally accepted that long-term potentiation is the result of the induction stimulus engaging processes that drive additional GluA1 AMPA receptors into the dendritic spines. One might expect that if memory formation depends on the synaptic changes that support LTP, then behavioral experiences that produce memories also should traffic additional GluA1 AMPA receptors into spines. In a remarkable set of experiments, Roberto Malinow and his colleagues (Rumpel et al., 2005) provided evidence that this occurs. They used genetic engineering methods to create GluA1 AMPA receptors and then injected these receptors into the amygdala. Green fluorescent protein was also expressed by the receptors and allowed neurons that contained these receptors to be visualized (Figure 10.7). They used a fear-conditioning procedure to establish a memory—the rats received several pairings of an auditory CS with shock. After the rats were tested for their fear response, they were sacrificed and slices of brain tissue from the **basolateral amygdala (BLA)** were prepared to determine if the behavioral training had driven GluA1 receptors into the spines.

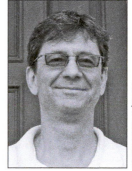

Courtesy of Roberto Malinow

Roberto Malinow

FIGURE 10.7 LTP studies have shown that GluA1 AMPA receptors are inserted into the plasma membrane of dendritic spines in response to synaptic activity. Malinow and his colleagues used a special technique to insert modified glutamate receptors, GluA1, into the lateral amygdala. (A) These receptors were labeled with a fluorescent molecule and could be visualized. (B) Rats with these fluorescent-tag AMPA receptors were tested for fear of a tone paired with shock or tested for fear of a tone unpaired with shock. Rats in the paired condition displayed fear to the tone. The rats were then sacrificed and slices were taken from their brains. An analysis of these slices revealed fear conditioning had driven the GluA1 AMPA receptors into the spines. (C) Schematic representation of the distribution of the GluA1 receptors prior to training. (D) After the training, rats in the paired condition had more GluA1 receptors trafficked into the plasma membrane than rats in the unpaired condition. These results indicate that a behavioral experience that produces fear conditioning also drives AMPA receptors into the synapse. (B–D after S. Rumpel et al. 2005. *Science* 308: 83–88.)

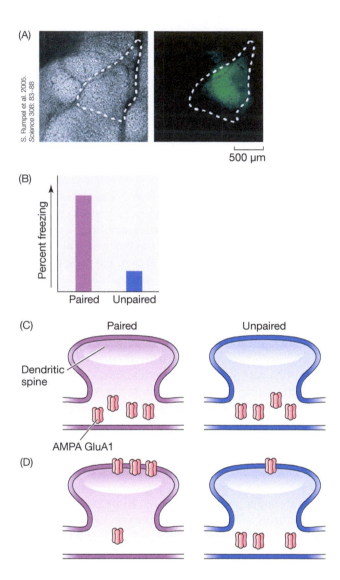

Malinow's group was able to detect the presence of these receptors in synapses because when glutamate binds to them electrical current can be detected that is slightly different from that produced by endogenous GluA1 receptors. To activate these synapses they stimulated the auditory pathway in the thalamus that projects to the amygdala. These experiments revealed that the conditioning experience had driven the GluA1 receptors into the dendritic spines because they were able to detect an increase in the signature response of synapses belonging to the neurons that fluoresced.

Preventing AMPA Receptor Trafficking Impairs Fear Conditioning

If the GluA1 AMPA receptor plays a critical role in the support of the fear memory, then it follows that if trafficking this receptor into the spine is prevented, the fear memory should be weak. Malinow's group also used genetic engineering to test this hypothesis. They created and injected a nonfunctional version of the GluA1 subunit receptor that would compete with the functional receptors for delivery to the membrane. This nonfunctional unit could be driven into the spine but would not respond properly to glutamate release. It might be thought of as a dummy receptor. The experiments revealed that rats with neurons that contained nonfunctional receptors displayed a reduced fear memory (Figure 10.8). This means that the memory for the fear experience, as measured by the rat's freezing response, depends on trafficking AMPA receptors with functional GluA1 subunits into the membrane.

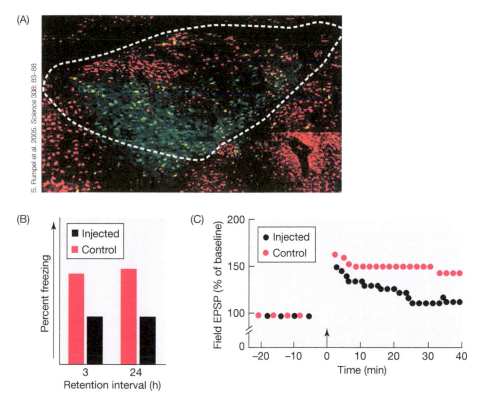

FIGURE 10.8 (A) Modified nonfunctional GluA1 receptors are injected into the lateral amygdala. These modified receptors compete with endogenous functional GluA1 receptors for trafficking into spines. (B) Rats injected with this receptor display impaired fear conditioning to a tone paired with shock. (C) Slices from animals injected with the modified receptor cannot sustain LTP induced in the lateral amygdala. (B, C after S. Rumpel et al. 2005. *Science* 308: 83–88.)

Ampakines and Cognitive Enhancement

AMPA receptors play a critical role in initiating the processes that strengthen synapses. The resulting upregulation of these receptors that also occurs is largely responsible for the enhanced synaptic response recorded as LTP (Figure 10.9). The empirical facts behind these conclusions have made AMPA receptors attractive candidates for the development of therapeutics designed to enhance memory and other complex forms of cognition. Gary Lynch and his colleagues have developed a class of drugs called **ampakines** that may enhance cognitive function (Baudry et al., 2012; Lynch and Gall, 2006).

Ampakines cross the blood–brain barrier and bind to a site on the AMPA receptor. However, they function as neither agonists nor antagonists. Their influence is observed when glutamate binds to the receptor. As previously learned, when glutamate binds to an AMPA receptor a channel opens and Na^+ enters the cell. Normally this channel rapidly closes. However, when an ampakine also binds to the AMPA receptor it slows down the deactivation or closure of the channel. Functionally, what this means is that when an ampakine is present there will be a prolonged current flow and enhanced synaptic

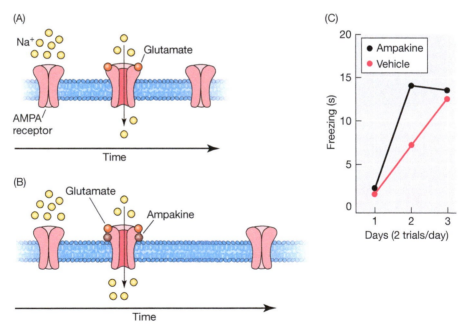

FIGURE 10.9 (A) When glutamate binds to AMPA receptors the conductance channel is briefly opened and this allows positive ions to enter. (B) When ampakines and glutamate both bind to the AMPA receptor, the channel stays open longer and therefore more ions enter and the synaptic response is enhanced. (C) Ampakines enhance the rate of auditory fear conditioning. (C from M. T. Rogan et al. *J Neurosci* 17: 5928–5935. © 1997 Society for Neuroscience.)

responses. Thus, the neuron will more likely depolarize (which should facilitate the opening of the NMDA receptor channel) and will also be more likely to release neurotransmitters onto other neurons to which it is connected.

There are a number of reports that ampakines can enhance learning (see Lynch and Gall, 2006 for a review). For example, Rogan et al. (1997) treated rats with an ampakine prior to fear conditioning to a tone paired with very mild shock. They reported that it enhanced the rate at which conditioned fear was established (see Figure 10.9C). There is also evidence that ampakines may be used to ameliorate mild memory impairments that develop with age.

NMDA and AMPA Receptors: Acquisition and Retrieval

When the NMDA receptor's contribution to LTP was discovered in the hippocampus, researchers found that APV, the NMDA receptor antagonist, blocked the induction but not the expression of LTP (see Chapter 2). This means that when APV was administered prior to the induction stimulus it prevented LTP, but when it was administered after LTP was established it had no effect. In contrast, AMPA receptors have been shown to be important in both the induction and expression of LTP.

In the context of building memories, these findings suggest that NMDA and AMPA receptors might make different contributions to the acquisition and retrieval of memories. Specifically, as suggested earlier, NMDA receptors should be critical for the acquisition of the memory but not for its retrieval. AMPA receptors, however, should be important for both the acquisition and retrieval of the memory.

Morris and his colleagues (Day et al., 2003) used a clever one-trial memory task to test this hypothesis. Training occurred in a large open arena that featured two landmarks, a pyramid and a stack of golf balls (Figure 10.10). Rats were first allowed to learn the layout of the arena. The floor of the arena had many small holes that could be filled either with just sand or sand and a food pellet. During the acquisition phase of training, the rat was released into the area twice. Each time it explored the area until it found an uncovered sand well that contained a distinctive food pellet (for example, a banana or cinnamon flavored pellet). The rat's task was to remember the location of the sand wells and the flavor of the pellets they contained.

To determine if the rat remembered the sand-well locations that contained the pellets, it was returned to one of four release points and fed one of the pellets (for example, banana). It was released into the arena, where the two sand wells that had contained food pellets in the acquisition phase were uncovered. Digging in the sand well that contained banana pellets, it would be rewarded with another banana pellet. However, digging in the other sand well would not yield a food pellet. Each day a new set of flavors was used, and the rats easily learned to dig in the sand well that contained the flavor pellet that they were fed at the release point. About 2 hours separated the acquisition and retrieval phase of the experiment.

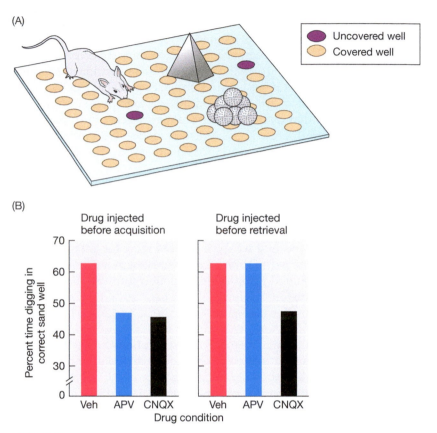

FIGURE 10.10 (A) This graphic is a schematic of the arena Morris and his colleagues used to study the role of glutamate receptors in the acquisition and retrieval of a memory for the location of flavored food pellets. On the retrieval test, the two sand wells that contained the flavored pellets on the acquisition trial were uncovered. The rat was fed one of the pellets in the release point. Its task was to remember which sand well contained that pellet during acquisition. (B) When given before acquisition, both APV and CNQX interfered with establishing the food-location memory. However, only CNQX, the AMPA receptor antagonist, interfered with the retrieval of the memory. Key: Veh = vehicle. (After M. Day et al. 2003. *Nature* 424: 205–209.)

After the rats had learned the task, Morris evaluated the role of NMDA and AMPA receptors in the acquisition and retrieval of the memory of the flavor location. To do this, either the NMDA antagonist APV or the AMPA receptor antagonist CNQX was injected into the hippocampus. These drugs were injected either before the acquisition phase or before the retrieval phase of the experiment.

Morris found that APV impaired performance when it was injected before the acquisition phase but had no effect when it was injected prior to the retrieval phase (Day et al., 2003). Note that because the rats were not impaired when APV was injected prior to retrieval, one can be confident that the drug did not impair sensory, motor, or motivational processes that are essential to performance. In contrast, CNQX impaired performance when it was injected both prior to the acquisition phase and prior to the retrieval phase. Recall that Winters and Bussey (2005) reported that AMPA receptors were critical to both the acquisition and retrieval of memories for objects. These results indicate that NMDA and AMPA glutamate receptors can play a role in the acquisition and retrieval of a memory similar to the role they play in the induction and expression of LTP. Specifically, NMDA receptors are critical only for acquisition, while AMPA receptors contribute both to acquisition and retrieval.

CaMKII and Memory Formation

Studies of synaptic plasticity suggest that NMDA and AMPA receptors are important because the opening of the NMDA calcium channel allows a spike of Ca^{2+} to enter the spine. Ca^{2+} is a second messenger that activates another messenger protein, calmodulin, which binds to the kinase CaMKII. This protein plays a critical role in establishing LTP, so one would expect that it also plays an important role in memory formation. Much of what is known about what CaMKII contributes to memory formation comes from studies with genetically engineered mice. The general strategy has been to either remove the CaMKII gene or overexpress the active form of CaMKII.

The first application of genetic engineering to the study of memory molecules was directed at CaMKII. Alcino Silva and his colleagues successfully deleted the CaMKII gene (Silva, Paylor et al., 1992; Silva, Stevens et al., 1992). LTP could not be induced in the CaMKII knockout mice (CaMKII KO) and these mice were severely impaired in both the visible-platform and place-learning versions of the Morris water-escape task (Figure 10.11). These were exciting results. Nevertheless, this pioneering work was also criticized for not completely ruling out the possibility that the mutation caused sensory motor impairments that were responsible for their poor performance.

Preventing Autophosphorylation of CaMKII Impairs Learning

One of the important properties of CaMKII is its capacity to autophosphorylate and remain in an active state in the absence of Ca^{2+}/calmodulin. Given the importance of autophosphorylated CaMKII to synaptic plasticity, Peter Giese and his colleagues (Giese et al., 1998; Irvine, Danhiez et al., 2011; Irvine, Maunganidze et al., 2011; Irvine et al., 2006) have studied mice that have been genetically engineered to be deficient in autophosphorylation. Synaptic plasticity studies of these animals indicate that LTP cannot be induced in the CA1 field by stimulating the Schaffer collateral fibers but that it can be induced in the dentate gyrus by stimulating the perforant path (Cooke et al., 2006; Irvine, Danhiez et al., 2011; Irvine, Maunganidze et al., 2011).

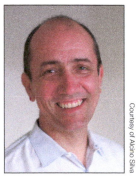

Alcino Silva

Courtesy of Alcino Silva

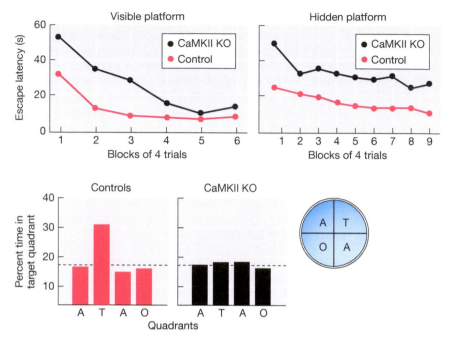

FIGURE 10.11 The CaMKII-deficient mouse (CaMKII KO) can learn to swim to the visible platform but cannot learn the location of the hidden platform. Note that control mice selectively search the target quadrant on a probe trial but that the defective CaMKII KO mice do not. (After A. J. Silva et al. 1992. *Science* 257: 206–211.)

Under limited training conditions (one trial), these autophosphorylation-deficient mice showed a deficit in inhibitory avoidance learning and in contextual and auditory-cue fear conditioning. However, if they were given only a few extra trials, they were completely normal (Figure 10.12). Thus, suppressing the autophosphorylation of CaMKII has a significant but limited effect on the formation of memories that support these behaviors (Irvine, Danhiez et al., 2011; Irvine, Maunganidze et al., 2011; Irvine et al., 2006). The finding that with additional training these animals acquired a memory for these tasks suggests that the one-trial impairment is unlikely due to sensory or motor impairment. One important implication of this work is that the autophosphorylation of CaMKII may be critical for the rapid (one-trial) formation of a memory but that other processes can compensate for this contribution (see Radwanska et al., 2011) when multiple training trials occur. It should be noted, however, that even though mice deficient in CaMKII autophosphorylation can learn under certain conditions, they are not normal.

CaMKII and Fear Memories

Sarina Rodrigues and her colleagues (Rodrigues et al., 2004) have provided some of the most convincing evidence that CaMKII can play a critical role in the formation of a fear memory. These researchers found that CaMKII was present

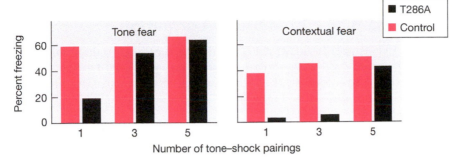

FIGURE 10.12 Autophosphorylation is critical for rapid formation of a fear memory but not essential for memories produced with multiple training trials. In this experiment, mice genetically engineered to impair autophosphorylation of CaMKII (T286A) and control mice received 1, 3, or 5 pairings of a tone and shock. Control mice acquired fear to the context and to the tone after only one pairing; however, the defective mice required several pairings to acquire the fear memory. (After E. E. Irvine et al. 2006. *Trends Neurosci* 8: 459–465.)

in synapses with NMDA receptors that contained GluN2B subunits. They then found that fear conditioning increased the presence of phosphorylated CaMKII in dendritic spines, indicating that the conditioning experience activated this kinase. In addition, they observed that a drug (KN-62) that inhibits CaMKII activation blocked the acquisition of both contextual and auditory fear conditioning and also prevented LTP in this region of the brain (Figure 10.13). This is exactly the pattern of results one would expect based on the role of CaMKII in synaptic plasticity. Note that the basolateral amygdala is believed to be a critical memory site for fear conditioning.

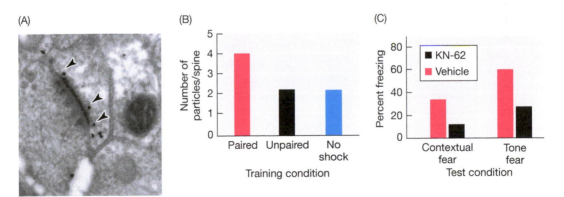

FIGURE 10.13 Fear conditioning produces increased phosphorylated CaMKII in dendritic spines in the amygdala. (A) A micrograph showing particles of phosphorylated CaMKII in a spine. (B) Rats that had received paired presentations of a tone and shock have more particles of phosphorylated CaMKII in spines than control animals that received either no shock or unpaired presentations of the tone and shock. (C) KN-62, which inhibits the phosphorylation of CaMKII, impairs both contextual and tone fear conditioning. (From S. M. Rodrigues et al. 2004. *J Neurosci* 24: 3281–3288. © 2004 Society for Neuroscience.)

Actin Dynamics and Memory Formation

Studies of LTP established that actin regulation is critical to the evolution of the synaptic changes that support LTP (see Chapters 3 to 8). Thus, it is not surprising that behavioral studies also reveal that actin regulation is critical for producing memories (see Lamprecht, 2011). Some evidence for this claim is described below.

A primary regulator of actin dynamics is cofilin (see Chapter 4). In its normal active state cofilin interferes with actin polymerization. In its phosphorylated state, however, the depolymerization property of cofilin is turned off. Given that synaptic changes supporting LTP require actin polymerization, one would expect that a behavioral experience that produces a memory would engage signaling pathways such as LIMK that would phosphorylate cofilin. This implication has been confirmed. For example, the training procedure used to produce an object-place recognition memory increases the ratio of phosphorylated cofilin to total cofilin in the hippocampus, a region of the brain that supports object-place recognition memory (Britta et al., 2012). Moreover, interfering with actin polymerization by infusing latrunculin into the hippocampus prevents the formation of the memory needed to perform the task.

Different regions of the brain support different types of memories. For example, the basolateral amygdala and prelimbic cortex provide critical support of fear memories but are not critical for a learned taste aversion that is acquired when one gets sick following the consumption of a novel food. Taste aversion memories are supported by neurons in the insular cortex. Thus, one would expect that the training procedure that produces a learned taste aversion would selectively activate actin regulation processes in the insular cortex but not in the basolateral amygdala. This predicted result has been confirmed. First, training that produces a learned taste aversion increases the length of the postsynaptic density in spines located in the insular cortex but has no effect on spines located in the basolateral amygdala or prelimbic cortex. Second, cytochalasin D, which interferes with actin polymerization, prevents the lengthening of the PSD in spines in the insular cortex and prevents the formation of the taste aversion memory (Bi et al., 2010).

Working and Reference Memory

At least since the writings of William James, memory researchers have been influenced by the idea that a memory trace induced by a new experience evolves in stages (see Chapter 1). An initial trace is formed that is labile and subject to rapid decay. However, during this period other processes are at work to yield a more enduring and stable trace that represents the information contained in the experience. This idea informs the chapters on synaptic plasticity and is further explored in Chapter 11.

It is also the case that everyday experiences support the idea that information can intentionally be held in memory and manipulated to solve a particular problem or achieve a particular goal. For example, you enter a grocery store with the intent of purchasing a few items (bread, milk, eggs, coffee, cheese, steak, and cake). Assuming you did not create a written list, you will have to maintain this information in memory until you complete your shopping. Once your shopping is complete there is no further need to maintain this information in memory. Psychologists refer to this category of memory as **working memory** (Baddeley, 1986; Baddeley et al., 2009).

An Animal Model

Psychologists have developed a variety of tasks that can be used to study working memory in animals (see Sanderson and Bannerman, 2012). David Olton (Olton and Samuelson, 1976) introduced a methodology that has proven to be quite useful—the **radial arm maze**, called that because it has a number of arms radiating out from the center (Figure 10.14). To create a working memory task each arm is baited with a food reward and the rodent is released from the center and allowed to collect all of the rewards. Once visited, an arm is not rebaited. So

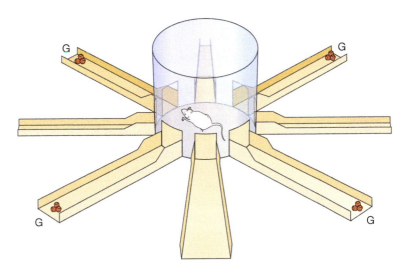

FIGURE 10.14   The radial arm maze can be used to study both working memory and reference memory. A trial begins when the rodent is placed in the center of the maze. It ends when the animal has retrieved the food reward from all baited arms. To do this only four of the eight arms are baited but the same four arms are baited on each trial. The rat has to learn which four arms are never baited (the reference memory component) and to remember which arms it previously visited (the working memory component). On a trial the rat can now make two types of errors: (1) a working memory error—it enters a previously sampled arm, and (2) a reference memory error—it enters an arm that was never baited.

the most efficient strategy is for the rodent to avoid reentering arms that have already have been visited. This requires that the animal "remember" the arms that no longer contain food—it is a working memory task. Radial arm mazes with up to 16 arms have been used, and rats are remarkably successful in this task. Once experienced with the procedure, rodents rarely revisit a previously sampled arm, thus not making a working memory error.

A variation of this task allows the researcher to study both working memory and what is called **reference memory**. In this variation the maze typically has eight arms but only four are baited. The same four arms are baited on each trial. Now the rat not only has to remember which arms it visited but also has to learn and remember which arms are baited and which are never baited. This is the reference memory component of the task. On a trial the rat can now make two types of errors: (1) a working memory error—it enters a previously sampled arm, and (2) a reference memory error—it enters arms that are never baited. Trained rats perform very well on this task, making almost no working or reference memory errors.

Critical Contributions of Glutamate Receptor Subunits

The availability of such tasks has allowed neurobiologists to discover some of the molecular events that support working and reference memory. Remarkably, the subunit composition of AMPA and NMDA receptors determines whether or not rodents are successful on working memory and reference memory tasks. However, before this evidence is discussed, it is useful to briefly return to the LTP experiment.

The point is made in Chapter 3 that the initial short-lasting, early phase of LTP depends on the rapid insertion of GluA1 AMPA receptors. Researchers using genetically altered mice have provided direct support for this view (Romberg et al., 2009). When a weak TBS is used, slices from control mice display a short-lasting LTP, but slices from mice that lack the gene for the GluA1 subunit (called GluA1 KO) do not express this short-lasting potential. Nevertheless, when stimulated by a stronger theta-burst protocol, slices from the GluA1 KO mice display an enduring LTP, equivalent to control mice, even though they do not display the early, short-lasting phase (Figure 10.15). These results indicate that GluA1 subunits are required for the initial early phase of LTP but not for the later developing phase, which likely requires GluA2 AMPA receptors. They also reveal that an enduring LTP can be established independent of any contribution from GluA1 receptors.

David Bannerman and his colleagues (Bannerman, 2009; Sanderson and Bannerman, 2012; Schmitt et al., 2003) have studied the performance of GluA1 KO mice in the radial arm maze. Unlike control mice they made numerous working memory errors, revisiting the previously baited arms. This result implies that synaptic changes that support working memory require the rapid addition of GluA1 receptors into the postsynaptic density. Additional support for this conclusion is that both the LTP impairment and the working memory impairment

(A)

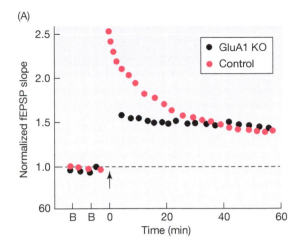

FIGURE 10.15   (A) GluA1 knockout (KO) mice do not express early-phase, short-lasting LTP but do express late-phase, enduring LTP. (B) The GluA1 KO mice do not differ from control mice in learning the reference memory component of the radial maze task but display severely impaired working memory. (A after C. Romberg et al. 2009. *Eur J Neurosci* 29: 1141–1152; B after W. B. Schmitt et al. 2003. *J Neurosci* 23: 3953–3959. © 2003 Society for Neuroscience; D. J. Sanderson and D. M. Bannerman. 2012. *Hippocampus* 22: 981–994.)

(B)

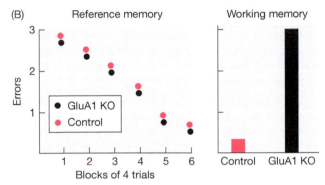

displayed by GluA1 KO mice can be rescued by transferring a GluA1 expression system into these mice (Schmitt et al., 2005). This form of genetic engineering restores the ability of some neurons to express the gene for the GluA1.

To master the reference memory component of the task—learning to discriminate which set of arms are baited and which are not—requires many training trials. Mice lacking GluA1 receptors learn this discrimination. This fact suggests that the synaptic changes that support this learning depend on some of the processes that produce the enduring form of LTP that the GluA1 KO mice display. One might speculate that repeated training can engage the processes that traffic GluA2 AMPA receptors.

Different subunits of the NMDA receptor also contribute selectively to working and reference memory. Specifically, the NMDA receptors composed of the GluN1 and GluN2A subunits are required for working memory but not for reference memory. Given this pattern of results, one might speculate that calcium influx through NMDA receptors composed of GluN1–GluN2A subunits contributes to the rapid insertion of GluA1 AMPA receptors. It is not yet clear just what if any NMDA receptor subunit combination is needed to support reference memory (Bannerman, 2009). However, there is no evidence that it depends on the GluN1–GluN2B subtype. The fact is that very little is yet known about how repeated training alters the basic processes involved in learning and memory.

The general conclusion from this discussion of working and reference memory is that the subunit composition of both AMPA and NMDA receptors is critical for working memory. It depends on processes that rapidly insert GluA1 AMPA receptors into the synapse. The insertion of these receptors depends in part on NMDA receptors composed of GluN1 and GluN2A subunits. In contrast, neither enduring LTP nor reference memory requires GluA1 receptors. Given the established role of GluA2 AMPA receptors in the maintenance of LTP, it is reasonable to speculate that reference memory depends on processes that regulate the trafficking of these receptors.

Summary

Studies of synaptic plasticity have strongly implicated glutamate receptors (NMDA and AMPA receptors) and CaMKII as major components in the signaling cascades that lead to strengthening of synapses. Both pharmacological and genetic engineering methodologies have been used to determine if these molecules are also critical to memory formation.

There are a large number of reports that NMDA receptors make a critical contribution to the acquisition, but not the retrieval, of some forms of memory. Such studies have revealed that interfering with the contribution of these receptors can impair memory formation, while enhancing the NMDA calcium channel function can enhance memory formation.

Studies of AMPA receptors have revealed that they play a critical role in both the acquisition and retrieval of memories. Particularly striking is that just as they can be driven into synapses by high-frequency stimulation used in LTP experiments, they can also be driven into spines by fear conditioning. Moreover, if normal AMPA receptors are not driven into spines, the acquisition of a fear memory is impaired. In addition, delaying the closure of AMPA receptor channels with ampakines appears to provide a potential therapy for enhancing the laying down of memory traces.

The regulation of actin that is so critical to each stage of LTP is also critical to the initial construction of memory traces that support learned behaviors. Behavioral experiences that generate new memories also engage processes that regulate actin, and construction of these memory traces is impaired when actin polymerization is prevented.

Studies of working and reference memory have revealed that these two types of memory depend on different subunit composition of AMPA and NMDA receptors. Working memory requires the rapid insertion of GluA1 AMPA receptors and this depends on NMDA receptors composed of GluN1 and GluN2A subunits. Reference memory does not require GluA1 AMPA receptors but may depend on AMPA receptors containing GluA2 subunits.

References

Baddeley, A. D. (1986). *Working Memory*. New York: Oxford University Press.

Baddeley, A., Eysenck, M. J., and Anderson, M. C. (2009). *Memory*. Hove and New York: Psychology Press.

Bannerman, D. M. (2009). Fractionating spatial memory with glutamate receptor subunit-knockout mice. *Biochemical Society Transactions, 37*, 1323–1327.

Bannerman, D. M., Rawlins, J. N., and Good, M.A. (2006). The drugs don't work—or do they? Pharmacological and transgenic studies of the contribution of NMDA and GluR-A-containing AMPA receptors to hippocampal-dependent memory. *Psychopharmacology, 8*, 533–566.

Baudry, M., Kramar, E., Xu, X., Zadran, H., Moreno, S., Lynch, G., Gall, C., and Bi, X. (2012). Ampakines promote spine actin polymerization, long-term potentiation, and learning in a mouse model of Angelman syndrome. *Neurobiology of Disease, 47*, 210–215.

Bi, A. L., Wang, Y., Li, B. Q., Wang, Q. Q., Ma, L., Yu, H., Zhao, L., and Chen, Z. Y. (2010). Region-specific involvement of actin rearrangement-related synaptic structure alterations in conditioned taste aversion memory. *Learning and Memory, 17*(9), 420–427.

Britta, S., Nelson, A., Christine, F., Witty, A., Elizabeth, A., Williamson, A., Jill, M., and Daniel, A. (2012). A role for hippocampal actin rearrangement in object placement memory in female rats. *Neurobiology of Learning and Memory, 98*(3), 284–290.

Cain, D. P. (1997). LTP, NMDA, genes and learning. *Current Opinion in Neurobiology, 7*, 235–242.

Cain, D. P., Saucier, D., and Boon, F. (1997). Testing hypotheses of spatial learning: the role of NMDA receptors and NMDA-mediated long-term potentiation. *Behavioral Brain Research, 84*, 179–193.

Campeau, S., Miserendino, M. J., and Davis, M. (1992). Intra-amygdala infusion of the N-methyl-D-aspartate receptor antagonist AP5 blocks acquisition but not expression of fear-potentiated startle to an auditory conditioned stimulus. *Behavioral Neuroscience, 106*, 569–574.

Cooke, S. F., Wu, J., Plattner, F., Errington, M., Rowan, M., Peters, M., Hirano, A., Bradshaw, K. D., Anwyl, R., Bliss, T. V., and Giese, K. P. (2006). Autophosphorylation of αCaMKII is not a general requirement for NMDA receptor-dependent LTP in the adult mouse. *Journal of Physiology, 574*, 805–818.

Day, M., Langston, R., and Morris, R. G. (2003). Glutamate-receptor-mediated encoding and retrieval of paired-associate learning. *Nature, 424*, 205–209.

Fanselow, M. S. and Kim, J. J. (1994). Acquisition of contextual Pavlovian fear conditioning is blocked by application of an NMDA receptor antagonist D,L-2-amino-5-phosphonovaleric acid to the basolateral amygdala. *Behavioral Neuroscience, 108*, 210–212.

Giese, K. P., Fedorov, N. B., Filipkowski, R. K., and Silva, A. J. (1998). Autophosphorylation at Thr286 of the α calcium-calmodulin kinase II in LTP and learning. *Science, 279,* 870–873.

Irvine, E. E., Danhiez, A., Radwanska, K., Nassim, C., Lucchesi, W., Godaux, E., Ris, L., and Giese, K. P. (2011). Properties of contextual memory formed in the absence of αCaMKII autophosphorylation. *Molecular Brain, 28,* 4–8.

Irvine, E. E., Maunganidze, N. S., Pyza, M., Ris, L., Szymańska, M., Lipiński, M., Kaczmarek, L., Stewart, M. G., and Giese, K. P. (2011). Mechanism for long-term memory formation when synaptic strengthening is impaired. *Proceedings of the National Academy of Sciences USA, 108,* 18471–18475.

Irvine, E. E., von Hertzen, L. S., Plattner, F., and Giese, K. P. (2006). AlphaCaMKII autophosphorylation: a fast track to memory. *Trends in Neurosciences, 8,* 459–465.

Keith, J. R. and Rudy, J. W. (1990). Why NMDA receptor-dependent long-term potentiation may not be a mechanism of learning and memory: reappraisal of the NMDA receptor blockade strategy. *Psychobiology, 18,* 251–257.

Lamprecht, R. (2011). The roles of the actin cytoskeleton in fear memory formation. *Frontiers in Behavioral Neuroscience, 5,* 39.

Lynch, G. and Gall, C. M. (2006). Ampakines and the threefold path to cognitive enhancement. *Trends in Neurosciences, 10,* 554–562.

Matus-Amat, P., Higgins, E. A., Sprunger, D., Wright-Hardesty, K., and Rudy, J. W. (2007). The role of dorsal hippocampus and basolateral amygdala NMDA receptors in the acquisition and retrieval of context and contextual fear memories. *Behavioral Neuroscience, 12,* 721–731.

Morris, R. G., Anderson E., Lynch, G. S., and Baudry, M. (1986). Selective impairment of learning and blockade of long-term potentiation by an N-methyl-D-aspartate receptor antagonist, AP5. *Nature, 319,* 774–776.

Morris, R. G., Davis, S., and Butcher, S. P. (1990). Hippocampal synaptic plasticity and NMDA receptors: a role in information storage? *Philosophical Transactions of the Royal Society B: Biological Sciences, 329,* 187–204.

Nakazawa, K., Sun, L. D., Quirk, M. C., Rondi-Reig, L., Wilson, M. A., and Tonegawa, S. (2003). Hippocampal CA3 NMDA receptors are crucial for memory acquisition of one-time experience. *Neuron, 38,* 305–315.

Niewoehner, B., Single, F. N., Hvalby, O., Jensen, V., Borgloh, S. M., Seeburg, P. H., Rawlins, J. N., Sprengel, R., and Bannerman, D. M. (2007). Impaired spatial working memory but spared spatial reference memory following functional loss of NMDA receptors in the dentate gyrus. *European Journal of Neuroscience, 25,* 837–846.

Olton, D. S. and Samuelson, R. J. (1976). Remembrance of places passed: spatial memory in rats. *Journal of Experimental Psychology: Animal Behavior Processes, 2,* 97–116.

Radwanska, K., Medvedev, N. I., Pereira, G .S., Engmann, O., Thiede, N., Moraes, M. F., Villers, A., Irvine, E. E., Kaczmarek, L., Stewart, M. G., and Giese, K. P. (2011).

Mechanism for long-term memory formation when synaptic strengthening is impaired. *Proceedings of the National Academy of Sciences USA, 108*, 18471–18475.

Rodrigues, S. M., Farb, C. R., Bauer, E. P., LeDoux, J. E., and Schafe, G. E. (2004). Pavlovian fear conditioning regulates Thr286 autophosphorylation of Ca^{2+}/calmodulin-dependent protein kinase II at lateral amygdala synapses. *Journal of Neuroscience, 24*, 3281–3288.

Rogan, M. T., Stäubli, U. V., and LeDoux, J. E. (1997). AMPA receptor facilitation accelerates fear learning without altering the level of conditioned fear acquired. *Journal of Neuroscience, 17*, 5928–5935.

Romberg, C., Raffel, J., Martin, L., Sprengel, R., Seeburg, P. H., Rawlins, J. N., Bannerman, D. M., and Paulsen, O. (2009). Induction and expression of GluA1 (GluR-A)-independent LTP in the hippocampus. *European Journal of Neuroscience, 29*, 1141–1152.

Rumpel, S., LeDoux, J. E., Zador, A., and Malinow, R. (2005). Postsynaptic receptor trafficking underlying a form of associative learning. *Science, 308*, 83–88.

Sanderson, D. J. and Bannerman, D. M. (2012). The role of habituation in hippocampus-dependent spatial working memory tasks: evidence from GluA1 AMPA receptor subunit knockout mice. *Hippocampus, 22*, 981–994.

Saucier, D. and Cain, D. P. (1995). Spatial learning without NMDA receptor-dependent long-term potentiation. *Nature, 378*, 186–189.

Schmitt, W. B., Deacon, R. M., Seeburg, P. H., Rawlins, J. N., and Bannerman, D. M. (2003). A within-subjects, within-task demonstration of intact spatial reference memory and impaired spatial working memory in glutamate receptor-A-deficient mice. *Journal of Neuroscience, 23*, 3953–3959.

Schmitt, W. B., Sprengel, R., Mack, V., Draft, R. W., Seeburg, P. H., Deacon, R. M., Rawlins, J. N., and Bannerman, D. M. (2005). Restoration of spatial working memory by genetic rescue of GluR-A-deficient mice. *Nature Neuroscience, 8*, 270–272.

Silva, A. J., Paylor, R., Wehner, J. M., and Tonegawa, S. (1992). Impaired spatial learning in alpha-calcium-calmodulin kinase II mutant mice. *Science, 257*, 206–211.

Silva, A. J., Stevens, C. F., Tonegawa, S., and Wang, Y. (1992). Deficient hippocampal long-term potentiation in alpha-calcium-calmodulin kinase II mutant mice. *Science, 257*, 201–206

Stote, D. L. and Fanselow, M. S. (2004). NMDA receptor modulation of incidental learning in Pavlovian context conditioning. *Behavioral Neuroscience, 118*, 253–257.

Tang, Y. P., Shimizu, E., Dube, G. R., Rampon, C., Kerchner, G. A., Zhuo, M., Liu, G., and Tsien, J. Z. (1999). Genetic enhancement of learning and memory in mice. *Nature, 401*, 63–69.

Tayler, K. K., Lowry, E., Tanaka, K., Levy, B., Reijmers, L., Mayford, M., and Wiltgen, B. J. (2011). Characterization of NMDAR-independent learning in the hippocampus. *Frontiers of Behavioral Neuroscience, 5*, 1–12.

Tsien, J. Z., Huerta, P. T., and Tonegawa, S. (1996). The essential role of hippocampal CA1 NMDA receptor-dependent synaptic plasticity in spatial memory. *Cell, 87,* 1327–1338.

Wiltgen, B. J., Royle, G., Gray, E. E., Abdipranoto, A., Thangthaeng, N., Jacobs, N., Saab, F., Tonegawa, S., Heinemann, S. F., O'Dell, T. J., Fanselow, M. S., and Vissel, B. (2010). A role for calcium-permeable AMPA receptors in synaptic plasticity and learning. *PLOS ONE, (5)*9, e12818.

Winters, B. D. and Bussey, T. J. (2005). Glutamate receptors in perirhinal cortex mediate encoding, retrieval, and consolidation of object recognition memory. *Journal of Neuroscience, 25,* 4243–4251.

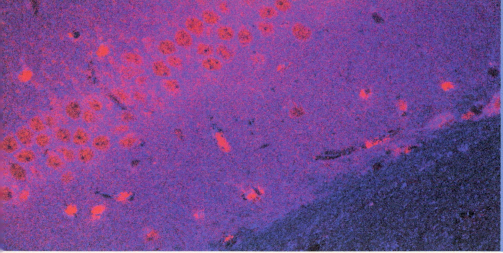

Memory Consolidation

The initial creation of a memory is rapid and depends only on post-translation processes. However, it is unlikely to endure unless other processes are recruited and continue long after the initiating behavioral experience. The perspective introduced in Chapter 9 has guided neurobiologists attempting to uncover the molecular processes that create enduring memories (Figure 11.1). It assumes that a behavioral experience quickly establishes a short-term memory (STM) trace that can evolve into a long-term memory (LTM) trace.

The evolution and consolidation of the LTM trace requires time and depends on processes that operate for hours following the initiating behavioral experience. The goal of this chapter is to describe some of the consolidation processes (translation and transcription) that establish long-term memories. Three important principles emerge.

1. Enduring memories require that the behavioral experience initiate processes that generate new proteins and thus depend on translation and transcription.

2. These consolidation processes occur in multiple waves that can continue for at least 24 hours.

3. These processes are sustained by an autoregulatory positive feedback loop that ensures a continuous supply of synaptic mRNAs for local translation.

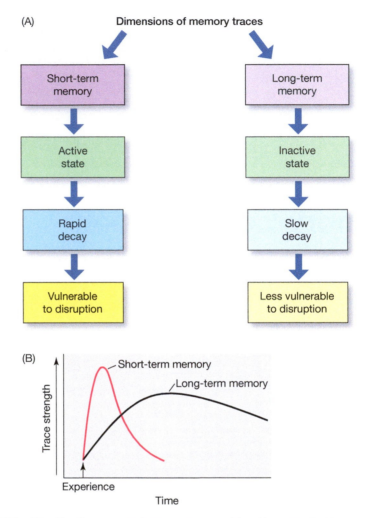

FIGURE 11.1 Shortly after an experience, memory retrieval is supported by an active short-term trace. As this trace decays, a more stable, long-term memory trace is generated that can support memory retrieval for a much longer period of time.

To understand the empirical basis of these principles it is necessary to describe the logic of the research paradigm used to investigate the consolidation period and address the question, *how do we define a long-term memory?*

The Research Paradigm

Researchers often use the experimental strategy described in Figure 11.2 to uncover the molecular–cellular processes that contribute to memory consolidation. Typically, the subject is trained on a task such as fear conditioning or inhibitory

FIGURE 11.2 This figure illustrates the generic research design for determining the contribution of a particular molecule(s) to memory storage. A drug or gene is evaluated by assessing its effect on memory at two retention intervals—a short interval (1–2 hours) designed to assess short-term memory (STM) and a longer interval, usually about 24 hours, designed to assess long-term memory (LTM).

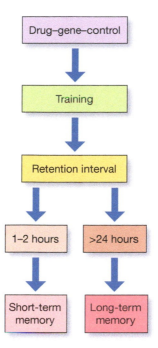

avoidance learning. Two variables are included in the experiment. The first is a pharmacological or genetic manipulation designed to influence some target molecule that has been hypothesized as important for memory; a drug treatment can be delivered either before or after training. The second variable is called the **retention interval**—the time between the training experience that establishes the memory and the test used to retrieve the memory. The assumption is that performance at short retention intervals (usually fewer than 4 hours) is supported by the short-term memory but that test performance at longer retention intervals requires a consolidated long-term memory.

The logic of this strategy can be further understood by considering a hypothetical experiment in which a drug is used to evaluate the contribution of some particular molecule (M_x) to memory consolidation. The drug is thought to degrade the contribution M_x makes to memory consolidation and, in this case, is infused into the brain prior to training. Figure 11.3 shows two possible outcomes produced by the drug. The outcome in Figure 11.3A indicates that the drug impaired performance

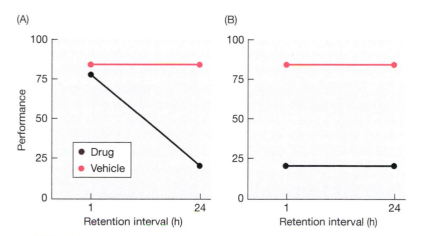

FIGURE 11.3 (A) The drug targeted at M_x impaired performance at the 24-hour retention interval but had no effect at the 1-hour retention interval. This result is consistent with the hypothesis that M_x is important for the consolidation of the long-term memory trace and is not critical for the short-term memory trace. (B) The treatment impaired performance at both the 1-hour and 24-hour retention intervals. This result is consistent with the hypothesis that M_x contributes to both short-term and long-term memory but is also consistent with other interpretations.

at the long, 24-hour retention interval but had no effect on performance at the short, 1-hour retention interval. These results would be consistent with the hypothesis that M_x contributes to the consolidation of the long-term memory trace. They also support an even stronger conclusion—that the short-term memory trace did not depend on a contribution from M_x. This is because the drug did not impair retention at the short interval. Thus, the results shown in Figure 11.3A will be the signature pattern required to support the hypothesis that a targeted molecule or signaling cascade contributes to memory consolidation and not to memory formation. This pattern has been observed in many experiments.

In contrast, Figure 11.3B shows that the drug impaired performance at both the short and long retention intervals. These data are more difficult to interpret. They could mean that the generation of both the STM and the LTM traces requires a contribution from M_x. However, these data are also consistent with the hypothesis that the drug used to influence M_x interfered with how the animal normally sampled the environment (see Chapter 9). If one repeated the experiment but infused the drug immediately after training and obtained the same result, then this interpretation could be ruled out.

Criterion for When the Memory is Consolidated

Generally speaking neurobiologists want to answer two questions: *how long does it take to consolidate a memory?* and *what are the critical molecular events that contribute to the outcome?* The answer to the first question requires specifying a criterion for when the memory is consolidated. This is a somewhat controversial issue (Dudai, 2004). However, the criterion consistent with the overall theme of this chapter is that *a memory is consolidated when it is no longer vulnerable to pharmacological–molecular treatments that interfere with the translation and transcription events initiated by the memory-producing behavioral experience.* Based on this criterion, a general answer is that the duration of the consolidation period depends on how long the memory can be retained. A memory that endures for many days requires a long consolidation period with multiple waves of protein synthesis contributing to the outcome, whereas a memory that lasts only a day or so will depend on a much shorter period. The sections that follow describe the basis of these conclusions and how these answers emerge.

Inhibiting Protein Synthesis

The classic approach to studying memory consolidation begins with evaluating the effect of inhibiting protein synthesis on memory retention. Typically, a broadscale inhibitor such as the antibiotic anisomycin is used to interfere with translation (see Bourtchouladze et al., 1998; Davis and Squire, 1984). More recently Cristina Alberini's laboratory provided a comprehensive assessment of the effects of protein synthesis inhibition on consolidation (Bambah-Mukku et al., 2014) that offers a basis for analysis. In their experiments, rats were trained on an inhibitory avoidance task and anisomycin

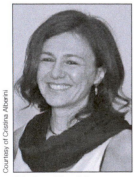

Cristina Alberini

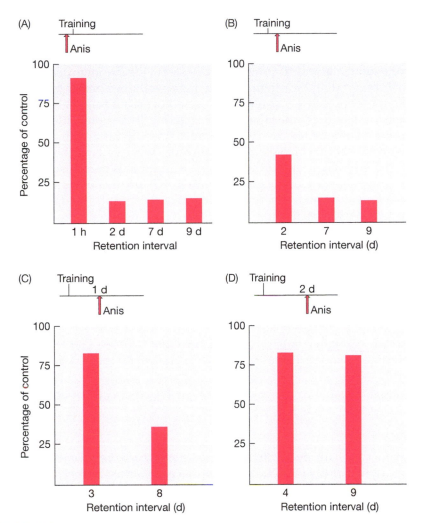

FIGURE 11.4 Inhibiting protein synthesis by delivering anisomycin (Anis) reveals two waves of consolidation. (A) Anisomycin delivered prior to training has no effect on short-term memory (1-hour retention) but prevents the consolidation of long-term memory (2-, 7-, 9-day retention). (B) Delivering anisomycin shortly after training allows the development of a memory that can endure for 2 days but then decays. (C) Delivering aniso-mycin 1 day following training has no effect on retention 3 days after training but impairs retention 8 days after training. (D) Anisomycin delivered 2 days following training has no effect on memory retention. To simplify the data, the results for animals infused with anisomycin are presented as percentage of control animals' performance. Thus, a low percentage means poor memory retention. (After D. Bambah-Mukka et al. 2014. *J Neurosci* 34: 12547–12599.)

was infused into the hippocampus to inhibit protein synthesis. An important feature of these experiments is that both the timing of the infusion and the retention interval were varied. A summary of their results is presented in Figure 11.4.

Figure 11.4A shows that inhibiting translation prior to training has almost no effect on memory retention 1 hour later, but the memory does not persist at the longer retention intervals. This result is consistent with the idea that short-term memory (observed at the 1-hour retention interval) does not depend on new protein but new protein is required for the memory to endure. In Figure 11.4B, anisomycin was infused immediately after training. This would allow for some local protein synthesis to be initiated because it would take a few minutes for the drug to have its effect. Note that the memory was available 2 days following training but that by day 7 the memory was gone. When anisomycin was infused 1 day following training (see Figure 11.4C) the memory was present at least 3 days following training but had decayed significantly by day 8. Finally, when the anisomycin infusion was delayed until 2 days after training it had no effect on the long-term retention of the memory (see Figure 11.4D).

Several important conclusions are supported by these results.

- A short-term memory can be established that does not require new protein.
- Preventing the initiation of protein synthesis prior to training prevents the memory from enduring.
- Allowing protein synthesis to occur for about 5–10 minutes following training can support a memory that can endure for about 2 days.
- For the memory to endure for more than 3 days requires a second wave of protein synthesis that takes place about a day following training.
- By about 2 days following training the memory is consolidated in the hippocampus.

Collectively the results indicate that it takes somewhere between 1–2 days for the memory to be fully consolidated and that at least *two waves of protein synthesis are required*. One wave is initiated immediately following training and a second wave about 1 day following training.

Molecular Basis of Consolidation

Although these data provide information about the temporal parameters of consolidation, they tell us nothing about the underlying molecular events that are engaged to produce the outcome. In this section, some of the key molecular events are identified.

Local Protein Synthesis: The First Wave

Recall that mRNAs and translation machinery are present in the dendritic spine region and synaptic activity can stimulate the **BDNF** → **TrkB** → **mTOR** → **TOP** pathway to rapidly upregulate the translation capacity of stimulated spines (see Chapter 6). Given this arrangement, one could hypothesize that the initial wave of protein synthesis is the result of engaging the molecules that generate **local protein synthesis** and this wave is responsible for the memory that persisted for about 2 days when anisomycin was administered a few minutes after training (see Figure 11.4B). The local protein synthesis hypothesis makes a number of interesting predictions, some of which are described as follows.

MTOR   Activation of the protein mTOR is a critical outcome of BDNF signaling. It is responsible for upregulation of the translation machinery (ribosomal complexes) in the dendritic spine region. Interfering with mTOR activation *prior to training* should prevent memory consolidation (which depends on protein synthesis) but should have no effect on short-term memory, which does not require new protein. In contrast, delaying the interfering event until a few minutes after training should have no effect on long-term memory because local translation is initiated rapidly and the new proteins will be in place before mTOR is inhibited. These predictions have been confirmed.

In another set of experiments, Alberini's group used rapamycin to prevent the activation of mTOR, which would prevent the initiation of local protein synthesis (see also Bekinschtein et al., 2007; Jobim et al., 2012). As shown in Figure 11.5, when rapamycin was infused into the hippocampus prior to training there was no memory retention either 2 or 7 days later, yet short-term memory was not affected. In contrast, when the infusion of rapamycin was delayed until a few minutes after training, it had no effect on memory retention. In addition to supporting the hypothesis that the molecular effects that support local protein synthesis are responsible for the initial wave of protein synthesis, these data imply that unless local protein synthesis occurs *there will be no second wave.*

The protein mTOR is more complex than previously described. It forms two functionally distinct multiple protein complexes. One complex, called mTOR complex 1 (mTORC1),

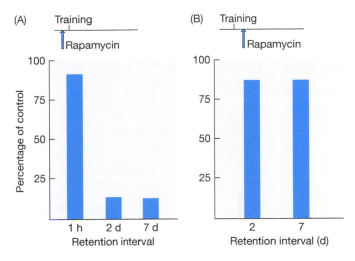

FIGURE 11.5 Disrupting mTOR activation by rapamycin reveals that local protein synthesis is responsible for the first wave of consolidation. (A) Rapamycin infused into the hippocampus prior to inhibitory avoidance training has no effect on short-term memory (1-hour retention) but prevents the consolidation of long-term memory (2- and 7-day retention). (B) Rapamycin infused just after training has no effect on memory consolidation. These results indicate that in the absence of local protein synthesis neither the first or second wave of consolidation will occur but permitting local protein synthesis to occur allows not only for the first wave but also the second wave. To simplify the data, the results for animals infused with rapamycin are presented as the percentage of control animals' performance. Thus, a low percentage means poor memory retention. (After D. Bambah-Mukka et al. 2014. *J Neurosci* 34: 12547–12599.)

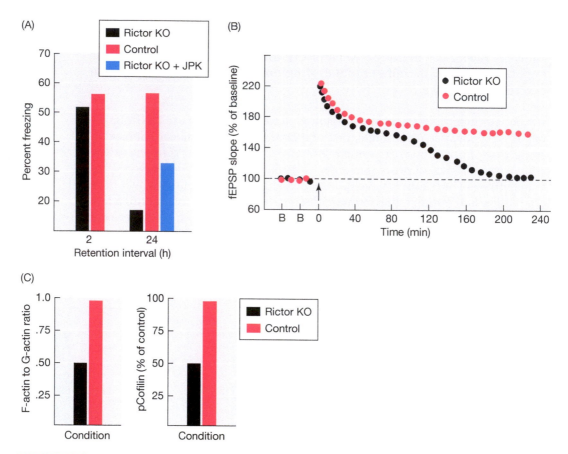

FIGURE 11.6 Studies of rictor KO mice found that mTORC2 contributes to long-term memory but does not influence short-term memory. (A) When experiencing contextual fear conditioning, rictor KO mice display normal short-term memory (2-hour retention test) but impaired long-term memory (24-hour retention test). This impairment is partially rescued by infusing an agent, jasplakinolide (JPK), which promotes actin polymerization. (B) Theta-burst stimulation (4 × 100Hz) induces early-phase, short-lasting LTP in rictor KO mice but does not induce the late-phase, long-lasting LTP in these mice. (C) The regulation of actin dynamics and signaling is disrupted in rictor KO mice. The ratio of F-actin to G-actin is a measure of the level of actin polymerization. It is reduced in the rictor KO mice. Phosphorylated cofilin (pCofilin) is required for actin polymerization. It is reduced in the rictor KO mice. These data indicate that the long-term but not short-term memory depends on signaling cascades regulated by mTORC2. Impaired long-term memory and LTP are due in part to impaired actin regulation in the rictor KO mice. (After W. Huang et al. 2013. *Nature Neurosci* 16: 441–448.)

is sensitive to (inhibited by) rapamycin, while the other, mTOR complex 2 (mTORC2), is insensitive to rapamycin.

The rapamycin-sensitive mTORC1 complex is important for local protein synthesis; it regulates mRNA translation through activating downstream targets such as p70s6 kinase and the elongation-factor-binding protein 4E-BP (see Hoeffer and Klann, 2010 for a review). The mTORC2 complex is insensitive to rapamycin and has been studied by genetic deletion in neurons in the forebrain of one of its components, called **rictor** (*r*apamycin-*i*nsensitive *c*ompanion of *TOR*). This deletion reduces the activity of mTORC2. Studies of mice with this genetic deletion (called rictor KO) found that mTORC2 contributes to long-term memory but does not influence short-term memory (Huang et al., 2013). These results were obtained using both fear conditioning (Figure 11.6A) and Morris place-learning tasks. Moreover, a rapidly emerging short-lasting LTP could be generated in slices from rictor KO mice but a long-lasting LTP could not be produced (Figure 11.6B). Huang et al. (2013) also found that deletion of rictor disrupted signaling cascades that are critical to actin polymerization (such as phosphorylation of cofilin) and the ratio of F-actin to G-actin (Figure 11.6C). In addition, treatments that directly promote actin polymerization partially rescue the memory deficit associated with the rictor KO factor.

In summary, signaling cascades regulated by the mTOR protein complex contribute to memory consolidation in two ways: (1) mTORC1 regulates signaling cascades that increase local protein synthesis, whereas (2) mTORC2 regulates processes that contribute to the regulation of actin. Disrupting either of these functions will impair the development of long-term memory but have no influence on the formation of a short-term memory (Figure 11.7).

BDNF   The activation of mTOR is a downstream outcome of BDNF–TrkB signaling. Thus, one should expect that BDNF activation also will be critical for consolidation. Indeed, a large literature indicates that BDNF plays a prominent role in the consolidation of memories (see Berkinschtein et al., 2007; Rattiner, Davis, French et al., 2004; Rattiner, Davis, and Ressler, 2004; Tyler et al., 2002).

It has been known for some time that BDNF protein levels in the BLA dramatically increase during the first hour following auditory-cue fear conditioning but then return to baseline (Ou and Gean, 2006; Rattiner, Davis, and Ressler, 2004). However, Po-Wu

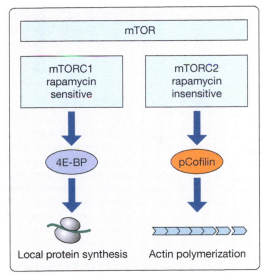

FIGURE 11.7   This figure illustrates mTOR's two distinct protein complexes and their sensitivity to rapamycin. The mTORC1 complex removes the inhibitory influence of the TOP protein 4E-BP to initiate local protein synthesis. The mTORC2 complex contributes to continuation of actin polymerization. (After C. A. Hoeffer and E. Klann. 2010. *Trends Neurosci* 33: 67–75.)

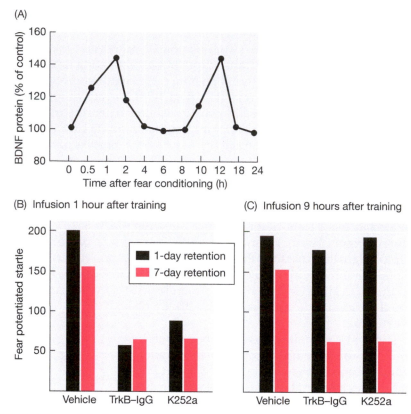

FIGURE 11.8 (A) BDNF protein levels peak at 1 and 12 hours following fear conditioning. (B) Impairing BDNF function 1 hour after training with either the BDNF scavenger TrkB–IgG or the TrkB antagonist K252a impairs the fear response at both the 1-day and 7-day retention intervals. (C) In contrast, administering these treatments 9 hours after training impairs the fear response only on the 7-day retention test. The measure of fear was the fear-potentiated startle response. Rats startle more to a brief loud noise in the presence of a fear stimulus. These results indicate that the first peak of BDNF is critical for the memory expressed on both the 1- and 7-day retention tests. However, the second peak is required only to support the memory expressed on the 7-day retention test. (After L. C. Ou et al. 2009. *Neurobio Learn Mem* 93: 372–382.)

Gean and his colleagues (Ou et al., 2009) expanded the time period over which BDNF was measured and discovered two distinct peak levels of BDNF expression. One peak of BDNF occurred 1 hour after training but the other did not occur until 12 hours later, and BDNF did not return to its pre-training baseline level until 30 hours after training (Figure 11.8A).

To determine if these peaks were functionally significant, Ou et al. (2009) infused the BDNF scavenger TrkB–IgG or the TrkB receptor antagonist K252a into the BLA, either 1 or 9 hours prior to fear conditioning. TrkB–IgGs are nonfunctional TrkB receptors that compete with endogenous TrkB receptors for BDNF. Their presence depletes the availability of extracellular BDNF to bind to the functional TrkB receptors. Rats were tested at two retention intervals—1 day or 7 days after training. Interfering with BDNF function by either method impaired the development of long-term memory. Interference 30 minutes before training markedly reduced the fear expressed at both the 1-day and 7-day retention test. However, eliminating BDNF function 9 hours after training only reduced the fear expressed 7 days after training (Figure 11.8B,C).

These results are important because they indicate that (a) the processes needed to secure this long-lasting fear memory (for at least 7 days) operate for 9 hours and perhaps longer, and (b) separate BDNF-dependent processes support retention at the 1- and 7-day retention intervals. The processes that support 1-day retention do not depend on BDNF expressed 12 hours after training, but the processes that support 7-day retention depend on BDNF translated during both peak periods.

Genomic Signaling: The Second Wave

The BDNF → TrkB → mTOR → TOP signaling cascade is the basis for the initial wave of protein synthesis and supports memories that can endure for a couple of days. However, for memories to endure a week or more requires a second wave of protein synthesis. How is the second wave generated? To answer this question requires a brief discussion of genomic signaling.

AN AUTOREGULATORY LOOP   A behavioral experience (such as inhibitory avoidance learning) that initiates local protein synthesis also initiates genomic signaling. For example, inhibitory avoidance training leads to an increase in phosphorylation of the transcription factor CREB (Bambah-Mukku et al., 2014; Taubenfeld et al., 2001) that can endure for 20 hours.

There is a large literature indicating that CREB activation is critical to the production of long-lasting memories (Alberini, 2009; Alberini and Kandel, 2014; Bourtchouladze et al., 1994; Rao-Ruiz et al., 2019; Silva et al., 1998). For instance, John Guzowski (Guzowski and McGaugh, 1997) used the antisense methodology (see Chapter 6) to disrupt CREB protein level. Antisense oligodeoxynucleotides (ODNs) that interfere with the translation of particular proteins can be injected into regions of the brain thought to be memory storage sites. The rationale is that if the antisense is administered long enough before a behavioral experience, less CREB protein will be available to target the transcription of the new mRNAs needed to produce the enduring memory. Guzowski infused antisense ODNs for CREB into the dorsal hippocampus and 6 hours later trained rats on the place-learning version of the Morris water-escape task. He reasoned that if memory genes are targeted by CREB protein, then reducing available CREB by blocking its translation should impair LTM but not STM. Consistent with this reasoning,

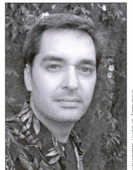

John Guzowski

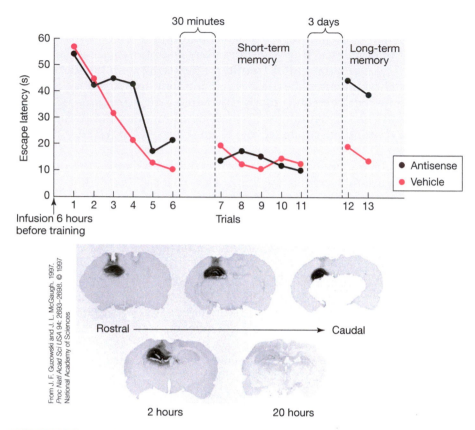

FIGURE 11.9 Infusing an antisense that blocks CREB translation leads to impaired long-term memory for place learning in the Morris water-escape task, but does not affect short-term memory. Note that rats injected with the antisense performed as well as the control rats when the retention interval was only 30 minutes but displayed much longer escape latencies than controls when the retention interval was 3 days. The photograph shows the extent and duration of the antisense. Note that the antisense was no longer present 20 hours after training. (After J. F. Guzowski and J. L. McGaugh. 1997. *Proc Natl Acad Sci USA* 18: 2693–2698. © 1997 National Academy of Sciences.)

his rats were normal when tested 30 minutes after training but were markedly impaired when tested 3 days after training (Figure 11.9).

BDNF signaling is required for phosphorylation of CREB. Interfering with it dramatically reduces levels of phosphorylated CREB (Bambah-Mukku et al., 2014; Chen et al., 2012). Once phosphorylated, CREB targets the transcription of mRNAs for many synaptic proteins (Alberini, 2009; Rao-Ruiz et al., 2019). However, a key part of the consolidation story is that CREB also targets the transcription of another transcription factor called C/EBPβ. An important feature of the CREB–C/EBPβ relationship is shown in Figure 11.10. Note that levels of phosphorylated CREB increase almost immediately following inhibitory

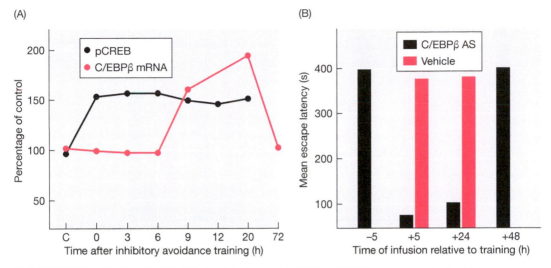

FIGURE 11.10   (A) Increased levels of phosphorylated CREB (pCREB) are present in the hippocampus shortly after training and remain high for at least 20 hours. In contrast, increased levels of C/EBPβ mRNA are not observed until 9 hours after training. (B) C/EBPβ antisense (AS) infused into the hippocampus 5 and 24 hours after training impaired retention of the inhibitory avoidance memory. Rats were tested 48 hours after training. These results indicate that C/EBPβ-protein-dependent processes operate at least 24 hours following training. (A after S. M. Taubenfeld et al. 2001. *J Neurosci* 21: 84–91. © 2001 Society for Neuroscience; B after S. M. Taubenfeld et al. 2001. *Nature Neurosci* 4: 813–818.)

avoidance training but detectable levels of C/EBPβ do not emerge until about 9 hours later. Moreover, antisense to C/EBPβ injected at 5 and 24 hours following training prevents the consolidation of the inhibitory avoidance memory. These observations suggest that C/EBPβ protein may be a critical contributor to the second wave of protein synthesis, *but how?*

Alberini's laboratory also revealed that C/EBPβ targets BDNF for transcription. Specifically, antisense to C/EBPβ 5 hours after training completely blocked the late expression of BDNF and memory consolidation. Remarkably, the memory impairment associated with antisense to C/EBPβ could be rescued by injecting BDNF into the hippocampus within 5 hours after training but not if injected 2 days after training (Figure 11.11). So not only is BDNF a target of C/EBPβ, its expression is critical to the second wave.

The important conclusions from this set of experiments are illustrated in Figure 11.12.

- A behavior that can produce an enduring long-term memory rapidly activates post-translation processes that establish a short-term memory that can endure for a few hours.

- Within minutes, the activation of the BDNF → TrkB → mTOR → TOP cascade initiates local protein synthesis (the first wave).

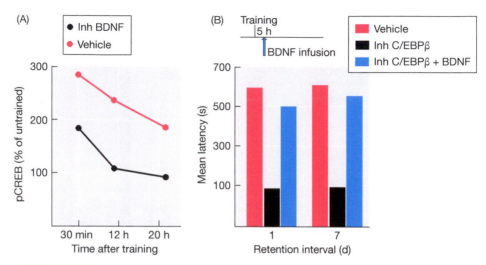

FIGURE 11.11 (A) Inhibiting BDNF signaling dramatically reduces phosphorylated CREB associated with avoidance training. (B) Infusing BDNF into the hippocampus 5 hours following training restores the memory impairment produced by inhibiting C/EBPβ. These results indicate that not only is BDNF a target of C/EBPβ, but also its expression is critical to the second wave of consolidation. (After D. Bambah-Mukka et al. 2014. *J Neurosci* 34: 12547–12599.)

- In addition, BDNF initiates genomic signaling that leads to phosphorylating CREB.
- CREB targets transcription of genes for synaptic protein to be transported to the stimulated dendritic spines.
- In addition, it targets the transcription factor C/EBPβ for expression.
- C/EBPβ in turn targets the transcription of BDNF, which is transported back to the stimulated spines to support the second wave of consolidation.
- In essence, the second wave of consolidation is supported by what Alberini and colleagues (Bambah-Mukku et al., 2014) call an autoregulatory **BDNF → CREB → C/EBPβ → BDNF** positive feedback loop that operates for about 48 hours.

SLEEP AND REACTIVATION PROCESSES   It should be appreciated that processes that support the second wave of protein synthesis operate across the sleep–wake cycle So it is possible that processes occurring during sleep are involved in memory consolidation. In fact, for over a century it has been recognized that sleep benefits memory retention (Rasch and Born, 2013). The primary basis for this statement is that (a) subjects who are allowed to sleep after learning show less forgetting than those allowed to remain awake and (b) disrupting normal

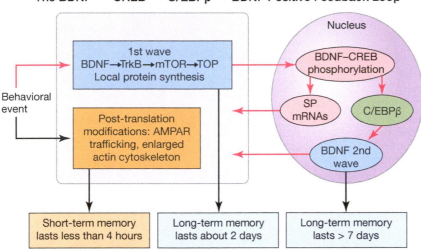

FIGURE 11.12 A memory-producing behavioral experience such as inhibitory avoidance training immediately activates a set of post-translation modifications in the dendritic spine compartment that produces a short-term memory. It also activates BDNF signaling to initiate local protein synthesis that can support a long-term memory that can last about 2 days. BDNF signaling also leads to the phosphorylation of CREB in the nucleus, which targets the transcription of mRNAs for synaptic protein as well as the transcription factor C/EBPβ. C/EBPβ targets BDNF for transcription. Synaptic protein mRNAs and BDNF are transported back to the dendritic spine to replenish the supply of synaptic proteins (SP). This positive autoregulatory BDNF → CREB → C/EBPβ → BDNF feedback loop (represented by the red arrows) lasts over a day and is responsible for the second wave of consolidation, which supports memories that can endure for over a week.

sleep patterns impairs retention of learned material (Rasch and Born, 2013; Jenkins and Dallenbach, 1924).

Historically, the beneficial effect of sleep was interpreted through the lens of what is called the **interference theory of forgetting**. The basic idea is that forgetting results from learning new information that interferes with or overwrites the old memory traces. Sleep after learning is important because it acts as a "temporary shelter" that simply postpones the effect of interference and thereby passively maintains the memory trace (Ellenbogen et al., 2006). While there is validity to this idea, the discovery that the benefits of sleep are associated with different stages of sleep moved the field toward the idea that during sleep intrinsic neural processes are at play that might actively contribute to memory consolidation (Rasch and Born, 2013). There now exists an enormous literature on this topic that is far beyond what can be discussed here (see Abel et al., 2013; Havekes and Abel, 2017; Rasch and Born, 2013).

It is useful to consider the widely accepted idea that during sleep there is intrinsic neural activity that results in the *reactivation or replay* of neuronal

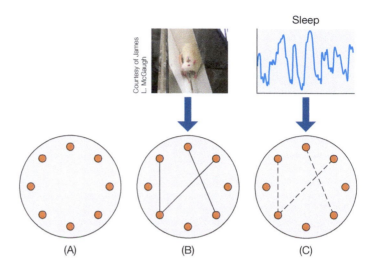

FIGURE 11.13 This figure illustrates a potential role for sleep in memory consolidation. (A) This circuit represents a set of weakly connected neurons. (B) A learning experience such as inhibitory avoidance learning strengthens synaptic connections among the set of neurons activated during learning. (C) During sleep, intrinsic neural activity reactivates this circuit with the consequence that new proteins are synthesized from the replacement protein provided by the positive autoregulatory BDNF → CREB → C/EBPβ → BDNF feedback loop to support the second wave of consolidation.

(A)   (B)   (C)

Sleep

ensembles recently established during learning (Buzsáki, 2015; Giri et al., 2019; Rasch and Born, 2013; Wilson and McNaughton, 1994). This fact is important because the autoregulatory positive feedback loop described above leaves an important question unanswered. It tells us that over many hours BDNF and other synaptic protein mRNAs are replenished, but how are they called into play to further strengthen the memory trace? Perhaps this is a consequence of the memory reactivation processes that occur during sleep. This idea is developed below and illustrated in Figure 11.13.

The initial wave of protein synthesis is initiated by behavior. Together with a large number of post-translation processes, synaptic proteins translated locally strengthen synaptic connections linking the members of the neuronal ensemble representing the memory. Translation and transcription processes embedded in the autoregulatory loop discovered by Alberini replenish these proteins, including BDNF. During sleep intrinsic neural activity then reactivates this ensemble to initiate additional rounds of local protein synthesis. In essence one can think of this intrinsic reactivation as a recapitulation of the initial learning experience. It is another learning experience that initiates another round of local protein synthesis.

There is little direct experimental evidence available to evaluate this idea. Several findings, however, support it. For example, if intrinsic activity during sleep recapitulates the behavioral activation of local protein synthesis, then one should expect the effects of sleep on memory consolidation should depend on mTOR, which initiates local synthesis. Consistent with this hypothesis, Ted Abel's laboratory (Tudor et al., 2016) found that sleep deprivation, which is associated with impaired memory consolidation, resulted in impaired mTOR function and impaired object-recognition memory. Moreover, restoring mTOR functioning by enhancing the downstream target of mTOR, 4EBP2, rescued the memory impairment.

Protein Degradation Processes

Just as there is evidence that protein degradation contributes to establishing long-lasting LTP (see Chapter 6), a case can be made that protein degradation mediated by the ubiquitin proteasome system (UPS) is critical for establishing enduring memories.

Several lines of evidence indicate that the UPS is involved in memory consolidation. First, behavioral experiences that induce lasting memories increase ubiquitination and proteasome activity (Artinian et al., 2008; Lopez-Salon et al., 2001). Fred Helmstetter's group (Jarome et al., 2011) found that fear conditioning rapidly ubiquitinates scaffolding proteins in the postsynaptic density of neurons in the amygdala. Moreover, antagonizing NMDA receptors prevents ubiquitination, suggesting that the UPS operates in parallel with the calcium-dependent processes needed to generate new protein (Figure 11.14A).

Second, drugs that block proteasome activity also prevent long-term memory formation (Artinian et al., 2008; Jarome et al., 2011; Lopez-Salon et al., 2001). For example, Jarome et al. (2011) reported that inhibiting the proteasome function (thereby preventing degradation of ubiquitin-tagged proteins) in the amygdala

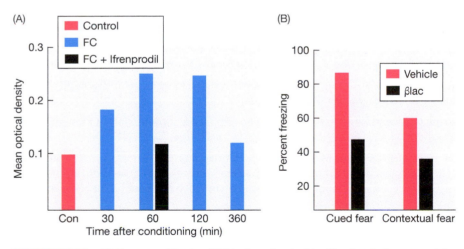

FIGURE 11.14   (A) Fear conditioning (FC) induced polyubiquitination in the amygdala. This process was prevented by the NMDA antagonist ifrenprodil. (Control rats received no conditioning.) (B) The proteasome inhibitor βlactone (βlac) impaired both cued and contextual fear conditioning. These results indicated that protein degradation is critical for consolidating long-term fear memories. (After T. J. Jarome et al. 2011. *PLOS ONE* 2011: 6:e24349. DOI: 10.1371/journal.pone.24349.)

impaired long-term memory for both cued and contextual fear (Figure 11.14B). Similarly, Lopez-Salon et al. (2001) reported that blocking proteasome function in the hippocampus prevented the formation of a long-term memory for an inhibitory avoidance experience. Based on studies of LTP (see Chapter 6), it is likely that this is because inhibiting the UPS prevents it from degrading proteins that repress protein translation and transcription.

Summary

Memories evolve in overlapping stages. A behavioral experience that produces a memory initiates a set of post-translation processes that rapidly traffic AMPA receptors into the postsynaptic density and create a stable actin cytoskeleton (see Chapter 4) that can support short-term memory. It also initiates BDNF signaling that leads to local protein synthesis, which is the basis for the first consolidation wave. BDNF signaling also leads to the phosphorylation of CREB. CREB targets the transcription of mRNAs for synaptic proteins and the transcription factor, C/EBPβ. C/EBPβ targets BDNF for transcription. This positive-feedback, autoregulatory loop (BDNF → CREB → C/EBPβ → BDNF) supports an additional wave of consolidation. Intrinsic neural activity during sleep potentially provides another "learning experience" that initiates another round of local protein synthesis that supports the second wave of consolidation. In addition to the generation of new protein, the degradation of some proteins by the UPS is critical to the creation of enduring memories.

References

Abel, T., Havekes, R., Saletin, J. M., and Walker, M. P. (2013). Sleep, plasticity and memory from molecules to whole-brain networks. *Current Biology, 23,* 774–788.

Alberini, C. M. (2009). Transcription factors in long-term memory and synaptic plasticity. *Physiological Reviews, 89,* 121–145.

Alberini, C. M. and Kandel, E. R. (2014). The regulation of transcription in memory consolidation. *Cold Spring Harbor Perspectives in Biology, 7,* a021741.

Artinian, J., McGauran, A. M., De Jaeger, X., Mouledous, L., Frances, B., and Roullet, P. (2008). Protein degradation, as with protein synthesis, is required during not only long-term spatial memory consolidation but also reconsolidation. *European Journal of Neuroscience, 11,* 3009–3019.

Bambah-Mukku, D., Travaglia, A., Chen, D. Y., Pollonini, G., and Alberini, C. (2014). A positive autoregulatory BDNF feedback loop via C/EBPβ mediates hippocampal memory consolidation. *Journal of Neuroscience, 34,* 12547–12599.

Bekinschtein, P., Katche, C., Slipczuk, L. N., Igaz, L. M., Cammarota, M., Izquierdo, I., and Medina, J. H. (2007). mTOR signaling in the hippocampus is necessary for memory formation. *Neurobiology of Learning and Memory, 87,* 303–307.

Bourtchouladze, R., Abel, T., Berman, N., Gordon, R., Lapidus, K., and Kandel, E. R. (1998). Different training procedures recruit either one or two critical periods for contextual memory consolidation, each of which requires protein synthesis and PKA. *Learning and Memory, 5*, 365–367.

Bourtchuladze, R., Frenguelli, B., Blendy, J., Cioffi, D., Schutz, G., and Silva, A. J. (1994). Deficient long-term memory in mice with a targeted mutation of the cAMP-responsive element-binding protein. *Cell, 79*, 59–68.

Buzsáki, G. (2015). Hippocampal sharp wave-ripple: a cognitive biomarker for episodic memory and planning. *Hippocampus, 25*, 1073–1188.

Chen, D. Y., Bambah-Mukku, D., Pollonini, G., and Alberini, C. M. (2012). Glucocorticoid receptors recruit the CaMKIIα–BDNF–CREB pathways to mediate memory consolidation. *Nature Neuroscience, 15*, 1707–1714.

Davis, H. P. and Squire, L. R. (1984). Protein synthesis and memory: a review. *Psychological Bulletin, 96*, 518–559.

Dudai, Y. (2004). The neurobiology of consolidation, or, how stable is the engram. *Annual Review of Psychology, 55*, 51–86.

Ellenbogen, J. M., Payne, J. D., and Stickgold, R. (2006). The role of sleep in declarative memory consolidation: passive, permissive, active or none? *Current Opinion in Neurobiology, 16*, 716–722.

Giri, B., Miyawaki, H., Mizueki, K., Cheng, S., and Diba, K. (2019). Hippocampal reactivation extends for several hours following novel experience. *Journal of Neuroscience, 39*, 866–875.

Guzowski, J. F. and McGaugh, J. L. (1997). Antisense oligodeoxynucleotide-mediated disruption of hippocampal cAMP response element binding protein levels impairs consolidation of memory for water maze training. *Proceedings of the National Academy of Sciences USA, 18*, 2693–2698.

Havekes, R. and Abel, T. (2017). The tired hippocampus: the molecular impact of sleep deprivation on hippocampal function. *Current Opinion in Neurobiology, 44*, 13–19.

Hoeffer, C. A. and Klann, E. (2010). mTOR signaling: at the crossroads of plasticity, memory and disease. *Trends in Neuroscience, 33*, 67–75.

Huang, W., Zhu, P. J., Zhang, S., Zhou, H., Stoica, L., Galiano, M., Krnjević, K., Roman, G., and Costa-Mattioli, M. (2013). mTORC2 controls actin polymerization required for consolidation of long-term memory. *Nature Neuroscience, 16*, 441–448.

Jarome, T. J., Werner, C. T., Kwapis, J. L., and Helmstetter, F. J. (2011). Activity dependent protein degradation is critical for the formation and stability of fear memory in the amygdala. *PLOS ONE* 2011: 6:e24349. DOI: 10.1371/journal.pone.24349.

Jenkins, J. G. and Dallenbach, K. M. (1924). Obliviscence during sleep and waking. *The American Journal of Psychology, 35*, 605–612.

Jobim, P. F., Pedroso, T. R., Werenicz, A., Christoff, R. R., Maurmann, N., Reolon, G. K., Schröder, N., and Roesler, R. (2012). Impairment of object recognition memory by rapamycin inhibition of mTOR in the amygdala or hippocampus around the time of learning or reactivation. *Behavioral Brain Research, 228,* 151–158.

Lopez-Salon, M., Alonso, M., Vianna, M. R., Viola, H., Mello, E., and Souza, T. (2001). The ubiquitin-proteasome cascade is required for mammalian long-term memory formation. *European Journal of Neuroscience, 14,* 1820–1826.

Ou, L. C. and Gean, P-W. (2006). Regulation of amygdala-dependent learning by brain derived neurotrophic factor is mediated by extracellular signal-regulated kinase and phosphatidylinositol-3-kinase. *Neuropsychopharmacology, 31,* 287–296.

Ou, L. C., Yeh, S. H., and Gean, P-W. (2009). Late expression of brain-derived neurotrophic factor in the amygdala is required for persistence of fear memory. *Neurobiology of Learning and Memory, 93,* 372–382.

Rao-Ruiz, P., Couey, J. J., Marcelo, I. M., Bouwkamp, C. G., Slump, D. E., Matos, M. R., van der Loo, R. J., Martins, G. J., van den Hout, M., van ljcken, W. F., Costa, R. M., van den Oever, M. C., and Kushner, S. A. (2019). Engram-specific transcriptome profiling of contextual memory consolidation. *Nature Communications, 10,* 2232–2245.

Rasch, B. and Born, J. (2013). About sleep's role in memory. *Physiological Reviews, 93,* 681–766.

Rattiner, L. M., Davis, M., French, C. T., and Ressler, K. J. (2004). Brain-derived neurotrophic factor and tyrosine kinase receptor B involvement in amygdala-dependent fear conditioning. *Journal of Neuroscience, 24,* 4796–4806.

Rattiner, L. M., Davis, M., and Ressler, K. J. (2004). Differential regulation of brain-derived neurotrophic factor transcripts during the consolidation of fear learning. *Learning and Memory, 11,* 727–731.

Silva, A. J., Kogan, J. H., Frankland, P. W., and Kida, S. (1998). CREB and memory. *Annual Review Neuroscience, 2,* 127–148.

Taubenfeld, S. M., Milekic, M. H., Monti, B., and Alberini, C. M. (2001). The consolidation of new but not reactivated memory requires hippocampal C/EBPβ. *Nature Neuroscience, 4,* 813–818.

Tudor, J. C., Davis, E. J., Peixoto, L., Wimmer, M. E., van Tilborg, E., Park, A. J., and Abel, T. (2016). Sleep deprivation impairs memory by attenuating mTORC1-dependent protein synthesis. *Science Signaling, 9,* ra41.

Tyler, W. J., Alonso, M., Bramham, C. R., and Pozzo-Miller, L. D. (2002). From acquisition to consolidation: on the role of brain-derived neurotrophic factor signaling in hippocampal dependent learning. *Learning and Memory, 9,* 224–237.

Wilson, M. A. and McNaughton, B. L. (1994). Reactivation of hippocampal ensemble memories during sleep. *Science, 265,* 676–679.

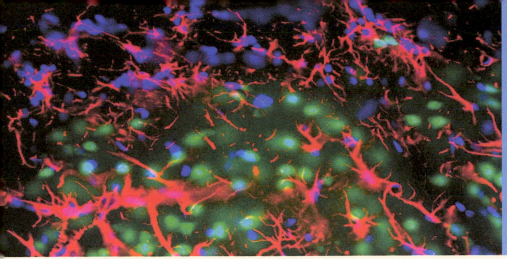

Courtesy of Heidi E. W. Day

Memory Modulation Systems

About 15 years ago my friend Wayne and I were out for a walk with his dogs. Basically, it was like any other walk—uneventful, filled with the usual banter. But that changed when suddenly one of the dogs, Poco, leaped in the air, followed by the sound of a rattlesnake. This was an arousing event. I vividly remember Poco's reaction and that we had to coax the dogs past this point in the road. This is one of the few things that I remember with any detail from our many walks. Something about arousing events makes them memorable.

The goal of this chapter is to provide an understanding of why this happens. It is organized around the idea that neural and hormonal processes that are activated by arousal can influence the cellular–molecular processes that consolidate memory. These neurohormonal events modulate the activity of neurons in the memory storage sites. First the memory modulation framework is described. Evidence is then presented that the basolateral region of the amygdala makes a critical contribution to memory modulation. Next, two general ways in which memory storage is influenced by the adrenal hormone **epinephrine** (released by the adrenal medulla) and its related neurotransmitter **norepinephrine** are described. The chapter ends with a brief discussion of how **glucocorticoids**, the other adrenal hormone, influence memory storage.

Memory Modulation Framework

The memory modulation framework illustrated in Figure 12.1 is the product of James L. McGaugh, his students, and his collaborators. The important assumptions of this framework follow.

1. A behavioral experience can have two independent effects: it can activate specific sets of neurons that represent and store the content of the experience, and it can activate hormonal and other neural systems that can influence the mechanisms that store the memory.

2. These hormonal and other neural systems are called **memory modulators**. They are not part of the storage system, but they can influence the synapses that store the memory.

3. Memory modulators have a time-limited role and influence only the storage of very recently acquired memories. They operate during a period of time shortly after the behavioral experience when the memory trace is being consolidated.

4. The neural systems that modulate memory strength are not necessary for the retrieval of the memory.

The basis for the memory modulation idea emerged when McGaugh was a graduate student (McGaugh, 1959, 2003; McGaugh and Petrinovich, 1959) and discovered that Karl Lashley (1917) had improved the rate at which rats learned a complicated maze by injecting them with a low dose of strychnine before training. Strychnine can be a lethal poison. However, at a low dose it is a stimulant and produces a state of arousal. McGaugh's insight was that the state of arousal created by strychnine might influence the processes that consolidate memory

FIGURE 12.1 The figure illustrates the memory modulation framework. Experience has two independent effects. It can initiate the acquisition and storage of the memory trace and it can activate the release of adrenal hormones that can modulate the processes that store the memory. (After J. L. McGaugh et al. 2000. *Science* 287: 248–251.)

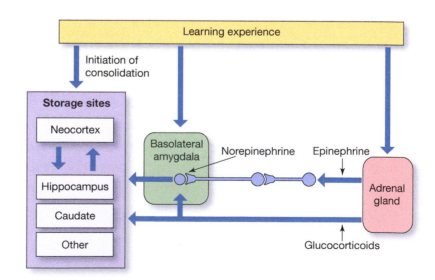

traces. To evaluate his idea, he injected the drug immediately after the rats had been trained and found improved retention performance. However, it had no effect on performance when administered before the retention test.

McGaugh and his colleagues subsequently found that strychnine given after training enhanced memories produced by a variety of behavioral experiences. The implication of these findings was unmistakable: *there is a brief period of time shortly after the memory-inducing behavioral experience when the strength of the memory trace can be modified.* McGaugh's early work was important because it established this idea.

The state of arousal generated by the behavioral experiences influences memory strength. This happens because arousing stimuli (such as encountering a rattlesnake) can stimulate the adrenal gland, specifically the adrenal medulla, to secrete a hormone or molecule into the blood stream called **adrenaline**. One general role of this hormone is to mobilize us for behavioral action. The expression "it gave me an adrenaline rush" relates to this effect. Adrenaline is often called epinephrine, and that is the name used in this discussion. Epinephrine belongs to a class of catecholamine hormones that bind to receptors called **adrenergic receptors**. It is closely related to norepinephrine, also secreted by the adrenal medulla but in much smaller quantities, which can act as a neurotransmitter in the brain. In addition to its energizing effects, epinephrine can have a second effect—it can influence the strength of a memory trace.

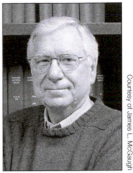

James McGaugh

The Great Modulator: The Basolateral Amygdala

The basolateral amygdala (BLA) is now thought to be the primary mediator of epinephrine's influence on memory (McGaugh, 2002, 2004). It has anatomical connections with many other regions of the brain that store memories, so it is in a position to influence the memory storage processes in these other regions (Figure 12.2). There is an extensive literature supporting this idea (see McGaugh, 2004; McIntyre et al., 2012). Some examples are described below.

To establish that the amygdala modulates memory storage in other regions of the brain, it must be shown that the amygdala is not itself a storage site for the memory. This means that the memory can be retrieved even if the amygdala is removed. For example, both the place-learning and

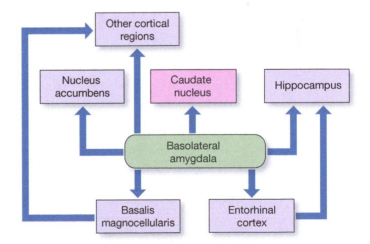

FIGURE 12.2 The amygdala is anatomically connected to many regions of the brain that are likely storage sites for different types of memories. Thus, it is in a position to influence or modulate storage processes in other regions of the brain. (After J. L. McGaugh. 2002. *Trends Neurosci* 25: 456–461.)

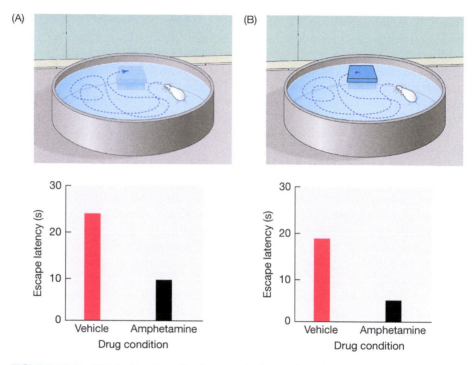

FIGURE 12.3 (A) Injecting the stimulant amphetamine into the amygdala following training on the place-learning version of the Morris water-escape task improved retention performance. (B) Injecting the amphetamine following training on the visible-platform task improved retention performance. (Short latency indicates better retention.) The hippocampus is thought to be a critical storage site for place learning and the caudate is thought to be critical for the visible-platform task. (After M. G. Packard and L. A. Teather. 1998. *Neurobiol Learn Mem* 69: 163–203.)

visible-platform versions of the Morris water-escape task can be learned and remembered even when the amygdala is significantly damaged (Sutherland and McDonald, 1990). Thus, the amygdala is not a critical storage site for these memories. Instead, the hippocampus is a key storage area for the place-learning memory, and the caudate is thought to be important for the acquisition and storage of the memory for the visible-platform task (the hippocampus and caudate are discussed in Part 3 chapters). Nevertheless, as shown in Figure 12.3, if d-amphetamine, a stimulant drug, is injected into the amygdala following training, retention performance on both versions of the task is enhanced (Packard et al., 1994; Packard and Teather, 1998). Thus, the amygdala facilitates the storage of these memories but is not needed to retain the memory.

The amygdala is not a unitary structure but consists of many subnuclei (Figure 12.4). Further research has revealed that neurons in the BLA are the critical mediator of the memory modulation properties of this region of the

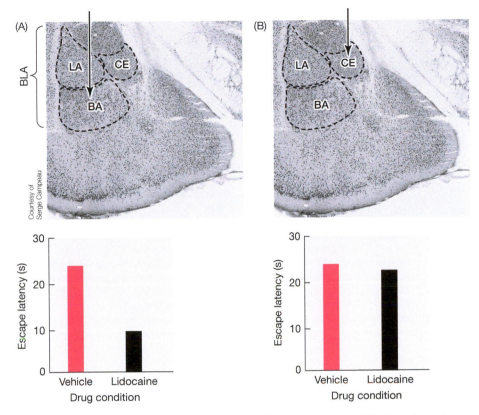

FIGURE 12.4   (A) An injection of lidocaine into the basal nucleus of the basolateral amygdala (BLA) following avoidance training impaired the retention of the inhibitory avoidance response. (B) Lidocaine had no effect when it was injected into the central nucleus of the amygdala. Key: LA = lateral nucleus; BA = basal nucleus; CE = central nucleus. (After M. B. Parent and J. L. McGaugh. 1994. *Brain Res* 66: 97–103.)

brain. This conclusion is based on experiments in which drugs that influence modulation were injected into specific subnuclei of the amygdala (McGaugh et al., 2000). For example, if lidocaine (a drug that temporarily suppresses neural activity) is injected into the basolateral nucleus, memory retention is impaired (see Figure 12.4A), but if it is injected into the central nucleus of the amygdala (see Figure 12.4B), it has no effect on retention (Parent and McGaugh, 1994). These data establish that the BLA is likely the major brain region mediating the effects of epinephrine.

The Role of Epinephrine

The adrenal medulla hormone epinephrine is now recognized as a major contributor to memory modulation processes. Paul Gold (Gold and Van Buskirk,

(A)

(B)

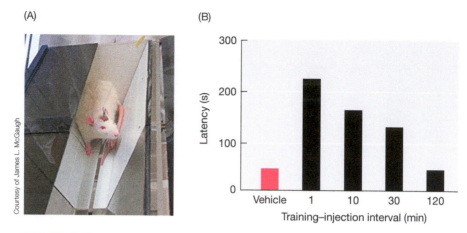

Courtesy of James L. McGaugh

FIGURE 12.5 On the training trial, rats received a mild shock when they crossed to the dark side of the apparatus. Compared to control rats injected with the saline vehicle, rats that were injected with a dose of epinephrine—calculated to mimic the level of epinephrine that would naturally be released from the adrenal gland if the animals had received a strong shock—displayed enhanced inhibitory avoidance. The enhancing effect of epinephrine, however, was time dependent. It was more effective when it was given shortly after the training trial. (After P. E. Gold and R. B. Van Buskirk. 1975. *Behav Biol* 13: 145–153.)

1975) provided the first direct evidence that it can strengthen memory traces. In this study, rats were given a single trial of inhibitory avoidance training with a low-intensity shock that was designed to be minimally arousing. These animals were then injected with epinephrine at different times after training. The basic idea was to inject a dose of epinephrine that would mimic what the adrenal gland would naturally release in response to a stronger, more arousing shock. Remarkably, the avoidance behavior of rats injected with the adrenal hormone was dramatically increased. The effect also was time dependent because the hormone had to be injected shortly after training (Figure 12.5). Epinephrine also influences the strength of human memories. Larry Cahill, for example, showed people a series of slides containing visual scenes (Cahill and Alkire, 2003). Some of these subjects were injected with epinephrine immediately following exposure to the scenes. A week later, these subjects were able to recall the scenes better than subjects injected with just the vehicle.

To influence neurons, molecules in the blood vesicles have to diffuse through the blood–brain barrier, which is designed to separate circulating blood from the brain's extracellular fluid. This barrier protects the brain from potentially harmful molecules. Even though they influence memory, epinephrine molecules are too large to cross the blood–brain barrier. So how does epinephrine released into blood vesicles influence amygdala function? The answer is that it exerts its influence on memory in two distinct ways. One path starts with epinephrine binding to receptors on the vagal nerve and ends with the release of the neurotransmitter norepinephrine into the BLA. The other path starts with epinephrine's influence on glucose released by liver cells. These two pathways and some of their influences are described in the sections that follow.

The Epinephrine Vagus Connection

In this section, the neurohormonal circuit linking epinephrine to the BLA is described and some of the supporting evidence is reviewed. The focus then turns to the influence of norepinephrine on memory processing. When epinephrine is released in the blood stream, it binds to adrenergic receptors located on a major cranial nerve, the **vagus** or vagal nerve (Figure 12.6). This nerve carries information about the body into the brain and synapses on a brain stem region called the **solitary tract nucleus** or **NTS** (Hassert et al., 2004; Miyashita and Williams, 2006). Neurons from the NTS synapse on a small collection of neurons (fewer than 2,000) in the brain stem called the **locus coeruleus** (**LC**). Neurons in the LC project widely to distant brain regions, including the forebrain, hippocampus, and amygdala. When activated, these neurons release the neurotransmitter

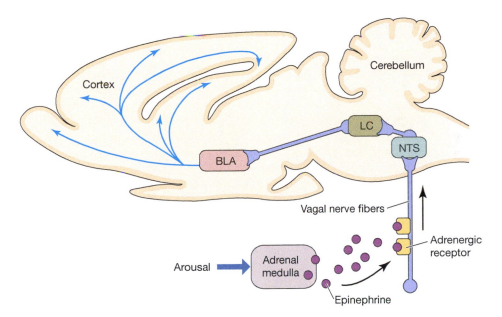

FIGURE 12.6 Epinephrine does not cross the blood–brain barrier. However, when it is released from the adrenal medulla it binds to adrenergic receptors on the vagal nerve. In response to activation, the vagal nerve releases glutamate on neurons in the solitary tract nucleus (NTS). Activated NTS neurons release glutamate onto neurons in the locus coeruleus (LC), which in turn release norepinephrine that binds to adrenergic receptors in the basolateral amygdala (BLA). Disrupting any component of this neurohormonal circuit will prevent arousal from enhancing memory.

(A)

(B)

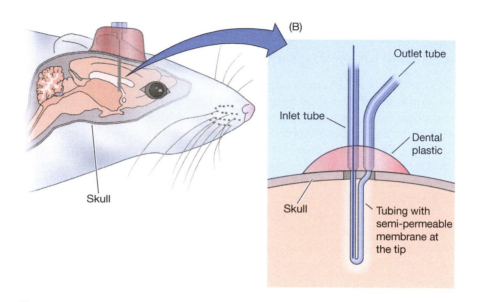

Outlet tube

Inlet tube

Dental plastic

Skull

Skull

Tubing with semi-permeable membrane at the tip

(C)

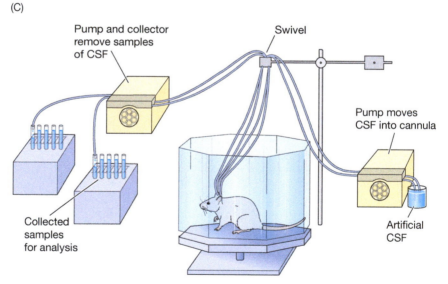

Pump and collector remove samples of CSF

Swivel

Pump moves CSF into cannula

Collected samples for analysis

Artificial CSF

FIGURE 12.7 Microdialysis allows extracellular fluid to be collected from deep within the brain. (A) A rat with a specially designed microdialysis probe implanted in the brain. (B) A detail of the microdialysis probe. (C) A freely moving rat connected to the instrumentation designed to extract a very small quantity of extracellular fluid. The content of this fluid can then be analyzed for its composition. Key: CSF = cerebral spinal fluid.

norepinephrine onto their target neurons. The release of norepinephrine into the BLA is the key outcome of the vagus connection (McIntyre et al., 2012).

Several lines of evidence support the existence of this neurohormonal circuit (see McIntyre et al., 2012). For example, when epinephrine is administered to anesthetized rats it activates the vagal nerve. However, this outcome is prevented by the beta-adrenergic receptor antagonist sotalol (Miyashita and Williams, 2006). This result supports the hypothesis that epinephrine binds to beta-adrenergic receptors on the vagal nerve. Epinephrine in the periphery also increases the firing rate of neurons in the LC, and the temporary inactivation of neurons in the NTS reduces memory enhancement by a peripheral injection of epinephrine (Williams and McGaugh, 1993). These results indicate that epinephrine in the periphery activates LC through the NTS.

Direct electrical stimulation of ascending vagal fibers increases glutamate levels in the NTS. Thus, as one might expect, antagonizing AMPA receptors (the mediators of synaptic transmission) in the NTS prevents epinephrine from enhancing memory (King and Williams, 2009). Finally, there is evidence that stimulating the ascending vagal fibers produces burst firing in neurons in the locus coeruleus (Dorr and Debonnel, 2006) and that stimulating the vagus nerve following inhibitory avoidance training can enhance the memory (Clark et al., 1998).

Training experiences that produce strong memories do so because epinephrine released from the adrenal gland ultimately results in release of norepinephrine into the BLA. If this is true one should be able to detect increases in the level of norepinephrine in the BLA when rats are shocked after crossing to the dark side of the avoidance apparatus. Quirarte and his colleagues (Quirarte et al., 1998) used a methodology called microdialysis (Figure 12.7) to observe this increase, which is shown in Figure 12.8A.

There is another interesting fact associated with this set of events. By itself, electric shock, the stimulus typically used to produce inhibitory avoidance learning, does not cause norepinephrine to be released in the amygdala. Rats

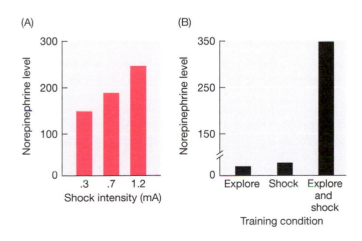

FIGURE 12.8 The microdialysis methodology was used to extract norepinephrine from the extracellular brain fluid. (A) The level of norepinephrine released into the extracellular fluid in inhibitory avoidance training is determined by the intensity of the shock. (B) Just shocking a rat or allowing it to explore the avoidance training apparatus does not increase the level of norepinephrine. That requires the rat both to explore the novel apparatus and to be shocked. (A after G. L. Quirarte et al. 1998. *Brain Res* 808: 134–140; B after C. K. McIntyre et al. 2002. *Eur J Neurosci* 16: 1223–1226.)

have to both explore the environment and then receive shock for norepinephrine to be released in the amygdala (McIntyre et al., 2002). It is as if the amygdala is designed to detect the coincidence of a novel behavioral experience and
an arousing event (Figure 12.8B).

Norepinephrine Enhances Memories

If LC neurons release norepinephrine into the amygdala and this event enhances memory storage, then one can make two predictions.

1. Injecting norepinephrine into the BLA following training should enhance
   the memory.
2. Injecting the beta-adrenergic receptor antagonist, propranolol, into the
   BLA should attenuate the memory resulting from an arousing behavioral
   experience.

These predictions have been confirmed. Figure 12.9A shows that injecting norepinephrine into the BLA following training on the place-learning version of
the Morris water task improves the rat's retention of the location of the hidden
platform. In contrast, injecting propranolol into the amygdala following training impairs retention of the platform location (Hatfield and McGaugh, 1999).
Figure 12.9B shows that injecting norepinephrine into the amygdala following
avoidance training with a weak shock enhances retention of the avoidance
response. However, if propranolol is injected after avoidance training with
an arousing strong shock, the avoidance response is reduced (Gallagher et al.,
1977; Liang et al., 1986).

Norepinephrine Enhances Glutamate Release and Arc Translation

Researchers now have a good understanding of the primary factors involved
in initiating amygdala-dependent memory modulation.

1. An arousing behavioral event induces the adrenal gland to release epinephrine into the blood stream.
2. Epinephrine binds to receptors on the vagal nerve.
3. The vagal nerve transmits a signal into the NTS that is conveyed to the
   amygdala as the release of norepinephrine from the locus coeruleus.

This sequence of events raises two questions: (1) how does the release of norepinephrine influence their target BLA neurons? and (2) what is the downstream
influence of BLA output on their target neurons, that is, how does this output
strengthen memories?

Neurons in the amygdala release glutamate. So the answers to these questions
center on how norepinephrine influences glutamate release and how it then influences the signaling mechanisms in the downstream target neurons that store
the memory. Adrenergic receptors in the amygdala are metabotropic—they are

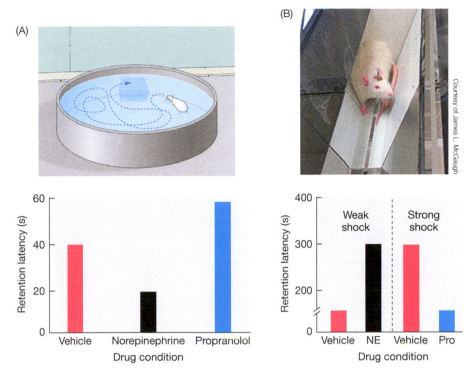

FIGURE 12.9 (A) The injection of norepinephrine into the amygdala following place learning enhanced the rat's retention of the platform location, but when propranolol was injected retention was impaired. (B) Norepinepherine (NE) injected into the amygdala following inhibitory avoidance training with a weak shock enhanced retention performance. Propranolol (Pro) injected into the amygdala following inhibitory avoidance training with strong shock impaired retention. (A after T. Hatfield and J. L. McGaugh. 1999. *Neurobiol Learn Mem* 71: 232–239; B after K. C. Liang et al.1986. *Brain Res* 368: 125–133.)

coupled to a G-protein complex. This complex becomes active and one of its protein subunits activates the effector protein, adenylyl cyclase, which then catalyzes the formation of the second messenger cAMP (cyclic adenosine monophosphate). The kinase target of cAMP is PKA. The upshot of this cascade is that neurons in the BLA generate a sustained release of glutamate onto neurons in the target storage sites.

Given that glutamate receptors are a primary mediator of intracellular signaling events that alter synaptic strength, then one would expect that additional glutamate released by BLA neurons would enhance these signal events. This would most likely result from calcium released from endoplasmic stores. For example, additional glutamate would be expected to activate the mGluR → IP3 → IP3R pathway to release calcium from the endoplasmic reticulum and facilitate local protein synthesis (see Chapter 5).

(A)

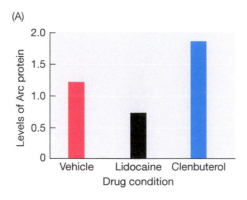

(B)

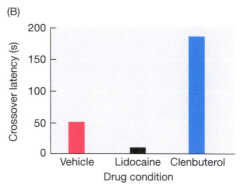

FIGURE 12.10 (A) This graph illustrates the effect of injecting lidocaine and clenbuterol into the BLA on the level of Arc protein in the hippocampus following inhibitory avoidance learning. (B) This graph illustrates the effect of these drugs on inhibitory avoidance learning. Note that lidocaine reduced the level of Arc protein in the hippocampus and decreased inhibitory avoidance learning. In contrast, clenbuterol increased the level of Arc protein and enhanced inhibitory avoidance learning. These results suggest that the BLA might modulate memory by influencing the level of Arc protein in the hippocampus. (After C. K. McIntyre et al. 2005. *Proc Natl Acad Sci USA* 102: 10718–10723.)

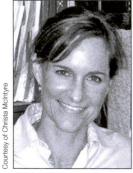

Christa McIntyre

Christa McIntyre and her colleagues were among the first to address the downstream effects of the BLA signal. For example, they reported that inhibitory avoidance training normally leads to the increased translation of Arc protein in the hippocampus (McIntyre et al., 2005). However, when lidocaine, a drug that inactivates neurons, is injected into the BLA prior to training, the level of Arc protein in the hippocampus is reduced and the memory for the inhibitory avoidance experience is impaired. In contrast, when clenbuterol, an adrenergic receptor agonist, is injected into the BLA, the level of Arc protein in the hippocampus is increased and the memory for the training experience is strengthened.

These results (Figure 12.10) indicate that activity in the BLA produced by inhibitory avoidance training modulates the level of Arc protein in another area of the brain, the hippocampus, and that the level of Arc protein correlates with the strength of the memory. Additional work from this group has extended this paradigm to show that (a) the amygdala signal enhances both Arc protein and CaMKII levels in another storage area (rostral anterior cingular cortex) for the inhibitory avoidance memory, and (b) inactivating the neurons in the BLA reduces memory and the expression of Arc and CaMKII (Holloway and McIntyre, 2011; Holloway-Erickson et al., 2012). McReynolds and McIntyre (2012) have described a variety of other ways in which the BLA signal can influence memory storages processes.

FIGURE 12.11   When norepinephrine is released into the hippocampus, PKA is activated and phosphorylates two sites (Ser 831 and Ser 845) on the GluA1 AMPA receptor subunit. This facilitates the trafficking of GluA1s into the dendritic spine and increases memory strength.

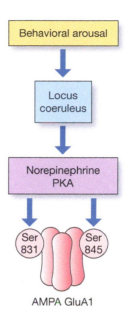

AMPA GluA1

The Norepinephrine Signal in Other Storage Areas

There is enhanced release of norepinephrine in the BLA as a result of the epinephrine → NTS → LC pathway (illustrated in Figure 12.6). However, LC neurons also project to other areas of the brain that store memories. For example, studies of LTP have reported that norepinephrine contributes to LTP in the hippocampus (Gelinas and Nguyen, 2005; Katsuki et al., 1997). Roberto Malinow and his colleagues (Hu et al., 2007) have discovered that norepinephrine facilitates LTP and memory of an explored context by facilitating trafficking of GluA1 AMPA receptors. This happens because when norepinephrine binds to adrenergic receptors the cAMP–PKA pathway is activated. PKA then phosphorylates two sites, Ser 831 and Ser 845, and facilitates trafficking of these receptors into the PSD, under weak training conditions (Figure 12.11)

The Epinephrine Liver–Glucose Connection

The second general way in which epinephrine can modulate memory storage, even though it does not cross the blood–brain barrier, is by its influence on the liver. The importance of this pathway is described below, beginning with a brief discussion of bioenergetics followed by a description of some of the evidence that glucose modulates memory storage and is especially important as we age. Finally, the influence of glucose levels on transcription is discussed.

Bioenergetics and the Brain

Translation and transcription processes that generate new protein and processes that distribute and arrange the new protein can last for many hours and require considerable energy. Initial changes in the underlying synapses are rapid and can rely on existing energy sources. However, available energy sources may not be sufficient to support transcription and translation processes that generate new protein. The flow of energy in cells is called **bioenergetics**, and the primary source of energy is glucose that enters the brain via the cerebral vasculature. Paul Gold and his colleagues have provided a large body of work that leads to the conclusion that epinephrine also enhances memory by its influence on glucose (Gold, 2005; Gold and Korol, 2012).

The most general function associated with the adrenal medulla is complementing the sympathetic nervous system in orchestrating the so-called "flight or fight" reaction. It contributes to this reaction by its interaction with the liver. A major function of the liver is to remove glucose from blood

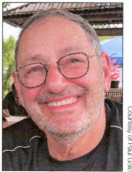

Paul Gold

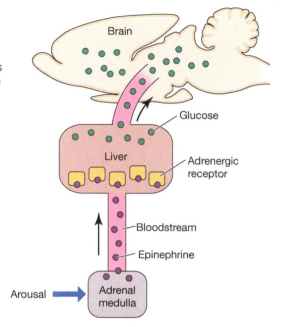

FIGURE 12.12 An arousing event activates the adrenal medulla to release epinephrine into the blood system where it binds to adrenergic receptors in the liver cell. This results in the liver secreting glucose into the blood where it enters the brain via the cerebral vasculature system.

and convert it to glycogen, where it is stored in preparation for future use. Cells in the liver contain adrenergic receptors. So when an arousing event is experienced, epinephrine is released and transported in blood to the liver where it binds to these receptors and initiates signaling that results in the liver secreting glucose into the blood (Figure 12.12). This increase in glucose provides energy to cells in the periphery that participate in the flight-or-flight response. In addition, glucose in the blood can enter the brain where it can be used to support the translation and transcription processes that strengthen the memory trace.

Glucose Modulates Memory

This framework makes a strong prediction: if epinephrine modulates memory strength through signaling the liver to secrete glucose, then one should be able to modulate the memory strength by directly increasing available glucose. There are numerous reports that injecting glucose systemically immediately following a training experience can do this (Gold, 2005; Messier, 2004). Figure 12.13 provides a useful example. It compares the effects of systemic glucose injections with a systemic injection of epinephrine on animals trained on an inhibitory avoidance task. Note that (a) in both cases the effect was dose dependent with both low and high doses having minimal effects, and (b) consistent with the modulation framework, when the interval separating training and injection was 1 hour, the optimal dose had no effect—the effect was time dependent. There also is evidence that glucose infused directly into memory storage sites enhances memory function (Gold and Korol, 2012).

(A)

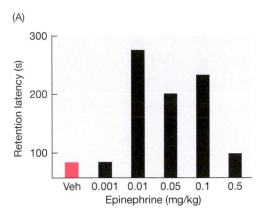

(B)

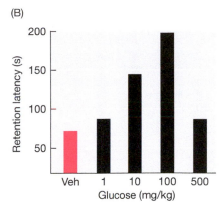

FIGURE 12.13   This figure illustrates that systemic injections of either epinephrine or glucose influence memory strength in a dose-dependent manner. These data support the view that epinephrine modulates memory by binding to adrenergic receptors on the liver cells causing them to release glucose. Key: Veh = vehicle. (A after P. E. Gold and R. B. Van Buskirk. 1975. *Behav Biol* 13: 145-153; B after P. E. Gold. 1986. *Behav Neur Biol* 45: 342–349.)

Glucose and Aging

An interesting change happens when animals age (Figure 12.14A,B)—arousing events generate the release of epinephrine in old animals but this increase is not accompanied by an increase in the level of blood glucose (Mabry et al., 1995). Moreover, even though old animals often can acquire memories, they forget more rapidly than younger animals (Gold, 2005). For example, when young rats acquire an inhibitory avoidance memory it remains stable for weeks, yet old rats lose the memory for this experience within several days.

Gold and his colleagues have advanced the hypothesis that the rapid forgetting seen in old animals is related to the failure of the liver to respond to epinephrine by secreting glucose. This hypothesis predicts that rapid forgetting by old animals can be prevented by a systemic injection of glucose. As predicted, injections of glucose reverse age-related rapid forgetting of memories established in several tasks. Figure 12.14C illustrates this outcome for rats trained on an inhibitory avoidance task. Note that old rats (24 to 25 months old) were severely impaired compared to young rats (3 to 4 months old) when the retention interval was 7 days. Remarkably, an infusion of glucose into the dorsal hippocampus following training completely reversed this impairment (Morris and Gold, 2013).

Glucose and Transcription

Long-lasting memories depend in part on genes targeted by the transcription factor CREB (see Chapter 11). Moreover, old rats display impaired CREB activation in response to memory-inducing behavioral training (Countryman and Gold, 2007; Kudo et al., 2005). There is evidence that impaired CREB activation is related in

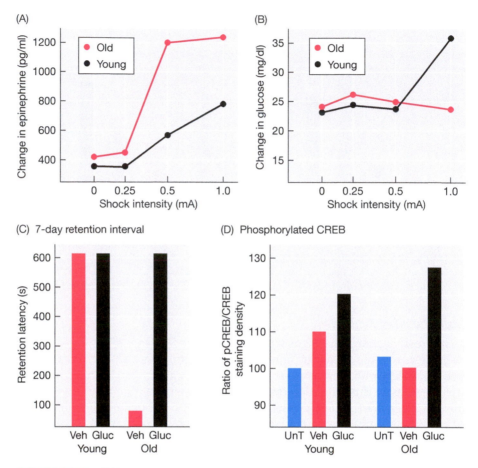

FIGURE 12.14 (A) In response to an arousing event (footshock), the adrenal gland releases epinephrine in both young and old rats. (B) Nevertheless, the liver of only young rats secretes glucose. (C) A systemic injection of glucose prevents forgetting in old rats tested 7 days after inhibitory avoidance training. (D) Enduring memories depend on new genes targeted by the transcription factor CREB (see Chapter 11). Avoidance training does not lead to CREB phosphorylation (pCREB) in old rats. However, if glucose is injected following training, pCREB is detected. Key: mA = milliamp; UnT = untrained; Veh = vehicle; Gluc = glucose. (A, B after T. R. Mabry et al. 1995. *Neurobiol Learn Mem* 64: 146–155; C, D after K. A. Morris and P. E. Gold. 2013. *Exp Geront* 48: 115–127.)

part to age-related changes in the adrenal response to arousal. This point is illustrated in Figure 12.14D, which shows that a systemic injection of either epinephrine or glucose following training increased phosphorylated CREB in the dentate gyrus region of the dorsal hippocampus of young rats. However, only glucose increased levels of phosphorylated CREB in old rats (Morris and Gold, 2013). Similar results were found when CREB activation was measured in the CA1 region of the dorsal hippocampus. This pattern is consistent with the view that enduring memories depend in part on the adrenal hormones and their targets—adrenergic receptors on the liver and vagal nerve—to support transcription and translation processes that produce the new protein needed to consolidate memories.

Gold and Korol (2012) have suggested another provocative conclusion. Given that glucose can reverse rapid forgetting in old rats, they propose that the underlying intracellular molecular machinery needed to consolidate memories may not be diminished. Instead, these translation and transcription processes require a contribution from the neuroadrenal hormonal modulation system. It is the age-related deficit in the adrenal medulla response to "arousing events" that is the problem. As they put it, "…in a sense, even seemingly salient events are non-emotional for aged rats and are not remembered well" (Gold and Korol, 2012, p. 6).

Glucocorticoids: The Other Adrenal Hormones

Highly arousing behavioral experiences can also cause the release by the adrenal cortex of the hormone corticosterone. Corticosterone is also classified as a **glucocorticoid** because it is involved in the metabolism of glucose. In contrast to adrenaline, glucocorticoids can directly enter the brain.

Glucocorticoids can also modulate memory (McEwen and Sapolsky, 1995; Roozendaal et al., 2006), and there is evidence that their influence depends on the BLA. If the synthetic glucocorticoid dexamethasone is administered systemically after inhibitory avoidance training, retention performance is enhanced. However, if the basolateral nucleus is lesioned, this effect is eliminated. In contrast, similar destruction of the central nucleus of the amygdala has no effect on the ability of dexamethazone to enhance retention. If RU 28362, a glucocorticoid receptor agonist, is injected into the basolateral nucleus following inhibitory avoidance training, retention performance is enhanced. No enhancement occurs, however, if it is injected into the central nucleus.

Glucocorticoids modulate memory but their influence depends on norepineprine binding to adrenergic receptors in the BLA. To illustrate this point, consider the experiment by Quirarte et al. (1997). They trained rats on the inhibitory avoidance task with weak shock. As expected, rats that were injected systemically with dexamethazone showed enhanced retention performance. However, if propranolol was directly injected into the BLA, dexamethazone did not enhance retention (Figure 12.15). Thus, it appears that the amygdala's ability to modulate memory storage depends on a coordinated adrenal gland response to a behavioral

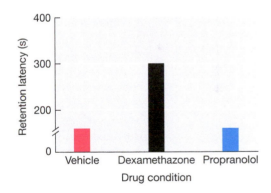

FIGURE 12.15 Dexamethazone is a synthetic glucocorticoid. When it is injected systemically following inhibitory avoidance training, it enhances retention. However, the effect of dexamethazone also depends on epinephrine being released in the amygdala, because when injected into the amygdala, propranolol prevents dexamethazone from enhancing retention. (After G. L. Quirarte et al. 1997. *Proc Natl Acad Sci USA* 94: 14048–14053.)

experience. Experiences that raise circulating levels of the two adrenal hormones, epinephrine and glucocorticoids, can result in a stronger memory. There is evidence that glucocorticoids influence memory by enhancing norepine-phrene's intiation of the cAMP–PKA signaling cascade (Roozandaal et al., 2006).

Summary

The discovery of a memory modulation system and its principal hormonal and neural components is one of the important achievements of biologically driven memory research. This work supports the importance of distinguishing between neural systems that store memories and neurohormonal systems that modulate storage circuits. This discovery also brings a whole-organism integrative perspective into the biological basis of memory. Specifically, memory consolidation is not just the product of the brain; it reflects the integration of behavioral influences on the brain and the adrenal gland component of the endocrine system.

Epinephrine is the principle memory-modulating hormone. Arousing stimulation causes the adrenal medulla to secrete it into the blood. However, it is too large to cross the blood–brain barrier, so its effects on the brain depend on two intermediary pathways.

One intermediary is the vagal nerve, where it binds to adrenergic receptors and ultimately signals the locus coeruleus to release norepinephrine into the BLA and other regions of the brain. Norepinephrine binds to adrenergic G-protein-coupled receptors and initiates the cAMP–PKA signaling cascade. This results in BLA neurons releasing glutamate onto neurons in storage areas and likely enhances release of endoplasmic reticulum calcium to facilitate the translation of local proteins, such as Arc and CaMKII.

The second intermediary is glucose. Epinephrine binds to adrenergic receptors on liver cells causing them to secrete glucose into the blood and the cerebral vascular system brings it into the brain. This sequence provides the brain with energy needed to carry out signaling cascades needed to activate transcription factors, such as CREB, to target memory genes (see Chapter 11) needed to produce a long-lasting memory. Old animals still mount an epinephrine response to arousing stimulation. However, this increase in epinephrine does not produce increased blood levels of glucose. The failure to mount a glucose response may be responsible for rapid forgetting by old animals. This is because systemic glucose injections following training enhance the level of phosphorylated CREB and prevent rapid forgetting.

Glucocorticoids can also modulate memory strength. This adrenal hormone crosses the blood–brain barrier and facilitates the action of norepinephrine, perhaps by augmenting its ability to engage the cAMP–PKA cascade.

Arousal usually signals that something important has happened that should be remembered. To ensure this outcome, multiple pathways exist by which the adrenal gland can influence neurons that store memories of arousing events.

References

Cahill, L. and Alkire, M. (2003). Epinephrine enhancement of human memory consolidation: interaction with arousal at encoding. *Neurobiology of Learning and Memory, 79,* 194–198.

Clark, K. B., Smith, D. C., Hassert, D. L., Browning, R. A., Naritoku, D. K., and Jensen, R. A. (1998). Posttraining electrical stimulation of vagal afferents with concomitant vagal efferent inactivation enhances memory storage processes in the rat. *Neurobiology of Learning and Memory, 70,* 364–373.

Countryman, R. A. and Gold, P. E. (2007). Rapid forgetting of social transmission of food preferences in aged rats: relationship to hippocampal CREB activation. *Learning and Memory, 14,* 350–358.

Dorr, A. E. and Debonnel, G. (2006). Effect of vagus nerve stimulation on serotonergic and noradrenergic transmission. *Journal of Pharmacology and Experimental Therapeutics, 318,* 890–898.

Gallagher, M., Kapp, B. S., Musty, R. E., and Driscoll, P. A. (1977). Memory formation: evidence for a specific neurochemical system in the amygdala. *Science, 198,* 423–435.

Gelinas, J. N. and Nguyen, P. V. (2005). Beta-adrenergic receptor activation facilitates induction of a protein synthesis-dependent late phase of long-term potentiation. *Journal of Neuroscience, 25,* 3294–3303.

Gold, P. E. (2005). Glucose and age-related changes in memory. *Neurobiology of Aging, 26,* 664.

Gold, P. E. and Korol, D. L. (2012). Making memories matter. *Frontiers in Integrative Neuroscience, 6,* Article 116.

Gold, P. E. and Van Buskirk, R. B. (1975). Facilitation of time-dependent memory processes with posttrial epinephrine injections. *Behavioral Biology, 13,* 145–153.

Hassert, D. L., Miyashita, T., and Williams, C. L. (2004). The effects of peripheral vagal nerve stimulation at a memory-modulating intensity on norepinephrine output in the basolateral amygdala. *Behavioral Neuroscience, 118,* 79–88.

Hatfield, T. and McGaugh, J. L. (1999). Norepinephrine infused into the basolateral amygdala posttraining enhances retention in a spatial water maze task. *Neurobiology of Learning and Memory, 71,* 232–239.

Holloway, C. M. and McIntyre, C. K. (2011). Post-training disruption of Arc protein expression in the anterior cingulate cortex impairs long-term memory for inhibitory avoidance training. *Neurobiology of Learning and Memory, 95,* 425–432.

Holloway-Erickson, C. M., McReynolds, J. R., and McIntyre, C. K. (2012). Memory-enhancing intra-basolateral amygdala infusions of clenbuterol increase Arc and CaMKIIa protein expression in the rostral anterior cingulate cortex. *Frontiers in Behavioral Neuroscience, 6,* 17.

Hu, H., Real, E., Takamiya, K., Kang, M. G., LeDoux, J., Huganir, R. L, and Malinow, R. (2007). Emotion enhances learning via norepinephrine regulation of AMPA receptor trafficking. *Cell, 131,* 160–173.

Katsuki, H., Izumi, Y., and Zorumski, C. F. (1997). Noradrenergic regulation of synaptic plasticity in the hippocampal CA1 region. *Journal of Neurophysiology, 77,* 3013–3020.

King, S. O. and Williams, C. L. (2009). Novelty-induced arousal enhances memory for cued classical fear conditioning: interactions between peripheral adrenergic and brainstem glutamatergic systems. *Learning and Memory, 16,* 625–634.

Kudo, K., Wati, H., Qiao, C., Arita, J., and Kanba, S. (2005). Age-related disturbance of memory and CREB phosphorylation in CA1 area of hippocampus of rats. *Brain Research, 1054,* 30–37.

Lashley, K. S. (1917). The effects of strychnine and caffeine upon the rate of learning. *Psychobiology, 1,* 141–170.

Liang, K. C., Juler, R. G., and McGaugh, J. L. (1986). Modulating effects of posttraining epinephrine on memory: involvement of the amygdala noradrenergic system. *Brain Research, 368,* 125–133.

Mabry, T. R., Gold, P. E., and McCarty, R. (1995). Age-related changes in plasma catecholamine and glucose response of F-344 rats to a single footshock as used in inhibitory avoidance training. *Neurobiology of Learning and Memory, 64,* 146–155.

McEwen, B. S. and Sapolsky, R. M. (1995). Stress and cognitive function. *Current Opinion in Neurobiology, 5,* 205–216.

McGaugh, J. L. (1959). Some neurochemical factors in learning. Unpublished PhD thesis, University of California, Berkeley.

McGaugh, J. L. (2002). Memory consolidation and the amygdala, a systems perspective. *Trends in Neurosciences, 25,* 456–462.

McGaugh, J. L. (2003). *Memory and Emotion.* New York: Columbia University Press.

McGaugh, J. L. (2004). The amygdala modulates the consolidation of memories of emotionally arousing experiences. *Annual Review of Neuroscience, 27,* 1–28.

McGaugh, J. L. and Petrinovich, L. (1959). The effect of strychnine sulfate on maze learning. *The American Journal of Psychology, 72,* 99–102.

McGaugh, J. L., Roozendaal, B., and Cahill, L. (2000). Modulation of memory storage by stress hormones and the amygdala complex. In M. S. Gazzaniga (Ed.), *The New Cognitive Neurosciences* (pp. 1981–1998). Cambridge, MA: MIT Press.

McIntyre, C. K., Hatfield, T., and McGaugh, J. L. (2002). Amygdala norepinephrine levels after training predict inhibitory avoidance retention performance in rats. *European Journal of Neuroscience, 16,* 1223–1226.

McIntyre, C. K., McGaugh, J. L., and Williams, C. L. (2012). Interacting brain systems modulate memory consolidation. *Neuroscience and Biobehavioral Reviews, 36,* 1750–1756.

McIntyre, C. K., Miyoshita, T., Setlow, B., Marjon, K. D., Steward, O., Guzowski, J. F., and McGaugh, J. L. (2005). Memory-influencing intra-basolateral amygdala drug infusions modulate expression of Arc protein in the hippocampus. *Proceedings of the National Academy of Sciences USA, 102,* 10718–10723.

McReynolds, J. R. and McIntyre, C. K. (2012). Emotional modulation of the synapse. *Reviews in the Neurosciences*, *23*, 449–461.

Messier, C. (2004). Glucose improvement of memory: a review. *European Journal of Pharmacology*, *490*, 33–57.

Miyashita, T. and Williams, C. L. (2006). Epinephrine administration increases neural impulses propagated along the vagus nerve: role of peripheral beta-adrenergic receptors. *Neurobiology of Learning and Memory*, *85*, 116–124.

Morris, K. A. and Gold, P. E. (2013). Epinephrine and glucose modulate training-related CREB phosphorylation in old rats: relationships to age-related memory impairments. *Experimental Gerontology*, *48*, 115–127.

Packard, M., Cahill, L., and McGaugh, J. L. (1994). Amygdala modulation of hippocampal-dependent and caudate nucleus-dependent memory processes. *Proceedings of the National Academy of Sciences USA*, *91*, 8477–8481.

Packard, M. G. and Teather, L. A. (1998). Amygdala modulation of multiple memory systems: hippocampus and caudate-putamen. *Neurobiology of Learning and Memory*, *69*, 163–200.

Parent, M. B. and McGaugh, J. L. (1994). Posttraining infusion of lidocaine into the amygdala basolateral complex impairs retention of inhibitory avoidance training. *Brain Research*, *66*, 97–103.

Quirarte, G. L., Galvez, R., Roozendaal, B., and McGaugh, J. L. (1998). Norepinephrine release in the amygdala in response to footshock and opioid peptidergic drugs. *Brain Research*, *808*, 134–140.

Quirarte, G. L., Roozendaal, B., and McGaugh, J. L. (1997). Glucocorticoid enhancement of memory storage involves noradrenergic activation in the basolateral amygdala. *Proceedings of the National Academy of Sciences USA*, *94*, 14048–14053.

Roozendaal, B., Okuda, S., Van der Zee, E. A., and McGaugh, J. L. (2006). Glucocorticoid enhancement of memory requires arousal-induced noradrenergic activation in the basolateral amygdala. *Proceedings of the National Academy of Sciences USA*, *103*, 6741–6746.

Sutherland, R. J. and McDonald, R. J. (1990). Hippocampus, amygdala, and memory deficits in rats. *Behavioural Brain Research*, *12*, 57–79.

Williams, C. L. and McGaugh, J. L. (1993). Reversible lesions of the nucleus of the solitary tract attenuate the memory-modulating effects of posttraining epinephrine. *Behavioral Neuroscience*, *6*, 955–962.

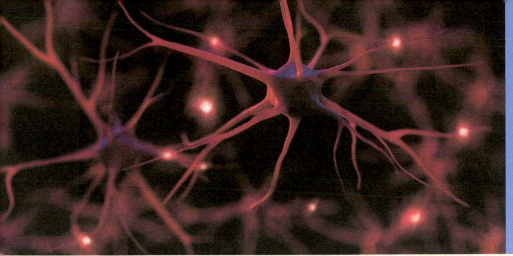

The Yin and Yang of Memory: Forgetting versus Maintenance

From the moment synaptic connections linking members of a neuronal ensemble that support a memory are strengthened, intrinsic neural processes are at work to weaken and return them to their prior baseline state. If one views these strengthened synapses as the fundamental basis of memory, then to the extent that they are weakened, memories will be forgotten (Hardt et al., 2013). From this perspective there are intrinsic neural events at work that actively degrade the synaptic basis of memory. However, from our subjective experience we know that memories can persist for very long periods of time. Thus, against intrinsic forces that actively degrade the synaptic basis of memories to produce forgetting, there also must be intrinsic forces at work to oppose this degradation and maintain the synapses that support memory. Hence the yin and yang of memory—forgetting versus maintenance. This chapter describes some of the neurobiological processes that work to promote the forgetting and maintenance of memories. It begins, however, with a discussion of how psychologists view forgetting.

Psychological View of Forgetting

This neurobiological view of forgetting is relatively new. Until quite recently the topic of forgetting belonged to psychology, and many psychologists found no reason to suppose such neuronal-based active forgetting existed. According to Medina (2018, p. 1) "…forgetting is referred to as the inability to recall something now that could be retrieved on an earlier occasion."

From a psychological perspective, almost all cases of amnesia (forgetting) stem from two sources: interference or retrieval failures. Interference can take two forms. One form derives from the empirical basis of Müller and Pilzecker's (1900) original theory of consolidation. They claimed that a second learning event could produce amnesia for a prior experience by interfering with the consolidation of the first, provided the second event was similar to the first and occurred shortly after it.

A second type of interference assigns forgetting to competition among similar memory traces for expression—a competing memory blocks or interferes with the expression of the target memory. This form of amnesia should also be considered the result of a retrieval failure (Baddeley et al., 2009; see Chapter 9 for a discussion of retrieval processes). The important signature of a retrieval failure is that amnesia is temporary and the memory can be recovered.

We all have experienced many instances of amnesia due to retrieval failures. Consider the modern problem: where did I put my cell phone? If you have good protective habits you will never have this problem because you put it in the same place every day but, if not, you have likely experienced retrieval failures. After a fruitless search you might then review the events of the day and finally recollect that you left the phone in the car. Moreover, at the same time you might also recover the memory of exactly where in the car you left the phone. So your memory for the phone's location was present, you just did not have the proper retrieval cues to access the memory.

In the realm of animal research, it has often been reported that lost memories can be recovered simply by exposing the animal to some aspects of the original training or even by stimulating them with some arousing pharmacological agent (Riccio and Richardson, 1984). Experimental psychologists have uncovered so many examples of amnesia due to retrieval failures that many of them see no reason to imagine that the synaptic underpinnings of memory may have been actively degraded. Thus, even today the idea of an active forgetting process is still controversial among many psychologists. Ricker et al. (2016), in their comprehensive review of the role of decay in forgetting, appear sympathetic to the decay idea. Ironically, however, in discussing the future of research on this topic they never imagined that studies of synaptic plasticity might have something to say about it.

Neurobiology of Forgetting: The Yin

The claim here is that there are identifiable cellular–molecular processes that control forgetting. The identification of these processes is a direct result of decades of work that have led to an understanding of the molecular basis of synaptic changes (discussed in Part 1). This claim makes two powerful predictions. If there are intrinsic processes that regulate forgetting, and we know what they are, then (1) forgetting can be prevented by interfering with these processes and (2) forgetting can be enhanced by activating these processes. In the following sections some of the evidence compelling the idea that active neural processes regulate forgetting is presented. The discussion is not comprehensive. There are a number of excellent reviews that provide more complete coverage (Davis and Zhong, 2017; Medina, 2018; Sachser et al., 2017).

Calcium Signaling Regulates Forgetting

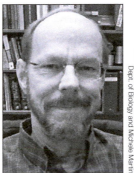

In a pioneering set of experiments, Brian Derrick's laboratory (Villarreal et al., 2002) provided the first evidence that forgetting is actively regulated. Previous studies had revealed that small amounts of calcium entering through NMDA receptors could depotentiate or reverse established LTP (Lee et al., 1998; Xiao et al., 1996). Based on these findings Derrick reasoned that both the depotentiation (decay) of LTP and forgetting could be blocked by chronically antagonizing NMDA receptors. Remarkably, systemic daily injections of an NMDA receptor antagonist prevented both the time-dependent reversal of LTP in the dentate gyrus and forgetting (Figure 13.1). Thus, not only are there

Brian Derrick

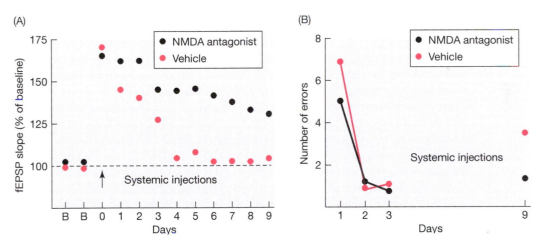

FIGURE 13.1 Inhibiting NMDA receptors prevents LTP decay and forgetting. (A) Theta-burst stimulation was applied to the perforant pathway to induce LTP in the dentate gyrus of intact rats. Within about 4 days it decayed to baseline in vehicle-treated rats, but this decay was prevented by daily systemic injections of an NMDA antagonist. (B) Rats learned a working memory task. After a 5-day retention interval, rats in the vehicle condition had forgotten the task as shown by their errors compared to controls. However, daily systemic injections of an NMDA antagonist prevented forgetting. These results support the hypothesis that active molecular events initiated by small amounts of calcium actively depotentiate the synapses that support the memory trace. (After D. M. Villarreal et al. 2002. *Nature Neurosci* 5: 48–52.)

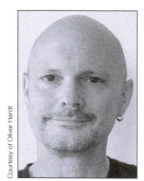

Oliver Hardt

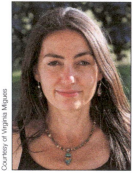

Virginia Migues

intrinsic neural events that actively produce forgetting but they are associated with NMDA calcium-dependent signaling.

AMPA Receptor Endocytosis

The persistence and strength of memory is positively correlated with the number of synaptic GluA2-containing AMPA receptors (Dong et al., 2015; Migues et al., 2010; Migues et al., 2014; Yao et al., 2008). If so, forgetting might be due to the gradual removal of these receptors over time. It follows that if one blocked the removal of AMPA receptors then forgetting could be prevented or greatly reduced.

Oliver Hardt and Virginia Migues provided a comprehensive evaluation of this hypothesis (Migues et al., 2016). To test the hypothesis, this group took advantage of the fact that synthetic peptides (for example, GluR23Y) are available that can prevent activity-dependent endocytosis of GluA2–AMPA receptors. They used several behavioral tasks to test the hypothesis (for example, object location and generalized contextual fear). In each task, infusion of these peptides into the dorsal hippocampus prevented forgetting (Figure 13.2). Thus, they speculated that preventing AMPA receptor endocytosis would preserve the memory indefinitely.

Mediators of Calcium Signaling

The above discussion establishes two important points: (1) calcium signaling contributes to forgetting and (2) the fatal outcome for forgetting is the removal of AMPA receptors. So what are some of the mediators of calcium signaling that lead to this outcome? Lucas de Oliveira Alvares and his colleagues (Sachser et al., 2016) confirmed and extended Derrick's basic findings and identified some of the downstream mediators of the effects of calcium signaling that contribute to forgetting. Inhibition of either NMDA receptors or voltage-dependent calcium channels (vdCCs) can prevent the forgetting of an object-location memory. This outcome suggests that both NMDA receptors and vdCCs combine to regulate forgetting. In addition, they identified the GluN2B-containing NMDA receptors (see Chapter 10) as the key NMDA receptor subtype mediating the decay of LTP and, by inference, forgetting.

The Hardt–Migues laboratory confirmed the importance of NMDA receptors in two important ways (Migues et al., 2019). They reported that (1) selectively inhibiting the GluN2B receptor prevented forgetting and (2) the infusion of the NMDA receptor co-agonist D-Serine, which would enhance NMDA activity, dramatically increased the rate of forgetting (Figure 13.3). These results support the idea that NMDA receptors can *bidirectionally regulate forgetting*. Inhibiting these receptors following training promotes retention, but increasing their activity promotes rapid forgetting.

CALCINEURIN   **Calcineurin** is the only phosphatase in the brain (recall that phosphatases remove phosphates) that is activated by calcium (Mansuy, 2003).

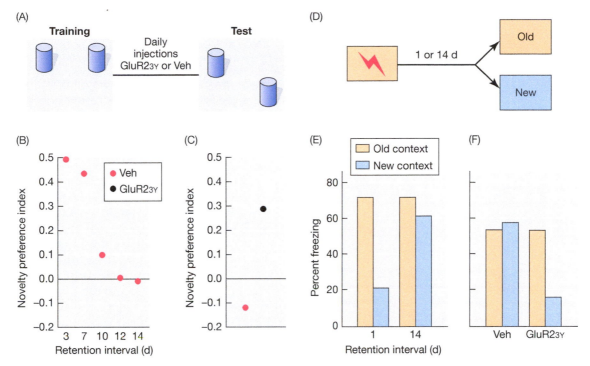

FIGURE 13.2   (A) During training animals explored two identical objects. In the test phase one object was moved to a new location. (B) Over a 14-day retention period rats forgot the location of the objects and explored the objects equally. (C) Daily injections of GluR23Y prevented forgetting. (D) Animals were shocked (conditioned) in a particular context; 1 or 14 days later they were tested either in the context where they were shocked or in a new but similar context. (E) When tested to each context 1 day after conditioning, animals displayed more fear to the old context than to the new. However, over the 14-day retention interval animals forgot exactly where they were shocked and displayed equivalent fear to both contexts; they generalized their fear of the old context to the new one. (F) Preventing AMPA endocytosis with GluR23Y prevented this forgetting. (After P. V. Migues et al. 2016. *J Neurosci* 36: 3481–3494.)

It has a large number of targets and has been shown to bidirectionally regulate both LTP and memory (Malleret et al., 2001; Mansuy, 2003). One target of calcineurin is stargazin (Tomita et al., 2005). In Chapter 3, stargazin, a transmembrane AMPA receptor regulatory protein (TARP), is identified as a central contributor to increasing the number of AMPA receptors in the postsynaptic density. When phosphorylated by CaMKII, stargazin is freed from the plasma membrane to be captured by traps provided by the scaffolding protein PSD-95 (see Figure 3.9). Tomita et al. (2005) reported that destabilizing the stargazin–PSD-95 interaction by dephosphorylating stargazin resulted in AMPA receptor removal. That being the case, Lucas de Oliveira Alvares (Sachser et al., 2016) hypothesized that the activation of calcineurin might be a downstream

(A)

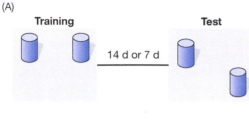

Training   **Test**

14 d or 7 d

(B)

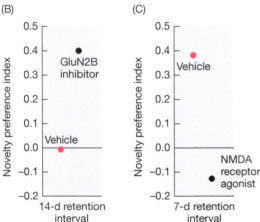

(C)

FIGURE 13.3 (A) In this object-location experiment rats explored two identical objects. During the 14-day retention interval a selective GluN2B receptor inhibitor was infused daily into the hippocampus. During the 7-day retention interval an NMDA receptor agonist was infused daily. (B) Selectively inhibiting GluN2B receptors prevented forgetting of the object's location. (C) An NMDA receptor agonist, in contrast, promoted rapid forgetting. These results indicate that NMDA receptors bidirectionally control forgetting. (After P. V. Migues et al. 2019. *Hippocampus* 29: 883–888.)

target of calcium that contributes to forgetting because dephosphorylating stargazin would liberate AMPA receptors from their PSD-95 traps. This event would then increase the likelihood of AMPA receptor endocytosis. If so, inhibiting either an NMDA receptor or calcineurin would prevent memory loss. Consistent with this idea, daily systemic injections of either an NMDA receptor inhibitor or a calcineurin inhibitor following object-location training preserved the memory for the location (Figure 13.4). This result was consistent with the hypothesis that calcineurin destabilizes the stargazin–PSD-95 interaction.

FIGURE 13.4 Inhibiting GluN2B NMDA receptors or the phosphatase calcineurin prevents forgetting of an object's location. (A) The animals were trained and tested on their memory for the location of an object. During the 7-day interval separating training and testing either an NMDA antagonist, a calcineurin inhibitor, or a vehicle (Veh) was infused into the hippocampus. During the test, vehicle-treated animals displayed a memory for the location of an object by exploring the object in the new location. (B, C) Vehicle-treated animals forgot the location of the objects and equally explored both objects. Inhibiting either NMDA receptors or calcineurin prevented forgetting; these animals preferentially explored the object in the new location. (After R. M. Sachser et al. 2016. *Sci Rep* 6: 22771.)

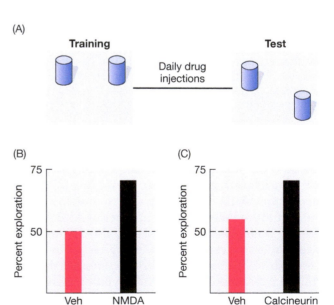

However, it is important to keep in mind that calcineurin has many other targets, so this is just one interpretation. A simple illustration of some of the events that lead to AMPA receptor endocytosis is shown in Figure 13.5.

STATE OF RAC1   **Rac1** is a member of the Rho family of GTPases and is thought to contribute to the regulation of actin dynamics (Heasman and Ridley, 2008). Evidence is accumulating that the state of Rac1 (active or inactive) following initial learning can determine the rate of forgetting. In its active state Rac1 often leads to rapid forgetting. If Rac1 is inactive, however, the rate of forgetting is markedly slower. The most systematic and compelling evidence for Rac1 as a regulator of forgetting comes from the study of memory in fruit flies (see Davis and Zhong, 2017 for a review of these findings). In rodents the virus-driven overexpression of Rac1 in the hippocampus accelerates forgetting of an object-recognition memory, whereas the expression of the dominant negative form (which reduces active Rac1) significantly enhances retention (Liu et al., 2016).

What determines the activity state of Rac1 is not well understood. Studies of protein trafficking in response to glutamate released onto single spines (Bosch et al., 2014; see Chapter 5) suggest that calcium signaling might be important. At the behavioral level, however, two variables have been identified: (1) stress produced by social isolation and (2) the interval separating training trials.

In the laboratory, mice are normally housed in small groups. Liu et al. (2016) reported that mice socially isolated for several days prior to learning show enhanced Rac1 activity. Moreover, these mice display impaired retention of what is called a **social-recognition memory** (the ability of the test mouse to remember an individual mouse with whom it recently interacted). This memory impairment was reversed, however, by inhibiting Rac1 activity in the hippocampus. Moreover, when previously isolated mice were resocialized, levels of Rac1 decreased back to normal and their social-recognition memory was restored to normal. In addition, if Rac1 activity was increased in the hippocampus then group-housed mice displayed impaired social-recognition memory. Thus, stress produced by social isolation can determine the activity state of Rac1.

As a general rule, when the learning experience involves multiple trials, spacing the trials produces better retention than if the trials are massed. For example, Jiang et al. (2016) reported that rats given massed trials (shocks delivered every 12 seconds) displayed rapid forgetting of contextual fear compared to rats given spaced trials (shocks delivered every 2 or 10 minutes). In addition, they reported that Rac1 levels were significantly reduced in the hippocampus of rats given spaced training. Supporting the idea

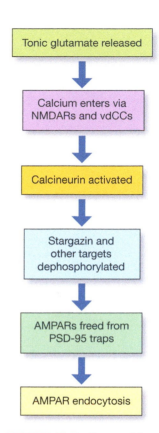

FIGURE 13.5 Some of the signaling events that lead to AMPA receptor (AMPAR) endocytosis. Following the strengthening of synapses that support memory there is tonic release of small amounts of glutamate. This leads to calcium entering spines and activating the phosphatase calcineurin which dephosphorylates the stargazin and other targets to liberate AMPA receptors from PSD-95 traps and allows their endocytosis.

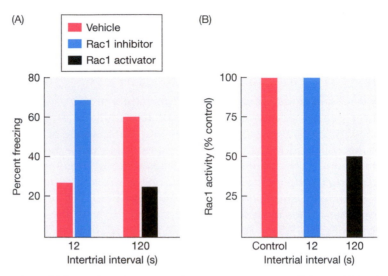

FIGURE 13.6 (A) Retention of a context fear memory was poor if the multiple shocks were separated by only 12 seconds. In contrast spaced presentations (120 seconds) of the shock resulted in no forgetting. When Rac1 was inhibited forgetting was prevented in animals in the 12-second condition, and when Rac1 was activated animals in the 120-second condition forgot the fear memory. (B) One hour after conditioning Rac1 levels in animals in the 12-second group remained high, whereas those in the 120-second condition were significantly lower than naïve control animals. These results suggest that the state of Rac1 can determine the rate of forgetting. (After L. Jiang et al. 2016. *Mol Neurobiol* 53: 1247–1253.)

that Rac1 activity was a determiner of forgetting, they reported that (a) if Rac1 was inhibited retention displayed by rats given massed trials was as good as rats in the spaced condition, and (b) forgetting was rapid if Rac1 was activated in rats in the spaced condition (Figure 13.6).

In summary, these results suggest that under some conditions the state of Rac1 during the retention period regulates forgetting. In the active state, Rac1 enhances the rate of forgetting whereas the inactive state favors retention. Just how the state of Rac1 influences retention is currently unknown. However, there is speculation that it does so by influencing actin dynamics. In support of this idea, Haruo Kasai's group (Hayashi-Takagi et al., 2015) demonstrated that the activation of Rac1 in single spines leads to their shrinkage and the activation of Rac1 in spines that have been enlarged by behavioral training results in forgetting.

Many cases of amnesia are due to competition for expression or retrieval failures. There is no doubt that forgetting, however, can be the result of cellular–molecular events that actively degrade the synaptic basis of memory. Given the power of these events one might wonder how memories can persist.

Memory Maintenance: The Yang

One way to view the temporal–sequential evolution of the synaptic basis of memory (generation, stabilization, and consolidation) is that at each successive stage processes are called into play that increase the resistance of the initial synaptic changes to disruption and protect the memory from decay. *Post-translation modifications* that include trafficking of AMPA receptors into the PSD and enlarging the actin cytoskeleton are sufficient to support memories that last a few hours. However, these initial changes do not resist active decay, so it is likely that these synapses are extremely vulnerable to post-learning calcium signals that initiate AMPA receptor endocytosis. Or it may be that in the immediate aftermath of these changes, Rac1, which may be part of the initial signaling cascade to increase actin polymerization, is left in an active state so that the seeds of forgetting are folded in with the molecular changes that originally strengthened the synapses (Davis and Zhong, 2017).

The construction of spines with enlarged actin cytoskeletons that occurs during the stabilization phase is not sufficient to buffer synapses against active decay over the long haul. However, it is reasonable to infer that it is a necessary intermediary event. Without the activation of actin polymerization processes and other actin management processes the critical events that support local protein synthesis cannot occur (see Chapter 6). In addition, large spines are typically the winners in the competition for the replacement synaptic proteins that spines need to endure. Thus, the creation of enlarged spines can be recognized as a structural–functional force against active decay.

The duration of memories is strongly associated with long-lasting multiple waves of consolidation (see Chapter 11). The critical question is, *what do these waves of protein synthesis bring to synapses (beyond replacement of synaptic proteins) that make them more resistant to forgetting?* In Chapter 7 the kinase PKMζ is discussed as a molecule that prevents decay of LTP. Given PKMζ's role in maintaining LTP, it should come as no surprise that it has been extensively investigated for its potential role in memory maintenance.

PKMζ Opposes Forgetting

Recall that PKMζ mRNA is present locally in the dendritic region where, in response to synaptic activity, it can be rapidly translated locally. It also lacks a regulatory domain, is always in the active catalytic state, and can self-perpetuate. As was the case for PKMζ's role in maintaining LTP, the primary strategy for memory maintenance has been to inactivate PKMζ with zeta inhibitory protein (ZIP). Given that ZIP reverses well established LTP, then the prediction is that it also should erase well consolidated memories. There is evidence that spatial memories, fear memories, inhibitory avoidance memories, instrumental-response memories, object-location memories, and taste-aversion memories have all been erased by injecting ZIP into the relevant storage sites

(Hardt et al., 2013; Kwapis et al., 2012; Pastalkova et al., 2006; Pauli et al., 2012; Sacktor, 2011; Serrano et al., 2008; Shema et al., 2007). Additional evidence is discussed below.

Interfering with PKMζ Erases a Taste-Aversion Memory

The work of Yadin Dudai and his colleagues provides an excellent example of the strategy of inactivating PKMζ with ZIP (Shema et al., 2007). They asked if the maintenance of the memory for an acquired taste aversion depends on PKMζ (Figure 13.7). They injected ZIP into the insular cortex, which previous studies had identified as a storage site for taste-aversion memories. A single injection of ZIP into the insular neocortex either 3, 7, or 25 days after training erased the memory. It is important to note that there was no time window constraining the effects of ZIP. The taste-aversion memory was erased even when it was 25 days old. In contrast, when it was injected into the hippocampus, which is not a storage site for the taste-aversion memory, ZIP had no effect. Moreover, even though ZIP erased old established taste memories, it did not alter the acquisition of a new taste aversion.

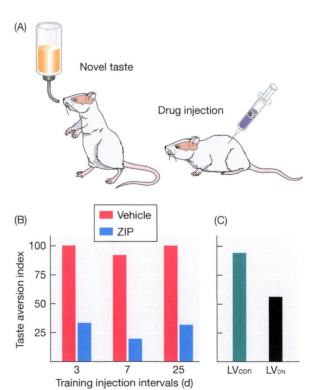

FIGURE 13.7 (A, B) Rodents will acquire an aversion to a novel taste that is followed by a drug that induces a temporary illness. A single injection of ZIP into the insular cortex will greatly reduce a well consolidated taste-aversion memory. (C) The lentivirus dominant negative PKMζ (LVDN) construct competes with PKMζ for expression. If it is injected into the insular cortex 5 days following the acquisition of a taste-aversion memory, the memory is weakened. Key: LVcon = lentivirus control. (A, B after R. Shema et al. 2007. *Science* 17: 951–953; C after R. Shema et al. 2011. *Science* 331: 1207–1210.)

Dudai's group (Shema et al., 2011) also confirmed the importance of PKMζ with another strategy. They infected neurons in the insular cortex with a lentivirus designed to transfect these neurons with a dominant negative gene (LVDN) that coded for an inactive form of PKMζ. This mRNA would compete with existing PKMζ for translation but the resulting protein would not be functional, so the predicted outcome was that rats treated with LVDN would not maintain an established taste-aversion memory. The virus was injected 5 days following the acquisition of the memory. Consistent with the prediction, rats injected with the virus displayed a markedly reduced taste aversion when tested 6 days later (see Figure 13.7C).

PKMζ Strengthens New Memories and Prevents Forgetting

Dudai's group also used the lentivirus approach to reveal that PKMζ *can enhance established memories*. In this case they asked two questions: could PKMζ convert a weak memory trace into a stronger one, and could it prevent the forgetting that normally occurs? To do this they designed lentiviruses to deliver the gene for PKMζ (LVPKMζ) or a control construct (LVcon) that did not contain the gene. To determine if PKMζ could strengthen a weak memory, rats were trained with a taste-aversion protocol designed to produce a weak taste aversion. Remarkably, injecting LVPKMζ into the insular cortex 5 days prior to this training enhanced the memory for that experience—it converted a weak memory into a strong one. To determine if PKMζ could rescue an older fading memory, rats were not tested until 9 days after training. Injecting LVPKMζ 6 days following training prevented normal forgetting.

PKMζ Prevents AMPA Receptor Endocytosis

As discussed above, a primary force producing forgetting is a calcium → calcineurin → stargazin signaling cascade that results in AMPA receptor endocytosis. Thus, it is important that Migues et al. (2010) provided evidence that PKMζ prevents forgetting by opposing endocytosis. They reasoned that if PKMζ maintains memory by preventing endocytosis, then (a) inhibiting PKMζ (by the polypeptide ZIP) should produce a memory loss accompanied by loss of synaptic AMPA receptors, and (b) both of these outcomes can be prevented if the peptide GluR23y which prevents endocytosis, is also infused into the same brain region. Their experiments supported these predictions (Figure 13.8).

The initial wave of consolidation begins with local protein synthesis and the translation of PKMζ, which can immediately resist the endocytotic process that removes AMPA receptors. However, for PKMζ to continue its role as a defender of synaptic changes supporting memory there must be a continuous supply of PKMζ mRNA available and it must be selectively delivered to the synapses supporting the memory trace. As noted in Chapter 7 the continuous supply of mRNA might be the result of a positive feedback loop whereby PKMζ translocates from the cytosol to the nucleus to phosphorylate CREB-binding protein and perhaps increase transcription of PKMζ mRNA (Ko et al., 2016). Selective

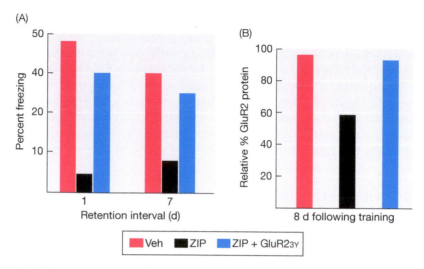

FIGURE 13.8 (A) Infusing the PKMζ inhibitor ZIP into the basolateral amygdala resulted in forgetting of conditioned fear. However, if GluR23Y was also infused, forgetting produced by ZIP was prevented. (B) Eight days following conditioning GluR2 protein in the PSD was reduced when ZIP was infused but not if GluR23Y also was infused. These results support the hypothesis that PKMζ counters forgetting by preventing AMPA receptor endocytosis. (After P. V. Migues et al. 2010. *Nature Neurosci* 13: 630–634.)

allocation of the mRNA could then be the result of enlarged spines with upregulated translation capacity capturing the mRNA. This is, of course, speculation.

Epilogue: Why Do We Forget or Remember?

This chapter describes some of the fundamental processes that underlie forgetting and support remembering. Why do we forget? One might suspect that forgetting is an adaptation that has evolved because of capacity limitation of our brains. By this view, we cannot always anticipate what events will subsequently prove to be important, so the default mode is to capture as much information as possible. However, much of it will prove to be of no importance. Active forgetting clears out unimportant memories, thereby making room for new memories and making it easier to retrieve important ones (see Hardt et al., 2013 for further discussion).

This may be an important consequence of forgetting but it may not be the underlying adaptation. A more fundamental answer may reside in the fact that in order for our brains to function, a proper balance between excitation and inhibition in the neural circuits must be maintained (Turrigiano, 2011). An array of homeostatic mechanisms evolved to regulate neuronal and circuit excitability (Turrigiano, 2011; Vitureira et al., 2013). The bidirectional modification of synapses (otherwise known as synaptic plasticity) may have evolved as one of these homeostatic mechanisms. It is very easy to potentiate synapses. In fact, spontaneous potentiation has been observed at the synaptic level (Hayashi-Takagi et al., 2015). Without countering processes, synapses would rapidly saturate in favor of too much excitation. From the perspective of the brain, processes that produce active forgetting at the psychological level may have evolved to help maintain the balance of excitatory and inhibitory inputs on a neuron. Thus, the stabilization, consolidation, and maintenance processes that support remembering may have evolved in order to selectively preserve synaptic changes that represent important events.

Summary

Potentiated synapses generated by behavioral events almost immediately encounter forces that depotentiate them (return them to their baseline condition). The fundamental principle associated with this outcome is that forgetting can be an active process brought about by these depotentiating forces. An important contributor to active forgetting is calcium-regulated AMPA receptor endocytosis. Removal of AMPA receptors promotes forgetting and preventing this event promotes remembering. The state of the GTPase Rac1 also has been identified as a regulator of forgetting. In its active state it promotes forgetting.

Left unopposed these forces will erase the synaptic basis of memory. One way to view the evolution of the synaptic basis of memory is that at each successive stage processes are called into play that increase the resistance of the initial synaptic changes to disruption and protect the memory from decay. Weak stimulation that only engages post-translation processes can generate synaptic changes that support memories. However, these synaptic changes are left unprotected from the processes (for example, AMPA receptor endocytosis) that produce active forgetting, hence only support a short-lasting memory. Stronger stimulation will activate actin management processes to generate an enlarged spine and local protein synthesis, including PKMζ, which will actively oppose AMPA receptor removal. The state of Rac1 is emerging as a regulator of forgetting. Just what determines its state and the downstream effects of its activation is not yet known.

The neurobiology of forgetting is a relatively new field. Some of the contributors of forgetting and maintenance have been identified but it is not yet clear if these processes will account for all types of forgetting or maintenance. There is still much to be learned in this young field and the developments described here give promise to an exciting future (see Awasthi et al., 2019).

References

Awasthi, A., Ramachandran, B., Ahmed, S., Benito, E., Shinoda, Y., Nitzan, N., and Dean, C. (2019). Synaptotagmin-3 drives AMPA receptor endocytosis, depression of synapse strength, and forgetting. *Science, 363*, eaav1483.

Baddely, A., Eysenck, M. W., and Anderson, M. C. (2009). *Memory*. New York: Psychological Press.

Bosch, M., Castro, J., Saneyoshi, T., Matsuno, H., Sur, M., and Hayashi, Y. (2014). Structural and molecular remodeling of dendritic spine substructures during long-term potentiation. *Neuron, 82,* 444–459.

Davis, R. L. and Zhong, Y. (2017). The biology of forgetting. *Neuron, 95,* 490–503.

Dong, Z., Han, H., Li, H., Bai, Y., Wang, W., Tu, M., Peng, Y., Zhou, L., He, W., Wu, X., Tan, T., Liu, M., Wu, X., Zhou, W., Jin, W., Zhang, S., Sacktor, T. C., Li, T., Song, W., and Wang, Y. T. (2015). Long-term potentiation decay and memory loss are mediated by AMPAR endocytosis. *Journal of Clinical Investigation, 125,* 234–247.

Hardt, O., Nader, K., and Nadel, L. (2013). Decay happens: the role of active forgetting in memory. *Trends in Cognitive Science, 17,* 111–120.

Hardt, O., Nader, K., and Wang, Y. T. (2014.) GluA2-dependent AMPA receptor endocytosis and the decay of early and late long-term potentiation: possible mechanisms for forgetting of short- and long-term memories. *Philosophical Transactions of the Royal Society London. Series B, Biological Sciences, 369,* 20130141.

Hayashi-Takagi, A., Yagishita, S., Nakamura, M., Shirai, F., Wu, Y. I., Loshbaugh, A. L., Kuhlman, B., Hahn, K. M., and Kasai, H. (2015). Labelling and optical erasure of synaptic memory traces in the motor cortex. *Nature, 525,* 333–338.

Heasman, S. J. and Ridley, A. J. (2008). Mammalian Rho GTPases: new insights into their functions from in vivo studies. *Nature Reviews Molecular Cellular Biology, 9,* 690–701.

Jiang, L., Mao, R., Zhou, Q., Yang, Y., Cao, J., Ding, Y., Yang, Y., Zhang, X., Li, L., and Xu, L. (2016). Inhibition of Rac1 activity in the hippocampus impairs the forgetting of contextual fear memory. *Molecular Neurobiology, 53,* 1247–1253.

Ko, H. G., Kim, J. I., Sim, S. E., Kim, T., Yoo, J., Choi, S. L., Baek, S. H., Yu, W. J., Yoon, J. B., Sacktor, T. C., and Kaang, B. K. (2016). The role of nuclear PKMζ in memory maintenance. *Neurobiology of Learning and Memory, 135,* 50–56.

Kwapis, J. L., Jarome, T. J., Gilmartin, M. R., and Helmstetter, F. J. (2012). Intra-amygdala infusion of the protein kinase Mzeta inhibitor ZIP disrupts foreground context fear memory. *Neurobiology of Learning and Memory, 98,* 148–153.

Lee, H. K., Kameyama, K., Huganir, R. L., and Bear, M. F. (1998). NMDA induces long-term synaptic depression and dephosphorylation of the GluR1 subunit of AMPA receptors in hippocampus. *Neuron, 21,* 1151–1162.

Liu, Y., Du, S., Lv, L., Lei, B., Shi, W., Tang, Y., Wang, L., and Zhong, Y. (2016). Hippocampal activation of Rac1 regulates the forgetting of object-recognition memory. *Current Biology, 26,* 2351–2357.

Malleret, G., Haditsch, U., Genoux, D., Jones, M. W., Bliss, T. V., Vanhoose, A. M., Weitlauf, C., Kandel, E. R., Winder, D. G., and Mansuy, I. M. (2001). Inducible and reversible enhancement of learning, memory, and LTP by genetic inhibition of calcineurin. *Cell, 140,* 675–686.

Mansuy, I. M. (2003). Calcineurin in memory and bidirectional plasticity. *Biochemical and Biophysical Research Communications, 311,* 1195–1208.

Medina, J. H. (2018). Neural, cellular and molecular mechanisms of forgetting. *Frontiers in Systems Neuroscience, 12,* 1–10.

Migues, P. V., Hardt, O., Finnie, P., Wang, Y. W., and Nader, K. (2014). The maintenance of long-term memory in the hippocampus depends on the interaction between N-ethylmaleimide-sensitive factor and GluA2. *Hippocampus, 24,* 1112–1119.

Migues, P. V., Hardt, O., Wu, D. C., Gamache, K., Sacktor, T. C, Wang, Y. T., and Nader, K. (2010). PKMzeta maintains memories by regulating GluR2-dependent AMPA receptor trafficking. *Nature Neuroscience, 13,* 630–634.

Migues, P. V., Liu, L., Archbold, G. E. B., Einarsson, E. O., Wong, J. X., Bonasia, K., Ko, S. H., Wang, Y. T., and Hardt, O. (2016). Blocking synaptic removal of GluA2-containing AMPA receptors prevents the natural forgetting of long-term memories. *Journal of Neuroscience, 36,* 3481–3494.

Migues, P. V., Wong, J., Lyu, J., and Hardt, O. (2019). NMDA receptor activity bidirectionally controls active decay of long-term spatial memory in the dorsal hippocampus. *Hippocampus, 9,* 883–888.

Müller, G. E. and Pilzecker, A. (1900). Experimentalle beitrage zur lehre vom gedachtinis. *Zeitschrift für Psychologie und Physiologie der Sinnesorgane, I,* 1–288.

Pastalkova, E., Serrano, P., Pinkhasova, D., Wallace, E., Fenton, A. A., and Sacktor, T. C. (2006). Storage of spatial information by the maintenance mechanism of LTP. *Science, 313,* 1141–1144.

Pauli, W. M., Clark, A. D., Guenther, H. J., O'Reilly, R. C., and Rudy, J. W. (2012). Inhibiting PKMζ reveals dorsal lateral and dorsal medial striatum store the different memories needed to support adaptive behavior. *Learning and Memory, 19,* 307–314.

Riccio, D. C. and Richardson, R. (1984). The status of memory following experimentally induced amnesia: gone, but not forgotten. *Physiological Psychology, 12,* 59–72.

Ricker, T. J., Vergauwe, E., and Cowan, N. (2016). Decay theory of immediate memory: from Brown (1958) to today (2014*). Quarterly Journal of Experimental Psychology, 9,* 1969–1995.

Sachser, R. M., Haubrich, J., Lunardi, P. S., and de Oliveira Alvares, L. (2017). Forgetting of what was once learned: exploring the role of postsynaptic ionotropic glutamate receptors on memory formation, maintenance, and decay. *Neuropharmacology, 112,* 94–103.

Sachser, R. M., Santana, F., Crestani, A. P., Lunardi, P., Pedraza, L. K., Quillfeldt, J. A., Hardt, O., and de Oliveira Alvares, L. (2016). Forgetting of long-term memory requires activation of NMDA receptors, L-type voltage-dependent Ca^{2+} channels, and calcineurin. *Scientific Reports, 6,* 22771.

Sacktor, T. C. (2011). How does PKMζ maintain long-term memory? *Nature Reviews Neuroscience, 12,* 9–15.

Serrano, P., Friedman, E. L., Kenney, J., Taubenfeld, S. M., Zimmerman, J. M., Hanna, J., Alberini, C., Kelley, A. E., Maren, S., Rudy, J. W., Yin, J. C., Sacktor, T. C., and Fenton, A. A. (2008). PKMζ maintains spatial, instrumental, and classically conditioned long-memories. *PLoS Biology, 6*, 2698–2706.

Shema, R., Haramati, S., Ron, S., Hazvi, S., Chen, A., Sacktor, T. C., and Dudai, Y. (2011). Enhancement of consolidated long-term memory by overexpression of protein kinase Mzeta in the neocortex. *Science, 331*, 1207–1210.

Shema, R., Sacktor, T. C., and Dudai, Y. (2007). Rapid erasure of long-term memory associations in cortex by an inhibitor of PKMζ. *Science, 317*, 951–953.

Tomita, S., Stein, V., Stocker, T. J., Nicoll, R. A., and Bredt, D. S. (2005). Bidirectional synaptic plasticity regulated by phosphorylation of stargazin-like TARPs. *Neuron, 45*, 269–277.

Turrigiano, G. (2011). Too many cooks? Intrinsic and synaptic homeostatic mechanisms in cortical circuit refinement. *Annual Review of Neuroscience, 34*, 89–103.

Villarreal, D. M., Do, V., Haddad, E., and Derrick, B. E. (2002). NMDA receptor antagonists sustain LTP and spatial memory: active processes mediate LTP decay. *Nature Neuroscience, 5*, 48–52.

Vitureira, N., Letellier, M., and Goda, Y. (2012). Homeostatic synaptic plasticity: from single synapses to neural circuits. *Current Opinion in Neurobiology, 22*, 516–521.

Xiao, M. Y., Niu, Y. P., and Wigstrom, H. (1996). Activity-dependent decay of early LTP revealed by dual EPSP recording in hippocampal slices from young rats. *European Journal of Neuroscience, 9*, 1916–1923.

Yao, Y., Kelly, M. T., Sajikumar, S., Serrano, P., Tian, D., Bergold, P. J., Frey, J. U., and Sacktor, T. C. (2008). PKMzeta maintains late long-term potentiation by N-ethylmaleimide-sensitive factor/GluR2-dependent trafficking of postsynaptic AMPA receptors. *Journal of Neuroscience, 28*, 7820–7827.

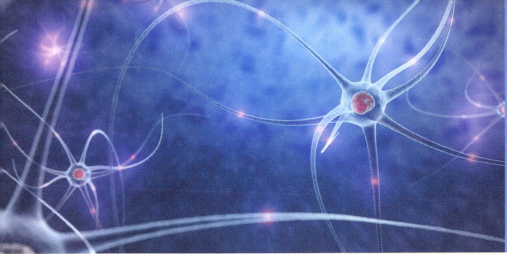

Hunting for Engrams

Neurobiologists have made significant progress toward understanding synaptic plasticity and in linking synaptic changes to the behavioral expressions of memory. Long before they dreamed of understanding these synaptic processes, however, they hoped it would be possible to find the physical substrate of memory in the brain (see Josselyn et al., 2017 for an interesting history). Methods developed in the last 10 years or so have brought the field closer to this goal. In this chapter some of the remarkable progress toward solving this problem is presented.

The search for the physical basis of memory immediately raises two big questions: what should one look for and where should one look? As noted in Chapter 2, memories from the brain's view are the changes in the connectivity among the collections of neurons responding to a particular experience. This view immediately rules out the idea that there is some dedicated place in the brain that is a warehouse or repository for our memories. Given that any particular experience will activate many different regions of the brain, this view also implies that the physical basis of a memory will be widely distributed. So the general answer to these questions is that one will have to look for collections of interconnected neurons that can be distributed widely across brain regions. This, of course, is a daunting proposition.

In his famous monograph, *In Search of the Engram*, Karl Lashley (1950) brought the term **engram** into memory vernacular to represent the persistent basis of memory. It was Richard Semon (1921), however, who invented the term (see Schacter, 1982). As elaborated in an excellent review by Josselyn et al. (2015), Semon's concept of the engram provides a useful framework for searching for the physical basis of memory. As detailed below, the engram has four properties: persistence, **ecphory**, content, and dormancy.

1. An engram is a *persistent* change in the brain that results from a specific experience or event.

2. An engram has the potential for *ecphory*—that is, an engram may be expressed behaviorally through interactions with retrieval cues, which could be sensory input, ongoing behavior, or voluntary goals. The term ecphory can be thought of as roughly equivalent to retrieval.

3. The *content* of an engram reflects what transpired at encoding and predicts what can be recovered during subsequent retrieval.

4. An engram may exist in a *dormant state* between the two active processes of encoding and retrieval (ecphory)—that is, an engram exists beyond the operations and processes required to form and recover it.

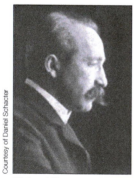

Courtesy of Daniel Schacter

Richard Semon

In thinking about these properties, it is important to note that *the engram is not the memory* but provides a physical basis for it. Memories emerge as a result of environmental or mental retrieval cues that activate the engram—or in Semon's words, when the process of ecphory "…awaken[s] the mnemic trace or engram out of its latent state into one of manifested activity…" (Semon, 1921, p. 12). In people, the manifested activity of an engram might reveal itself as vivid scenes and sounds of the past that we can identify as a memory. You can easily experience this state by remembering a recent party or family gathering. This would be a subjective state of mind, available only to you. However, in this chapter activation of an engram is identified with memory when its manifested activity can be linked to an observed change in behavior that can be attributed to past experience.

The concept of an engram assumes an underlying persistent change in the brain. It is remarkable that Hebb's (1949) idea—that modified connections among neurons belonging to *cell assemblies* are the basis of memory—remains the most generally accepted view of how the brain might support the persistent property of an engram (see Chapter 2). Today, cell assemblies are often called *neuronal ensembles* (Josselyn et al., 2015) but the fundamental idea is the same. So when modern neuroscientists are searching for engrams, they are looking for neurons that can be demonstrated to belong to cell assemblies–neuronal ensembles.

The Engram Search: A Story of Technical Advances

Since Lashley's pioneering studies, behavioral neuroscientists have been hunting for engrams. Early attempts were severely limited by the available research tools. Modern advances in locating engrams are intimately linked with the remarkable development of methods for identifying and manipulating "engram cells." Until recently, the primary tool of the engram hunters was lesion techniques (Josselyn et al., 2015). Such techniques ranged from the ablation of a large area of the brain, which contains many identifiable subregions, to more targeted lesions of specific anatomically distinct regions, to the use of neurotoxic chemicals to kill a large number of neurons within a defined anatomical region (Figure 14.1). The best one could hope for with such approaches was to find brain regions that contain cells that may be necessary for the behavioral

(A) (B)

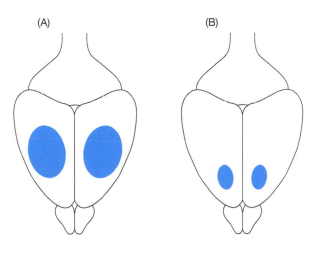

FIGURE 14.1 Until recently the hunt for engrams was restricted by available methods. (A) Ablation of a large cortical area. (B) Ablation of a smaller cortical area. (C, D) The use of stereotaxic surgery to target more specific regions such as the basolateral amygdala (BLA) or hippocampus for electrolytic or neurotoxic lesions. Key: LA = lateral nucleus; BA = basal nucleus; CE = central nucleus.

(C)

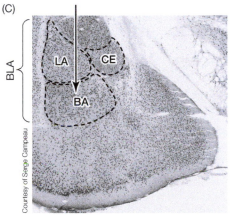

(D)

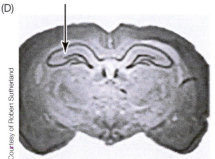

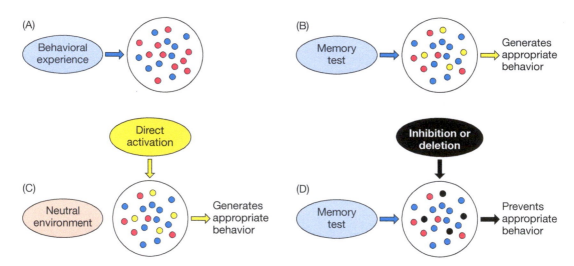

FIGURE 14.2 To conclude that neurons belong to an engram, the researcher must (A) be able to tag cells activated by the behavioral experience (red circles), (B) demonstrate that some of those cells are also activated by the memory test (yellow circles), (C) demonstrate that direct activation of these cells generates the appropriate behavior, and (D) demonstrate that inhibiting or ablating these specific cells (black circles) prevents the occurrence of the appropriate behavior.

expression of the engram. In spite of this limitation these approaches, combined with the work of neuroanatomists, have proven enormously valuable in generating hypotheses about where to look for engram cells and identifying the neural components of the various "memory systems" that are discussed in later chapters.

To move the field forward required methods that allowed identification of specific neurons that belong to the engram. Minimally, four criteria must be met (Figure 14.2).

1. The cells must be active both at the time of the learning experience and at the time of the memory test.
2. Their presence must be correlated with the generation of the appropriate memory.
3. When directly activated they can produce the behavioral expression of the memory.
4. When inhibited or deleted the behavioral expression of the memory will be prevented or reduced.

Neurons that meet these criteria are sometimes referred to as **engram cells**— they are members of the engram.

Immediate Early Genes

Fortunately, when a neuron depolarizes, the rise of intracellular calcium and other second-messenger pathways transiently activates the expression of **immediate early genes (IEGs)**, such as *c-Fos* and *Arc*. Such transient IEG activity can be used to mark a neuron that was activated by a behavioral experience. Paul Frankland's laboratory, for example, has used Fos expression to produce a brainwide mapping of neurons activated by the retrieval of a contextual fear memory (Wheeler et al., 2013).

When transcribed in the nucleus, *Arc* very quickly translocates to the cytoplasm. John Guzowski took advantage of this to successfully determine the correspondence between neurons activated when the rat explores the same environment on two different occasions (Guzowski et al., 1999). Thus, if the same neuron is activated by both experiences *Arc* should be present in *both* its nucleus and the cytoplasm, whereas cells activated by only the first or second experience would have *Arc* expressed only in *either* the nucleus or the cytoplasm (Figure 14.3).

IEG markers of cell activity are valuable but have a major limitation—they do not endure for very long (just a few minutes). This means that they cannot be used to determine if a cell is involved in an engram that supports a lasting memory. Methods were needed that could more permanently label cells activated at the time of a learning experience so that they could be compared with cells activated at the time of memory retrieval.

The TetTag Mouse

The development of a transgenic mouse called the **TetTag mouse** by Mark Mayford's group (Reijmers et al., 2007) provided an important step toward

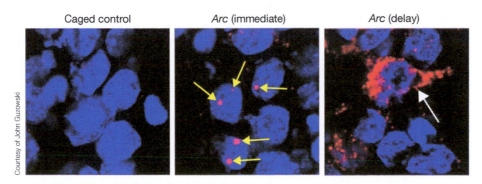

Caged control   *Arc* (immediate)   *Arc* (delay)

Courtesy of John Guzowski

FIGURE 14.3   The immediate early gene *Arc* has been used to identify cells that were activated by two experiences in the same context. *Arc* is immediately expressed in the nucleus but within about 15 minutes translocates to the cytoplasm. By comparing the location of *Arc* in cell populations following two experiences it is possible to tell which cells responded to both experiences. Such cells would contain *Arc* in both the nucleus and cytoplasm.

this goal. This mouse was genetically engineered so that it was possible to tag a recently activated neuron with a reporter gene *tau-LacZ* (LAC), which would fluoresce when exposed to light and serve as a mark or tag that the cell had been active. An important property of this tag is that it can endure for several days. How does this work?

Under normal circumstances when a cell is activated the IEG *c-Fos* will be expressed. The TetTag mouse was genetically engineered so that Fos promotes the expression of what is called the tetracycline–transactivator (tTA) system. When expressed, the tTA system has downstream effects that promote the expression of the reporter gene LAC. In order for the tTA system to be useful, however, the researcher must have *temporal control* over it—that is, it should promote LAC expression only when the animal is learning. The critical feature of the TetTag mouse is that it permits temporal control. To exert temporal control, Reijmers et al. (2007) used what is called a tTA OFF system. In this system, tTA's downstream effect on transcription is under the control of an antibiotic, doxycycline (DOX), that is in an animal's drinking water. As long as DOX is present the tTA system cannot promote the downstream effects that lead to LAC expression. However, when DOX is not present, Fos-promoted tTA expression will promote the expression of LAC. Thus, by controlling when DOX is present, the researcher can determine the temporal window when the reporter gene will be activated and thus tag the neuron with a visible marker for later identification (Figure 14.4).

Mayford's laboratory developed the TetTag mouse to find engram cells in the basolateral amygdala that might be produced by a contextual fear-conditioning experience. Just prior to the conditioning event, DOX was removed from the water so that the tTA system would drive the expression of the LAC reporter in cells activated by conditioning. DOX was then put back in the water so that no additional cells would be tagged with LAC during the fear test. To qualify as a putative engram cell, the cell had to contain both the reporter gene LAC (which marked cells activated at the time of learning) and a marker for an IEG, *Zif/Egr* (ZIF), which tagged cells activated by the test cues. Using this methodology, they were able to find cells active both at the time of conditioning and during the test. However, only a small number of cells (12%) tagged by the conditioning event contained both markers (see Figure 14.4).

Mayford's results are important because they demonstrated that it was possible to tag neurons that likely belonged to an engram supporting a fear memory. However, these active cells could only be identified in fixed tissue, which precluded the ability to study their functional properties—for example, whether their activation would produce a behavioral expression of memory and whether their inhibition would prevent the expression of the memory. Thus, one can only speculate that they may belong to the engram that supports the memory.

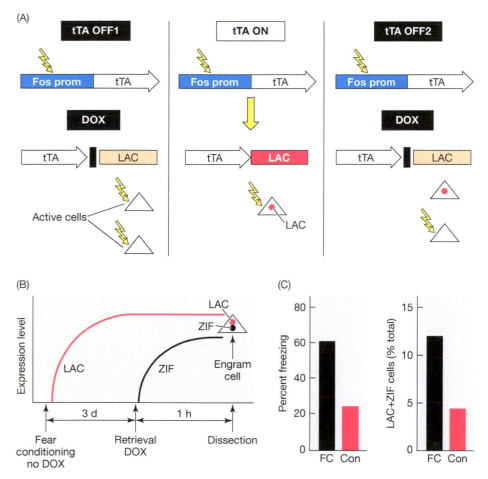

FIGURE 14.4 (A) The TetTag mouse is genetically engineered so that a reporter gene, *tau-LacZ* (LAC), will be expressed only in cells that are active at a particular time. In this system, in response to neural activity, the Fos promotor drives the expression of the tTA system, which then promotes the expression of LAC. Temporal control of expression of LAC is regulated through a tTA ON system. As long as doxycycline (DOX) is in the animal's drinking water (tTA OFF) the tTA system cannot drive LAC expression. When DOX is removed from the water, however, tTA expression promotes the transcription of LAC (tTA ON). This results in active cells being tagged with LAC. When DOX is returned to the drinking water (tTA OFF2), LAC will continue to be expressed in cells tagged during the tTA ON period but will not be expressed in other cells that might be active during this period. (B) Fear conditioning takes place with DOX removed, and cells that are active during this period are tagged with the LAC reporter, which persists for several days. Cells that are active during the retrieval test briefly express the IEG ZIF. Brains are then prepared for cell counts. Cells that are tagged with both LAC and the IEG marker ZIF are considered engram cells because they were activated by both the conditioning experience and the retrieval test. (C) Animals that were conditioned (FC) displayed more freezing behavior compared to controls (Con) and showed more LAC+ZIF co-labeled cells than controls. (Figure after L. G. Reijmers et al. 2007. *Science* 317: 1230–1233.)

Optogenetics

The ability to study the functional properties of neurons changed dramatically with the development of optogenetics (discussed in Chapter 9) and the ability to combine it with the tTA system and other methods for tagging cells (see DeNardo and Luo, 2017). In a ground-breaking set of experiments, Tonegawa's laboratory (Liu et al., 2012) used a virus to infect neurons in the dentate gyrus of the hippocampus with the gene for channelrhodopsin-2 (ChR2). Recall that this gene codes channels that conduct positive ions into the cell. Thus, when stimulated by blue light, action potentials would be generated in these neurons (see Chapter 9). The goal was to have neurons activated by a contextual fear conditioning event express these channels. If these cells belong to the fear engram then by stimulating them with blue light the behavioral expression of the fear memory—behavioral freezing—should occur. To achieve this goal the tTA system was used to provide temporal control over the expression of ChR2. So as long as the mice were on DOX, the Fos promotor could not activate the expression of ChR2. Therefore, prior to fear conditioning, DOX was removed from the drinking water so that the neurons activated by the conditioning event would express ChR2. Following training the mice were placed back on DOX to prevent any further expression of ChR2. Remarkably, when mice were later placed into a familiar nonaversive environment, applying blue light to these neurons produced the same behavior, freezing, that was elicited in the context where shock was delivered (Figure 14.5). This finding supports the conclusion

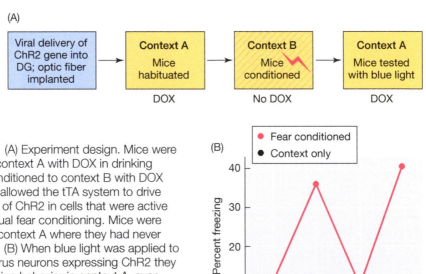

(A)

Viral delivery of ChR2 gene into DG; optic fiber implanted	→	Context A Mice habituated	→	Context B Mice conditioned	→	Context A Mice tested with blue light
		DOX		No DOX		DOX

FIGURE 14.5 (A) Experiment design. Mice were habituated to context A with DOX in drinking water, then conditioned to context B with DOX removed. This allowed the tTA system to drive the expression of ChR2 in cells that were active during contextual fear conditioning. Mice were then tested in context A where they had never been shocked. (B) When blue light was applied to the dentate gyrus neurons expressing ChR2 they displayed freezing behavior in context A, even though they were never shocked in that context. When the light was off they did not display freezing. Key: DG = dentate gyrus; DOX = doxycycline. (After X. Liu et al. 2012. *Nature* 484: 381–385.)

that the cells in the dentate gyrus expressing ChR2 were engram cells for the contextual fear memory (see Tonegawa et al., 2015 for a review).

Information is processed through the hippocampus via the trisynaptic circuit (see Chapter 2). Thus, one should expect to find that a contextual fear experience should tag neurons in both the dentate gyrus and CA3. Moreover, if such cells are part of the engram that supports the contextual fear memory, then inhibiting these cells in either the dentate gyrus or CA3 should interfere with the expression of the engram. This hypothesis was addressed and confirmed by Christine Denny in René Hen's laboratory (Denny et al., 2014). They developed a transgenic animal that permitted a comparison of cells activated during conditioning with those activated at the time of testing. They successfully identified very small populations of cells in both regions that were active at the time of both conditioning and training. In addition, using optogenetics to silence cells in either subfield at the time of testing greatly reduced the tendency of the animal to freeze. Notably, they also found that many of the cells active at the time of conditioning were not activated by the test. This finding strongly suggests that of the neurons that could potentially participate in the memory engram only a small subset is actually selected. This conclusion is explored further later in this chapter.

Dynamics of Engram Formation

The experiments just discussed demonstrated that engram cells can be identified, and by controlling their activity it is possible to control the behavioral expression of the engram. Activating identified cells produced the behavioral expression of the engram, and silencing these cells prevented the behavioral expression of the engram in the presence of natural retrieval cues. Such experiments tell us very little, however, about how engrams are assembled to represent a particular behavioral experience. It is of historical interest to consider Hebb's view of the matter.

> If some way can be found of supposing that a reverberatory trace might cooperate with the structural change, *and carry the memory until the growth change is made*, we should be able to recognize the theoretical value of the trace which is an activity only, without having to ascribe all memory to it. The conception of a transient, unstable reverberatory trace is therefore useful, if it is possible to suppose also that some permanent structural change reinforces it. (Hebb, 1949, p. 62)

Very recent advances in genetics and microscopy have enabled researchers to track the behavior of specific cells activated by a learning experience and observe their dynamics in the post-learning period, including sleep, and when the memory for the experience is retrieved. To do this requires the ability to (a) record the activity of cells in the field of interest and (b) discriminate cells that were activated by the learning experience from cells that were not activated. In a remarkable set of experiments Kaoru Inokuci's group (Gandour et al., 2019) were able to do this. To measure activity of cells, they created transgenic mice that permitted them to measure transient Ca^{2+} influxes in single neurons, which is a sign of a cell's activity. They measured this activity by a head-mounted miniature fluorescent microscope that was inserted into the brain region of interest—the CA1 field in the dorsal hippocampus.

To discriminate the engram cells from non-engram cells they used a viral system to deliver a photoconvertible fluorescent protein called Kikume Green Red whose expression was under the control of a tTA-regulated Fos promotor. The important feature of this system is that cells containing this protein fluoresce *green*, but when the animal is off of DOX and the cell is activated, thereafter the protein fluoresces *red*. This means that cells activated by the learning experience (theoretically engram cells) will fluoresce red but non-engram cells will fluoresce green.

Gandour et al. (2019) used this methodology to measure the activity of engram and non-engram cells (a) at the time of learning, (b) for several hours thereafter, and (c) at the time of retrieval. They were interested in tracking the development of an engram established when the animal explores a particular context—a contextual memory. Based on prior results they knew that the CA1 region of the dorsal hippocampus contained engram cells that supported the context memory. Several important findings emerged (Gandour et al., 2019).

- During exploration of the novel context (the learning phase), cells identified as engram cells fire much more repetitively than non-engram cells.
- During sleep the population activity of engrams remained similar to the activity observed during the learning session.
- The population activity of non-engram cells, in contrast, was more varied and became dissimilar to activity of non-engram cells during learning.
- The engram population is composed of several subensembles that replay the initial experience.
- Some of the subensemble activity present at the time of learning did not replay.
- Only subensembles activated during sleep were reactivated during retrieval.
- These ensembles were not activated when the mice were placed in a different context.

This pattern of results strongly suggests that repetitive synchronous activity among subensembles allows the engram to survive through the post-learning period and provide a basis for context memories (Figure 14.6). Hebb no doubt would be pleased by this finding.

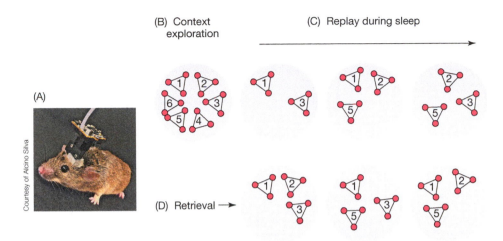

FIGURE 14.6 (A) A mouse with a head-mounted miniature fluorescent microscope. (B) Mice were genetically engineered so that cells activated by context exploration switched from fluorescing green to fluorescing red. Context exploration activated subassemblies of neurons. Each number represents a specific subassembly. (C) During sleep some but not all of these subassemblies replayed. In contrast, neurons that continued to fluoresce green did not display coherent activity patterns of replay (not illustrated). (D) During the retrieval period when the mice were returned to the context, only subassemblies that were replayed during sleep were activated. (B–D after K. Gandour et al. 2019. *Nat Commun* 10: 2637–2671.)

What Gets to Be an Engram Cell?

Recall that both Reijmers et al. (2017) and Denny et al. (2014) reported that many of the neurons active at the time of the learning event were not activated during the retrieval of the memory. They did not become engram cells. In addition, as just described, some of the subensembles activated by the learning event dropped out during sleep and were not activated by retrieval. Such observations raise an interesting question: given that the population of neurons that have the potential to become members of the engram far exceeds the number that actually do, *what determines which cells get selected to belong to an engram?*

The work of Sheena Josselyn and her colleagues has led the way to an answer (Josselyn, 2010; Josselyn and Frankland, 2018). The story begins with the discovery that the viral overexpression of the transcription factor CREB in neurons in the lateral amygdala rescued a long-term memory deficit in conditioned fear (Josselyn et al., 2001; Figure 14.7). This observation led to the hypothesis that the virally infected neurons overexpressing CREB were preferentially recruited to the fear engram. This hypothesis was confirmed by the finding that in response to the

Sheena Josselyn

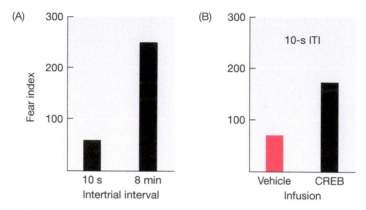

FIGURE 14.7 (A) This graph illustrates the results of a long-term memory test when the intertrial interval (ITI)—the time separating light–shock conditioning trials—was either 10 seconds or 8 minutes. Note that long-term memory was poor when the ITI was 10 seconds compared to when the ITI was 8 minutes. (B) This graph shows that injecting a virus that expresses CREB into the lateral amygdala (LA) prior to the conditioning trials can eliminate the impaired long-term memory normally found when the ITI is only 10 seconds. (After S. A. Josselyn et al. 2001. *J Neurosci* 21: 2404–2412.)

fear-generating cues, neurons overexpressing CREB also were more likely to express the IEG *Arc* (a marker of very recent cell activity) compared to the noninfected cells. Moreover, by co-infecting these CREB-expressing neurons with an inducible diphtheria toxic receptor, they were able to show that the CREB overexpressing cells belong to the engram. Diphtheria infused into the region selectively killed cells containing the receptor and this resulted in a loss of the memory (Figure 14.8).

What are the properties of neurons that overexpress CREB that favor their allocation into an engram? Given that CREB is a major transcription factor targeting memory genes, one might suppose that these cells are favored because genomic signaling initiated by synaptic activity would favor the consolidation of increases in synaptic strength that link members of the ensemble. This hypothesis, however, is wrong. It turns out that the *intrinsic excitability of neurons is increased in neurons that overexpress CREB*. This lowers the threshold for a neuron to fire action potentials in response to synaptic input, which in turn influences how it affects other neurons to which it is connected.

It is this increased excitability that allows CREB-expressing neurons to out-compete other neurons that potentially might become members of the engram. This happens because neurons in the population that could become part of the engram have inhibitory connections with other members. Thus, when potential engram cells are activated by the environmental experience (fear conditioning), the output from CREB-expressing neurons inhibits those neurons not expressing CREB and this prevents them from becoming part of the engram

(A) Some neurons (red) in the lateral amygdala are infected with CREB

(B) Fear conditioning selects neurons (blue) over-expressing CREB

(C) A neurotoxin designed to target cells that overexpress CREB erases the fear memory

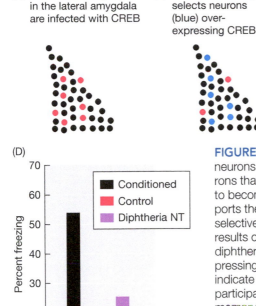

(D)

FIGURE 14.8   (A) Herpes simplex viral vector infects some neurons in the lateral amygdala with CREB. (B) These neurons that now overexpress CREB are preferentially selected to become part of the engram or memory trace that supports the fear memory. (C) Diphtheria neurotoxin (NT) selectively kills the neurons that overexpress CREB. (D) The results of the fear-conditioning experiment revealed that the diphtheria treatment that selectively killed neurons overexpressing CREB also erased the fear memory. These results indicate that (a) neurons in the lateral amygdala compete to participate in the neuron ensemble that supports the fear memory and (b) neurons expressing high levels of CREB at the time of fear conditioning win the competition. (After S. A. Josselyn. 2010. *J Psychiatry Neurosci* 35: 221–228.)

that supports the fear memory (Figure 14.9). Although this principle of engram allocation was discovered in the lateral amygdala, it also appears to operate in other brain regions, including the hippocampus, insular cortex, and piriform cortex (see Josselyn and Frankland, 2018).

(A) Potential engram cells

(B) Selected engram cells

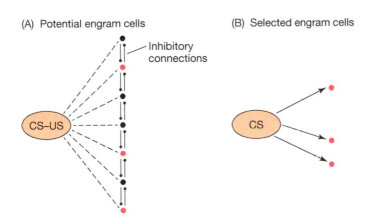

FIGURE 14.9   (A) Many cells have the potential to become engram cells. However, the excitatory threshold for cells expressing CREB (red circles) is lower than other cells. Because potential engram cells are reciprocally inhibitory, the CREB-expressing cells will inhibit other cells and prevent them from becoming engram cells. (B) This will result in only a subset of the cells activated by the learning experience becoming engram cells. Key: CS = conditioned stimulus; US = unconditioned stimulus.

Summary

For nearly 100 years memory researchers have engaged in the hunt for the properties of the brain that allow our experiences to persist and influence our thoughts and behavior. Semon's (1921) concept of the engram provides a framework to guide modern engram hunters. Advances in genetics, microscopy, and optics have made it possible for neurobiologists to identify engram cells, control their activity, study the dynamics of engram formation, and understand how they get allocated to the engram. Remarkably, Hebb's (1949) concept of cell assemblies and how they might be established through reverberating activity remains the most generally accepted view.

References

DeNardo, L. and Luo, L. (2017). Genetic strategies to access activated neurons. *Current Opinion in Neurobiology, 45*, 121–129.

Denny, C. A., Kheirbek, M. A., Alba , E. L., Tanaka, K. F., Brachman, R. A., Laughman, K. B., Tomm, N. K., Turi, G. F., Losonczy, A., and Hen, R. (2014). Hippocampal memory traces are differentially modulated by experience, time, and adult neurogenesis. *Neuron, 83*, 189–201.

Gandour, K., Ohlawa, N., Fukai, T., and Inokuci, K. (2019). Orchestrated ensemble activities constitute a hippocampal memory engram. *Nature Communications, 10*, 2637–2671.

Guzowski, J. F., McNaughton, B. L., Barnes, C. A., and Worley, P. F. (1999). Environment-specific expression of the immediate-early gene Arc in hippocampal neuronal ensembles. *Nature Neuroscience, 2*, 1120–1124.

Hebb, D. O. (1949). *Organization of Behavior.* New York: John Wiley & Sons.

Josselyn, S. A. (2010). Continuing the search for the engram: examining the mechanism of fear memories. *Journal of Psychiatry and Neuroscience, 35*, 221–228.

Josselyn, S. A. and Frankland, P. W. (2018). Memory allocation: mechanisms and function. *Annual Review of Neuroscience, 41*, 389–413.

Josselyn, S. A., Kohler, S., and Frankland, P. W. (2015). Finding the engram. *Nature Reviews Neuroscience, 16*, 521–534.

Josselyn, S. A., Kohler, S., and Frankland, P. W. (2017). Heroes of the engram. *Journal of Neuroscience, 37*, 4647–4657.

Josselyn, S. A., Shi, C., Carlezon, W. A. Jr., Neve, R. L., Nestler, E. J., and Davis, M. (2001). Long-term memory is facilitated by cAMP response element-binding protein overexpression in the amygdala. *Journal of Neuroscience, 21*, 2404–2412.

Lashley, K. S. (1950). In search of the engram. In J. F. Danielli and R. Brown (Eds.), *Symposium of the Society for Experimental Biology, IV* (pp. 454–482). Cambridge, UK: Cambridge University Press.

Liu, X., Ramirez, S., Pang, P. T., Puryear, C. B., Govindarajan, A., Deisseroth, K., and Tonegawa, S. (2012). Optogenetic stimulation of a hippocampal engram activates fear memory recall. *Nature, 484*, 381–385.

Reijmers, L. G., Perkins, B. L., Matsuo, N., and Mayford, M. (2007). Localization of a stable neural correlate of associative memory. *Science, 317*, 1230–1233.

Schacter, D. L. (1982). *Stranger Behind the Engram: Theories of Memory and the Psychology of Science*. Hillsdale, NJ: Erlbaum.

Semon, R. (1921). *The Mneme*. London: George Allen & Unwin. (Original work published 1904).

Tonegawa, S., Liu, X., Ramirez, S., and Redondo, R. (2015). Memory engram cells have come of age. *Neuron, 87*, 918–931.

Wheeler, A. L., Teixeira, C. M., Wang, A. H., Xiong, X., Kovacevic, N., Lerch, J. P., McIntosh, A. R., Parkinson, J., and Frankland, P. W. (2013). Identification of a functional connectome for long-term fear memory in mice. *PLOS Computational Biology, 9*, e1002853.

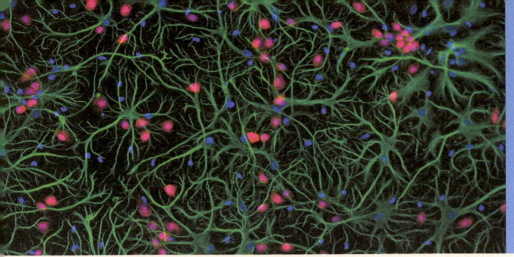

© iStock.com/jmimages

15

The Fate of Retrieved Memories

Engrams preserve our representations of the past and provide a link to the present. An engram's existence, however, can only be confirmed if sensory inputs from the present arouse it from its dormant state to influence behavior. This would be produced by Semon's process of ecphory or, in contemporary language, retrieval processes. In the experiments that we have discussed to this point, the function of retrieval was to determine the impact of some treatment on memory—did it enhance or impair the memory? However, the impact of retrieval extends far beyond merely serving as a readout for an established engram. Many researchers argue that a complete account of memory requires an understanding of how retrieval processes influence memory (Dudai, 2006; Frankland et al., 2019; Sara, 2010; Semon, 1921; Spear, 1973; Tulving and Thompson, 1973).

To provide some context for this view, consider two perspectives on retrieval functions. One perspective emerged in the 1960s when the consolidation hypothesis was being seriously evaluated by animal researchers. Specifically, a phenomenon called **cue-dependent amnesia** was reported (Lewis, 1972; Misanin et al., 1968). In essence the claim was that retrieving a memory returned it into a labile state that made it vulnerable to disruption. This is called the **destabilization function**.

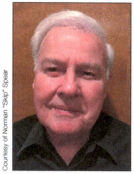

Norman Spear

Another view, articulated by Norman "Skip" Spear (1973), provides context for the second perspective. He argued that the brain may not honor the division between memory acquisition and memory retrieval. Acquisition and retrieval are terms used by researchers to describe experimental manipulations or phases of an experiment. From the brain's standpoint, however, the retrieval test is just another experience, which includes both retrieved information contained in the engram and new information provided by the present experience. In effect the brain does not know whether it is acquiring a new memory or retrieving an old one. The role of the brain is to assess this new content and integrate it with previously acquired information represented in the engram, which results in a *new engram that contains both the retrieved and new information*. This is called the **integrative function**. These two views of retrieval functions (destabilization and integration) provide a framework for addressing the question, *what is the fate of a retrieved memory?*

Historical Context

As noted in Chapter 9 initial evaluations of the consolidation hypothesis centered on the use of electroconvulsive shock (ECS) to "disrupt" consolidation. In many cases the delivery of ECS shortly after acquisition training did produce

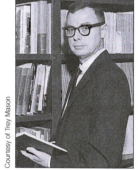

Donald J. Lewis

amnesia. However, debate centered on the source of the amnesia. Was the amnesia the result of a storage failure or was it due to a retrieval failure? Many results were consistent with the retrieval failure account because the memory could be recovered. For example, if the retention interval was increased, recovery from the amnesia sometimes was observed—the memory could be retrieved. It was also the case that a brief reminder cue, composed of some aspect of the original training (also called a **reactivation treatment**), given prior to the memory test could "restore the memory." In this context Donald Lewis (Misanin et al., 1968) discovered cue-dependent amnesia—amnesia produced when a retrieved memory is followed by a disrupting event such as ECS. The experiment was simple: instead of giving ECS after initial training he gave it after a reactivation treatment and this produced amnesia for the original memory.

Cue-Dependent Amnesia

In the Lewis study, a Pavlovian fear conditioning procedure was used to establish the fear memory trace (engram). Rats received a single pairing of a noise conditioned stimulus (CS) and a shock unconditioned stimulus (US). The next day, after the trace was "consolidated," some rats were brought to the training environment where the noise CS was presented for 2 seconds. This experience was designed to retrieve or reactivate the fear memory trace. To determine if the reactivated trace was vulnerable to disruption, some of these rats also received ECS immediately after the reactivation experience. Other

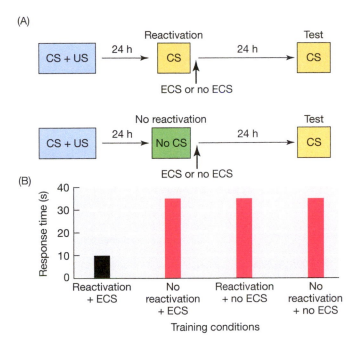

FIGURE 15.1 (A) Lewis used a fear-conditioning experiment to study the vulnerability of a reactivated memory—a noise CS was paired with a shock US. In one condition, 24 hours after fear conditioning, the CS was presented to reactivate the fear memory. Some animals received electroconvulsive shock (ECS), while others did not. In the second condition, the fear memory was not reactivated, but animals received either ECS or no ECS. All animals were tested for fear of the CS. (B) The results of the experiment. Note that when the memory trace was reactivated by briefly presenting the CS, ECS disrupted the memory for the CS shock experience. ECS had no effect when it was presented in the absence of shock. (After J. R. Misanin et al. 1968. *Science* 160: 554–558.)

rats also received ECS the next day, but without the reactivation experience. Rats that received both the reactivation treatment and ECS were extremely impaired when given a full test the next day, that is, they showed no fear in the presence of the noise (Figure 15.1). ECS had disrupted a fear memory trace that had already had time to consolidate and attain long-term memory status. These rats displayed cue-dependent amnesia.

Active Trace Theory

Recall from previous chapters that memory traces can be distinguished by their state of activation. When initially formed, memory traces are said to be in an active state and vulnerable to disruption but, with time, the trace becomes inactive and more resistant to disrupting events (see Chapter 9). In explaining cue-dependent amnesia, Lewis argued that retrieving an established memory

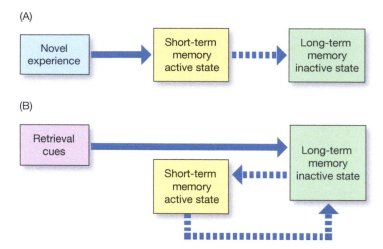

FIGURE 15.2 This figure illustrates the assumptions of Lewis's active trace theory. Memories exist in either a short-term memory (STM) active state or a long-term memory (LTM) inactive state. (A) A novel experience can create an active STM trace that will decay into the inactive LTM state. (B) Retrieval cues can retrieve an inactive LTM trace and place it in the active state that then will decay into the inactive LTM state. Memories in the active state are more vulnerable to disruption than memories in the inactive state.

returned it to an active state and temporarily increased its vulnerability to disruption (Lewis, 1972). The specific assumptions of this framework are as follows (Figure 15.2).

- Memories can exist in either a short-term memory active state or long-term memory inactive state.

- There are two ways a memory trace can be put into the short-term active state: (1) novel experiences generate new active memory traces, and (2) retrieving or reactivating existing long-term memory traces will return these traces to the short-term active state.

- Memories in the active state are vulnerable to disruption.

- Memory traces become inactive with time, and in the inactive state they are less vulnerable to disruption.

Lewis's results and theory were intriguing but also generated much controversy. Although some researchers replicated these results, others did not, and no one had any idea as to why this was the case. Two findings, however, brought the idea that reactivated memories are vulnerable to disruption out of hibernation and the second of these findings contributed to a new theoretical interpretation—**reconsolidation theory**.

Reconsolidation Theory

Susan Sara reported the first important result (Przybyslawski and Sara, 1997). Rats were first trained to solve a spatial-learning task. The researchers discovered that if an NMDA antagonist was systemically injected following the reactivation of this memory trace, the rats were not able to perform the task the next day. They also reported that memory was disrupted only if the drug was given within 90 minutes of reactivating the memory. This suggested the intriguing possibility that reactivated memories might need to be reconsolidated.

Shortly thereafter, Karim Nader and his colleagues (Nader et al., 2000) published their novel findings and the fate of retrieved memories and the concept of reconsolidation entered center stage. Nader's experiments were similar to the Lewis experiment (Misanin et al., 1968) with two exceptions.

1. Instead of delivering ECS, the protein synthesis inhibitor anisomycin was injected into the lateral nucleus of the amygdala following the reactivation of a Pavlovian conditioned, auditory-cue fear memory.

2. The rats were tested twice. One test was designed to measure the effect of anisomycin on short-term memory. The other test, at a longer retention interval, was designed to test anisomycin's effect on long-term memory.

Anisomycin had no effect on the short-term memory test but produced a large impairment on the long-term memory test (Figure 15.3).

(A)

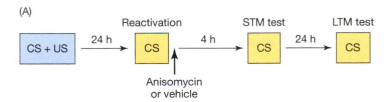

(B)

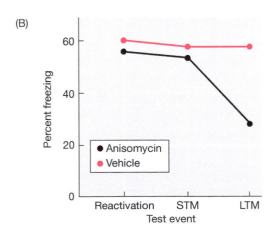

FIGURE 15.3   (A) The design of Nader's experiment. Rats were conditioned to an auditory-cue CS paired with a shock US. Following the reactivation of the fear memory, either the protein synthesis inhibitor anisomycin or the vehicle solution in which the drug was suspended was injected into the lateral nucleus of the amygdala. Rats were then given either a short-term memory (STM) test or a long-term memory (LTM) test. (B) Anisomycin disrupted the long-term retention of the reactivated fear memory but had no effect on the short-term retention of the memory. (After K. Nader et al. 2000. *Nature* 406: 722–726.)

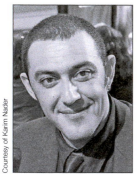

Karim Nader

It should be noted that many years prior to Nader's work, Judge and Quartermain (1982) reported that anisomycin could produce cue-dependent amnesia when given following a reactivation treatment. They concluded that the reactivation event made the memory vulnerable to the effects of anisomycin but did not speculate on just how it produced amnesia, even though it was known to inhibit protein synthesis.

Thus, neither the idea that active memory traces are vulnerable to disruption nor the idea that anisomycin could produce cue-dependent amnesia was new. The reason Nader's result captured the interest of neurobiologists was that he proposed a bold new idea called reconsolidation theory to explain the result (Nader, 2003). Nader's theory, which has two parts, is illustrated in Figure 15.4. First, he proposed that when a memory is retrieved *the synapses underlying the trace become unbound or weakened*. This means that retrieval itself can disrupt or destabilize an established memory trace and thereby produce amnesia. This thought is disconcerting. It implies that the very act of retrieval can potentially cause the memory to be lost. The reason this does not happen is explained by his second assumption—that *retrieval also initiates another round of protein synthesis so that the trace is "reconsolidated."* The new round of protein synthesis rescues the trace weakened by retrieval.

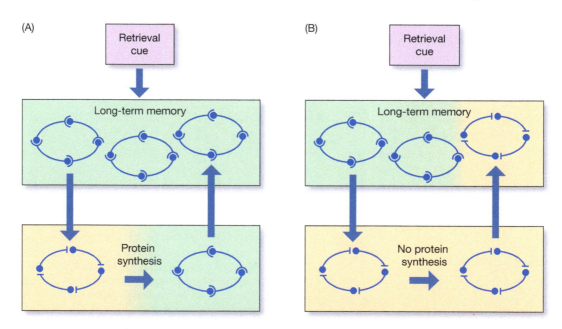

FIGURE 15.4 (A) A retrieval cue activates a well consolidated but inactive memory trace from long-term memory. The synaptic connections linking the neurons involved in the trace become unbound. However, retrieval also initiates protein synthesis and the memory trace is reconsolidated. Thus, when it returns to the inactive state it will be stable. (B) If protein synthesis is prevented, the memory trace will be weakened or lost when it returns to the inactive state.

Trace Destabilization

Perhaps Nader's most important and provocative claim is that *retrieving a memory itself will unbind or destabilize the synapses that support the memory.* If this is true then it should be possible to identify the cellular–molecular events that are responsible for trace destabilization. Some of the contributing events that have been uncovered are described below and illustrated in Figure 15.5.

Trace destabilization depends on a reactivating stimulus increasing dendritic spine levels of calcium, either by activating NMDA receptors, as is the case in the amygdala (Ben Mamou et al., 2006; Jarome et al., 2011) or through voltage-dependent calcium channels (vdCCs), as is the case in the hippocampus (Suzuki et al., 2008). If NMDA receptors or vdCCs are antagonized prior to reactivation, the trace does not destabilize and anisomycin has no influence on the reactivated memory.

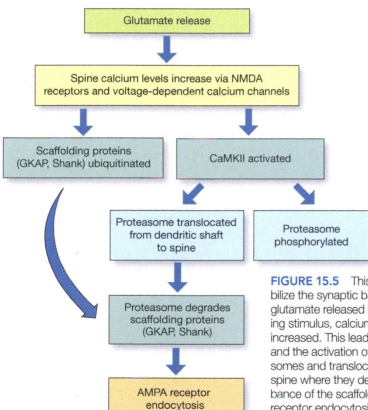

FIGURE 15.5 This figure illustrates key events that destabilize the synaptic basis of a memory trace. In response to glutamate released by neurons responding to the reactivating stimulus, calcium levels in the spine compartment are increased. This leads to ubiquitination of scaffolding proteins and the activation of CaMKII. CaMKII phosphorylates proteasomes and translocates them from the dendritic shaft to the spine where they degrade scaffolding proteins. The disturbance of the scaffolding complex could then lead to AMPA receptor endocytosis and depotentiation of the synapse. Consequently, new protein is required to restabilize the trace. However, if NMDA receptors (in the hippocampus) or voltage-gated calcium channels (in the BLA) are antagonized prior to reactivation, the trace will not destabilize. If the proteasome is inhibited, anisomycin will not affect the reactivated memory because new protein is not needed to restabilize the trace.

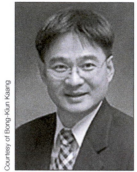

Bong-Kiun Kaang

Increased calcium levels contribute to trace destabilization by their influence on the ubiquitin proteasome system (UPS, see Chapter 6). The activation of the UPS is associated with two effects: (1) key scaffolding proteins (for example, GKAP and Shank) are ubiquitinated—tagged for degradation; and (2) CaMKII is activated and participates in activating proteasomes and translocating them from the dendritic shaft to the spine.

Bong-Kiun Kaang and his colleagues were the first to implicate the UPS as important for trace destabilization (Kaang and Choi, 2012; S. H. Lee et al., 2008). They demonstrated that reactivation of a contextual fear memory ubiquitinates scaffolding proteins in the dorsal hippocampus. These conditions set the stage for active proteasomes to degrade these proteins. One of these proteins, Shank, has been described as a master scaffolding protein that holds together other scaffolding proteins in the postsynaptic density (PSD) (Ehlers, 2003). Thus, degrading this protein would result in a major disruption of the PSD. One potential consequence of this disturbance would be the loss of the anchoring scaffolding protein, such as PSD-95, that traps AMPA receptors in the PSD. In this case there would be a decrease in the surface levels of these receptors, thereby depotentiating the synapse (see Figure 15.5). Thus, unless new protein is generated, the reactivated memory trace will not restabilize and the memory will be weakened.

If the above reasoning is correct, then it can be predicted that if the proteasome system is inhibited, scaffolding proteins will not be degraded and, therefore, new protein will not be needed to reconsolidate the memory. If so, inhibiting proteasome activity should prevent the memory loss normally produced by the protein synthesis inhibitor anisomycin. In support of this hypothesis, Kaang's group (S. H. Lee et al., 2008) reported that inhibiting proteasome activity in the hippocampus prevented the loss of a reactivated contextual fear memory (Figure 15.6) normally produced by anisomycin (see also Jarome et al., 2011).

(A)

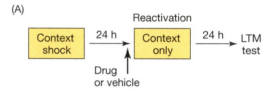

(B)

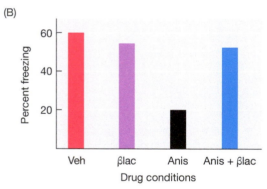

FIGURE 15.6   (A) The design of the Kaang experiment. (B) The protein synthesis inhibitor anisomycin infused prior to reactivation normally produces amnesia (reduced freezing). Inhibiting proteasome function with βlac, however, prevented destabilization of the synapses and protected against anisomycin-produced amnesia. The drugs or vehicle were injected into the hippocampus. Key: Veh = vehicle; Anis = anisomycin. (After S. H. Lee et al. 2008. *Science* 319: 1253–1256.)

What Triggers Destabilization?

It is disconcerting to think that our memory traces are destabilized when retrieved. It turns out that this is not always the case (Alberini et al., 2006; Lee, 2009; Sevenster et al., 2012). This raises the question, *what conditions of retrieval must be satisfied to destabilize the trace?* Many behavioral–reactivation training parameters have been employed to assess this question and there are reviews of this in the literature (see Exton-McGuinness et al., 2015; Rodriguez-Ortiz and Bermudez-Rattoni, 2017). Some of the major points are discussed below.

This research suggests that it is difficult to destabilize very strong memories or memories that are old (Inda et al., 2011), whereas memories established using weak training parameters appear to be more easily destabilized. This view has led to the **prediction error hypothesis** (Exton-McGuinness et al., 2015; Rodriguez-Ortiz and Bermudez-Rattoni, 2017). According to this hypothesis, a prediction error occurs if information retrieved from memory does not anticipate the current experience. This is sometimes called a mismatch. When a prediction error occurs it will activate the UPS system that destabilizes the trace.

An experiment from LeDoux's group (Diaz-Mataix et al., 2013) supports this idea. Using a Pavlovian fear conditioning procedure, they exposed rats to 10 pairings of an auditory-cue CS and a brief foot-shock US. The duration of the CS was 60 seconds. On every trial, the US occurred exactly 30 seconds following the CS onset. During the reactivation phase, one set of animals received the previously established CS–US training, with the US occurring 30 seconds following the CS onset. However, for another set this interval was changed and the US was presented 10 seconds following the CS onset. Note that this arrangement would create a prediction error—*the US occurred earlier than the retrieved engram would predict*. This should destabilize the engram. Anisomycin (to prevent protein synthesis and reconsolidation) or its vehicle was injected into the amygdala following the event. The result was that only rats experiencing both the prediction error and anisomycin displayed amnesia (reduced freezing) when they were tested the next day (Figure 15.7). This result strongly supports the hypothesis that prediction errors initiate processes that destabilize the engram (see Lee, 2010 for another example).

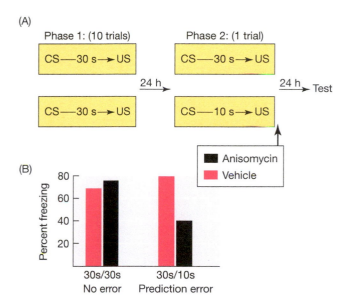

FIGURE 15.7 (A) The design of the LeDoux experiment. During phase 1 a shock unconditioned stimulus (US) was always delivered 30 seconds after the onset of the conditioned stimulus (CS). In phase 2 animals in the 30s/30s condition received one trial with the same 30-second interval separating CS onset and the presentation of US. To create a prediction error, animals in the 30s/10s condition received the shock 10 seconds after CS onset. The assumption is that these animals would predict that the US would occur 30 seconds after CS onset but this would be a prediction error because the US occurred sooner than predicted. (B) Creating the prediction error destabilized the engram so that anisomycin resulted in reduced fear. (After L. Diaz-Mataix et al. 2013. *Curr Biol* 23: 467–472.)

Destabilization, Repetition, and Integration

A basic principle of memory is that repetition of the same experience strengthens the memory. Perhaps for repetition to do this the *content of the repeated experience must be integrated into the engram representing the retrieved experience.* If this is true one might expect that the effect of repetition should depend on destabilization of the preexisting engram. Therefore, preventing destabilization should prevent the strengthening effect of repetition. Jonathan Lee (2008)

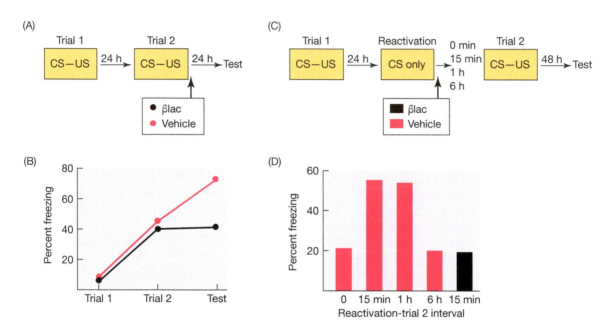

FIGURE 15.8 (A) The design of the Lee repetition experiment. (B) Additional learning normally produced by a second conditioning trial requires that the trace be destabilized because inhibiting proteasome activity by infusing βlac into the amygdala prevents the additional learning normally produced by the second trial. (C) Design of the Tay experiment. (D) Reactivating the engram produced by the first conditioning trial enhanced conditioning produced by the second trial, but only if the second trial occurred within a 15-minute to 1-hour window. This indicates that there is a temporal window of about 15 minutes to an hour during which the trace remains destabilized. This result depended on destabilizing the engram because it did not occur if proteasome activity was inhibited by βlac. (A, B after J. L. Lee et al. 2008. *Nature Neurosci* 11: 1264–1266; C, D after K. R. Tay et al. 2019. *J Neurosci* 39: 1109–1118.)

reported support for this idea (Figure 15.8). He gave rodents two contextual fear conditioning trials separated by 24 hours. To prevent destabilization, the proteasome inhibitor βlac was infused into the hippocampus prior to the second trial. As shown in Figure 15.8B, the animals infused with βlac did not benefit from the second trial. Thus, without destabilizing the engram there was no effect of the second context-shock training trial.

A slight variation of the just described experiment provides additional support for the destabilization hypothesis (Tay et al., 2019). In this case 15 minutes prior to a second context-shock trial the original memory was reactivated. The assumption was that reactivation (which did not include the shock) would destabilize the engram and facilitate the integration of the second conditioning experience into the representation of the first experience to strengthen the engram. Not only was this result obtained, preventing destabilization with βlac blocked the second conditioning trial from strengthening the engram. This experiment also revealed that there is a *temporal window* surrounding the effect of destabilization. No benefit was observed if the second conditioning trial occurred immediately following reactivation or 6 hours later. The window for integration opens about 15 minutes following reactivation and remains open for about an hour (see Figure 15.8C,D).

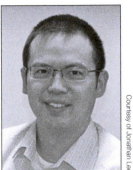

Jonathan Lee

Destabilization without Behavioral Expression

It was noted at the beginning of this chapter that an engram's existence can only be established if its retrieval produces a behavioral change appropriate to a test situation. However, it is interesting to ask, *can a destabilized engram be modified even if it does not produce a behavior*? There is a substantial literature that says it can be (see Rodriguez-Ortiz and Bermudez-Rattoni, 2017 for a review). Nader's laboratory (Ben Mamou et al., 2006) provided the seminal outcome supporting this idea. In their auditory-cue fear conditioning experiment an AMPA receptor antagonist (CNQX) was injected into the amygdala to prevent the auditory cue from evoking freezing—the behavioral expression of the memory. Nevertheless, the reactivation treatment still destabilized the fear engram because if anisomycin also was injected into the amygdala to prevent reconsolidation, the fear memory was reduced (Figure 15.9A,B). It is noteworthy, however, that blocking NMDA receptor function with the antagonist ifenpodil prevented destabilization and thus the need for reconsolidation, even though the reactivation treatment generated the freezing response (Figure 15.9C,D). These experiments established that the *fear engram exists independent of its ability to generate behavior*. This general conclusion applies to a variety of memories (Rodriguez-Ortiz and Bermudez-Rattoni, 2017).

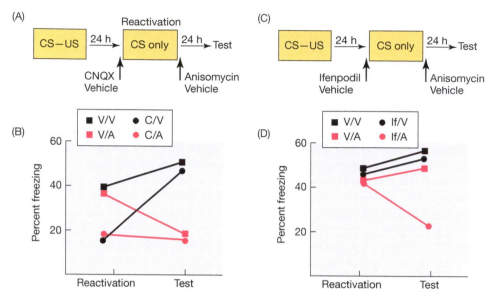

FIGURE 15.9 (A) The design of the Nader AMPA inhibition experiment. (B) Note that CNQX, an AMPA receptor antagonist, prevented the expression of the freezing response when the engram was reactivated. Nevertheless, anisomycin still produced amnesia (reduced freezing) on the test. (C) The design of the second Nader experiment. (D) Note that ifenpodil, an NMDA receptor antagonist, did not interfere with the expression of the freezing response when the engram was reactivated but it did prevent the amnesia normally produced by anisomycin (compare the If/A condition with V/A condition). Two conclusions are supported by the results: (1) the engram destabilizes even if the freezing behavior does not occur when the engram is reactivated, and (2) calcium-dependent processes initiated via NMDA receptors are essential to destabilize the engram. Key: A = anisomycin; C = CNQX; If = ifenpodil; V = vehicle. (Both experiments after C. Ben Mamou et al. 2006. *Nature Neurosci* 9: 1237–1239.)

Integration Theory and Amnesia

A strong case has been made that information contained in our current environment can become integrated into a retrieved engram. This conclusion also has implications for understanding amnesia. As noted, a classic debate centered on whether amnesia is a result of a storage failure or a retrieval failure. Proponents of the storage failure position argue that amnesia produced by reactivation coupled with some pharmacological treatment (such as anisomycin) represents a failure of the reactivated engram to be restored (reconsolidated). However, there is an alternative interpretation. Specifically, integration theorists Pascale Gisquet-Verrier and David Riccio (2018) argue that amnesia produced by this combination of events is a retrieval failure. Their argument centers around what is called the **encoding specificity principle** (Tulving and Thompson, 1973). The principle is that successful memory retrieval depends on a *match* *between the retrieval cues and the environmental stimulation encoded into the engram.* Retrieval failure will occur when key retrieval cues are missing. You have experienced amnesia due to retrieval failure many times, as when you initially can't remember where you put your phone but after providing yourself more retrieval cues you remember where it is.

To appreciate how this view can potentially explain amnesia associated with reconsolidation treatments, the phenomenon called **state-dependent learning** has to be introduced. The basic idea is that cues generated by our internal state at the time of a learning experience can become part of the engram, and these internal state cues need to be present at the time of retrieval to awaken the engram. As a simple example, if you are asked to memorize one list of words in a state of sadness and another list in the state of happiness, retrieval will be better if you are tested in the state you were in when you learned the list, for example happy–happy as opposed to happy–sad (Bower, 1981). Internal states induced by drugs are known to become part of the engram and thus are needed at the time of retrieval to activate the engram (Overton, 1991).

According to Gisquet-Verrier and Riccio (2018), when anisomycin or some other drug treatment is administered following reactivation of the memory, the internal conditions it produces become part of the engram and these internal conditions need to be part of the retrieval cue complex if the engram is going to be successfully retrieved. Thus, anisomycin does not produce amnesia because it prevented reconsolidating the engram—a storage failure. The amnesia is a retrieval failure because the internal state cues produced by anisomycin were not present when the animals were tested. Gisquet-Verrier and Riccio reviewed many experiments that support this interpretation. For example, if the protein synthesis inhibitor cycloheximide was injected systemically or into relevant brain structures following reactivation of an avoidance conditioning memory, avoidance performance was better if the cycloheximide was also administered prior to the test (Gisquet-Verrier et al., 2015).

Integration theory as articulated by Gisquet-Verrier and Riccio (2018) can provide an alternative account of some reconsolidation experiments. Perhaps of more importance is that their integration theory is based on the idea that information present in the current environment can become integrated into a destabilized–reactivated engram.

Memory Erasure: A Potential Therapy

Reactivated memories can be destabilized and modified. This fact has encouraged researchers to pursue the possibility that drug treatments given after reactivation might be successful in eliminating memories that are the basis of serious behavioral disorders. This strategy has been pursued to develop potential treatments for two important clinical problems: (1) drug addiction and relapse, and (2) debilitating fears such as those associated with post-traumatic stress disorder.

Cycle of addiction

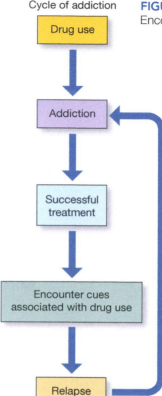

FIGURE 15.10 This figure illustrates the drug addiction–relapse cycle. Encountering cues associated with drug use can lead to relapse.

Drug Relapse

One of the major problems associated with drug addiction is relapse (Figure 15.10). Even after drug addicts have gone through what appears to be successful treatment, they often relapse into the addictive cycle. Environmental cues associated with drugs are one important contributor to relapse. When a drug such as cocaine is taken, the environmental cues become associated with some properties of the drug. This is another example of Pavlovian conditioning. When these cues are encountered, they induce or create a craving or urge to take the drug (Figure 15.11). This state is well documented in people (Childress et al., 1999). In some ways it is similar to the urge one experiences when encountering a bag of potato chips or the sight of chocolate candy. However, the urge associated with drug-related cues is much more potent and difficult to resist.

Imagine that a person with a specific drug addiction has gone through treatment and is now off the drug. Unfortunately, when he or she later encounters cues that were associated with the drug, the urge produced can be so powerful that relapse occurs and the individual reverts back to taking the drug. Given the power of these drug-related cues to evoke memories that produce relapse, it would be of enormous benefit to find treatment methods that could be used to attenuate or erase these memories. Some studies with rodents suggest that this might eventually be possible.

FIGURE 15.11 Cues associated with drug use induce a conditioned cocaine high, a craving for cocaine, and a wish to get high. The graph shows changes in the subjective state of recovering cocaine addicts after viewing a video showing simulated purchase, preparation, and smoking of crack cocaine. The subjects were patients in a treatment center and had not used cocaine for about 14 days. (After A. R. Childress et al. 1999. *Am J Psychiatry* 156: 11–18.)

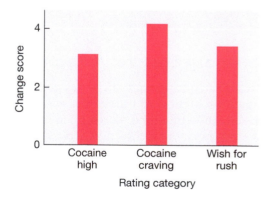

(A)

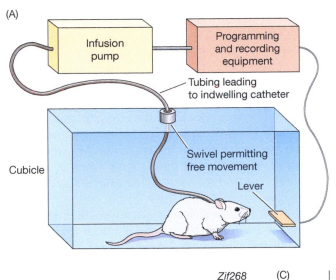

FIGURE 15.12   (A) The experimental methodology used to train a rat to press a lever
to self-administer a drug and become drug
addicted. A conditioned stimulus (CS) is also
presented when the drug is delivered. The
presentation of the drug-associated CS can
produce drug-seeking behavior (relapse) in
rats that have learned that lever pressing no
longer produces the drug. (B) The vehicle or
an antisense that blocks the translation of the
gene *Zif268* is delivered after repeated CS presentations. (C) This graph shows that during
the test for relapse the rats treated with *Zif268*
antisense made fewer bar presses than rats
who received the vehicle. This result suggests
that *Zif268* antisense prevented the reconsolidation of the drug memory associated with
the CS. (After J. L. Lee et al. 2005. *Neuron* 47:
795–801.)

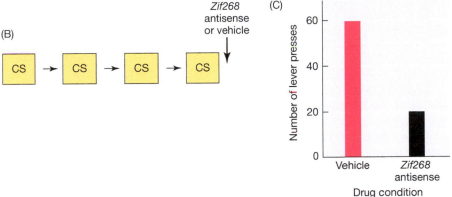

Preventing Relapse

Barry Everitt and his colleagues (Lee et al., 2005, 2006) have used the reactivation procedure to eliminate the ability of drug-related cues to produce relapse
in rats that have learned to self-administer cocaine. The exact procedures for
their experiments are complicated but basically entail training rats to learn a
lever-press response that produces an infusion of cocaine (Figure 15.12A). This
is the drug-seeking response. During this training the delivery of the cocaine
is also paired with a Pavlovian CS, the presentation of a light. The light is thus
associated with the drug. Theoretically, the light acquires the ability to evoke
an urge to take the drug and its presence can lead to relapse. To demonstrate
relapse, rats receive a session of training in which the response no longer produces the drug or the light. This results in the elimination of the drug-seeking

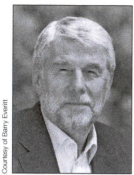

Barry Everitt

response. If these rats then receive presentations of the light CS, they will relapse into drug-seeking behavior.

Everitt's group asked if the reactivation procedure could be used to eliminate the memory evoked by the CS and thus prevent relapse. To do this they presented rats with multiple presentations of the CS without the drug. They then infused an antisense into the amygdala, which was designed to prevent translation of the immediate early gene *Zif268* that is known to play a role in reconsolidation. This protein is expressed in the amygdala in response to presentations of the drug-associated CS. Thus, Everitt reasoned that it might be involved in the reconsolidation of the reactivated drug memory. Remarkably, preventing the expression of the Zif268 protein completely eliminated the ability of the CS to induce relapse. The rats behaved as if the light–drug memory had been erased (Figure 15.12B).

There are many reports from animal models that disrupting their reconsolidation can impair drug-related memories. Moreover, many of the signaling pathways involved in reconsolidation of these memories have been identified. Unfortunately, as yet, there is no strong evidence that the tools of the reconsolidation procedure have been translated into clinical treatment programs (see Sorg, 2012).

Based on laboratory success it was hoped that the methods employed in the reconsolidation domain might be successfully applied in clinical settings to erase debilitating memories associated with drug addiction or post-traumatic stress disorders. Post-traumatic stress disorder is a severe anxiety disorder that can occur in a person who experiences one or more traumatic events. Although not conclusive, the evidence suggests that giving propranolol (the adrenergic receptor antagonist) during the post-trauma period may retard the development of this syndrome. Even if this treatment proves effective, however, it may not be applicable to people who have already developed the syndrome. Given the vulnerability of reactivated memories to disruption, there is some hope that it might be possible to develop therapies based on this methodology to treat people with existing debilitating fears.

The possible application of the reactivation procedure to help eliminate fear was explicitly recognized by Przybyslawski et al. (1999). They reported that the systemic administration of propranolol following the reactivation of an inhibitory avoidance memory greatly attenuated subsequent avoidance responding. Debiec and Nader (2004) also found that systemic injections of propranolol following the reactivation of the auditory-cue fear memory attenuated the rat's subsequent response to that cue.

Such experiments are far removed from clinical application, and unfortunately attempts at translating these tools to the clinical setting have been disappointing. In reviewing the current state of affairs, Roger Pitman concluded that "the translational gap to clinical application is huge" (Pitman, 2011, p.1) and described many of the difficulties that will have to be overcome if there ever will be clinical benefit from this work. So the promissory note is not yet fulfilled.

Rather than trying to erase debilitating memories by blocking their reconsolidation with pharmacological agents, some clinical researchers are now attempting to modify reactivated memories by taking advantage of the destabilization period to integrate counteracting experiences into the engram (Gisquet-Verrier and Riccio, 2018; Lee et al., 2017). It remains to be determined if this approach will be successful in a clinical setting (see Lee et al., 2017 for a review and assessment of this approach).

Summary

Two perspectives on retrieval processes, the *destabilization function* and the *integration function,* have contributed to our understanding of the fate of retrieved memories. The destabilization view originated with Don Lewis's report that reactivated memories are returned to an active state and might be vulnerable to disruption. He suggested that it is the state of the memory trace—active versus inactive—that makes it vulnerable to disruption. Interest in the destabilization function increased when Nader proposed the reconsolidation hypothesis—that retrieving a memory has two effects: (1) it unbinds/destabilizes the synapses that hold members of the engram together, and (2) it initiates a new round of protein synthesis that will ensure that the engram is restabilized.

The integration function perspective can be traced back to Semon (1921) and has modern proponents (Gisquet-Verrier and Riccio, 2018). Retrieval processes not only activate the engram they set conditions for the information contained in the present to be integrated with the information contained in the retrieved engram to create a new updated engram.

The destabilization and integrative perspectives emphasize different outcomes produced by retrieval processes. However, the research discussed in this chapter yields an important conclusion: *these two functions are intimately related.* The integration of new information into the retrieved engram appears to depend on retrieval processes destabilizing the engram, which does not always occur.

Destabilization is driven in part by a mismatch between information contained in the engram and what actually happens—a prediction error. When this happens a set of calcium-dependent processes is engaged to activate the ubiquitin–proteasome system to degrade scaffolding proteins that anchor AMPA receptors with a resulting loss of these receptors weakening of the engram. For about an hour (before the engram restabilizes) a window of opportunity exists that permits integration to occur. Because new information is now integrated into the engram, integration theorists note that this alters the conditions for subsequent retrieval. Unless the conditions of retrieval now match those represented in the new engram (the encoding specificity principle), amnesia resulting from a retrieval failure can occur. Future application of retrieval research to clinical problems likely will exploit the destabilization–integration functions to alter the engrams to contain information that counters behavioral pathologies.

References

Alberini, C. M., Milekic, M. H., and Tronel, S. (2006). Mechanisms of memory stabilization and de-stabilization. *Cell Molecular Life Science, 63*, 999–1008.

Ben Mamou, C., Gamache, K., and Nader, K. (2006). NMDA receptors are critical for unleashing consolidated auditory fear memories. *Nature Neuroscience, 9*, 1237–1239.

Bower, G. (1981). Mood and memory. *American Psychologist, 36*, 129–148.

Childress, A. R., Mozley, P. D., McElgin, W., Fitzgerald, J., Reivich, M., and O'Brien, C. P. (1999). Limbic activation during cue-induced cocaine craving. *American Journal of Psychiatry, 156*, 11–18.

Debiec, J. and Nader, K. (2004). Disruption of reconsolidation but not consolidation of auditory fear conditioning by noradrenergic blockade in the amygdala. *Neuroscience, 129*, 267–272.

Diaz-Mataix, L., Ruiz Martinez, R. C., Schafe, G. E., and LeDoux, J. E. (2013). Detection of a temporal error triggers reconsolidation of amygdala-dependent memories. *Current Biology, 23*, 467–472.

Dudai, Y. (2006). Reconsolidation: the advantages of being refocused. *Current Opinion in Neurobiology, 16*, 174–178.

Ehlers, M. (2003). Ubiquitin and the deconstruction of synapses. *Science, 302*, 800–801.

Exton-McGuinness, M. T., Lee, J. L., and Reichelt, A. C. (2015). Updating memories— the role of prediction errors in memory reconsolidation. *Behavioral Brain Research, 278*, 375–384.

Frankland, P. W., Josselyn, S. A., and Kohler, S. (2019). The neurobiological foundation of memory retrieval. *Nature Neuroscience, 22*, 1576–1585.

Gisquet-Verrier, P., Lynch, J. F., Cutolo, P., Toledano, D., Ulmen, A., Jasnow, A. M., and Riccio, D. C. (2015). Integration of new information with active memory accounts for retrograde amnesia: a challenge to the consolidation/reconsolidation hypothesis? *Journal of Neuroscience, 35*, 11623–11633.

Gisquet-Verrier, P. and Riccio, D. C. (2018). Memory integration: an alternative to the consolidation/reconsolidation hypothesis. *Progress in Neurobiology, 17*, 15–31.

Inda, M. C., Muravieva, E., and Alberini, C. M. (2011). Memory retrieval and the passage of time: from reconsolidation and strengthening to extinction. *Journal of Neuroscience, 31*, 1635–1643.

Jarome, T. J., Werner, C. T., Kwapis, J. L., and Helmstetter, F. J. (2011). Activity dependent protein degradation is critical for the formation and stability of fear memories in the amygdala. *PLOS ONE* 2011: 6:e24349. DOI: 10.1371/journal.pone.24349.

Judge, M. E. and Quartermain, D. (1982). Characteristics of retrograde amnesia following reactivation of memory in mice. *Physiology and Behavior, 4*, 585–590.

Kaang, B-K. and Choi, J-H. (2012). Synaptic protein degradation in memory reorganization. *Advances in Experimental Medicine and Biology, 970*, 221–240.

Lee, J. L. (2008). Memory reconsolidation mediates the strengthening of memories by additional learning. *Nature Neuroscience, 11,* 1264–1266.

Lee, J. L. (2009). Reconsolidation: maintaining memory relevance. *Trends in Neuroscience, 32,* 413–420.

Lee, J. L. (2010). Memory reconsolidation mediates the updating of hippocampal memory content. *Frontiers in Behavioral Neuroscience, 4,* 168.

Lee, J. L., DiCiano, P., Thomas, K. L., and Everitt, B. J. (2005). Disrupting reconsolidation of drug memories reduces cocaine-seeking behavior. *Neuron, 47,* 795–801.

Lee, J. L., Milton, A. L., and Everitt, B. J. (2006). Cue-induced cocaine seeking and relapse are reduced by disruption of drug memory reconsolidation. *Journal of Neuroscience, 26,* 5881–5887.

Lee, J. L., Nader, K., and Schiller, D. (2017). An update on memory reconsolidation updating. *Trends in Cognitive Sciences, 7,* 531–545.

Lee, S. H., Choi, J. H., Lee, N., Lee, H. R., Kim, J. I., Yu, N. K., Choi, S. L., Kim, H., and Kaang, B-K. (2008). Synaptic protein degradation underlies destabilization of retrieved fear memory. *Science, 319,* 1253–1256.

Lewis, D. J. (1972). Psychobiology of active and inactive memory. *Psychological Bulletin, 86,* 1054–1083.

Misanin, J. R., Miller, R. R., and Lewis, D. J. (1968). Retrograde amnesia produced by electroconvulsive shock after reactivation of a consolidated memory trace. *Science, 160,* 554–558.

Nader, K. (2003). Memory traces unbound. *Trends in Neurosciences, 26,* 65–72.

Nader, K., Schafe, G. E., and LeDoux, J. E. (2000). Fear memories require protein synthesis in the amygdala for reconsolidation after retrieval. *Nature, 406,* 722–726.

Overton, D. A. (1991). Historical context of state dependent learning and discriminative drug effects. *Behavioural Pharmacology, 2,* 253–264.

Pitman, R. K. (2011). Will reconsolidation blockade offer a novel treatment for posttraumatic stress disorder? *Frontiers in Behavioral Neuroscience, 5,* 11.

Przybyslawski, J., Roullet, P., and Sara, S. J. (1999). Attenuation of emotional and non-emotional memories after their reactivation: role of beta-adrenergic receptors. *Journal of Neuroscience, 19,* 6623–6238.

Przybyslawski, J. and Sara, S. J. (1997). Reconsolidation of memory after its reactivation. *Behavioural Brain Research, 84,* 241–246.

Rodriquez-Ortiz, C. J. and Bermudez-Rattoni, F. (2017). Determinants to trigger memory reconsolidation: the role of retrieval and updating information. *Neurobiology of Learning and Memory, 142,* 4–12.

Sara, S. J. (2010). Reactivation, retrieval, replay and reconsolidation in and out of sleep: connecting the dots. *Frontiers in Behavioral Neuroscience, 4,* 185.

Semon, R. W. (1921). *The Mneme*. London: G. Allen & Unwin. (Original work published 1904).

Sevenster, D., Beckers, T., and Kindt, M. (2012). Retrieval per se is not sufficient to trigger reconsolidation of human fear memory. *Neurobiology of Learning and Memory, 97*, 338–345.

Sorg, B. A. (2012). Reconsolidation of drug memories. *Neuroscience and Biobehavioral Reviews, 36*, 1400–1417.

Spear, N. E. (1973). Retrieval of memory in animals. *Psychological Review, 80*, 163–194.

Suzuki, A., Mukawa, T., Tsukagoshi, A., Frankland, P. W., and Kida, S. (2008). Activation of LVGRCCs and CB1 receptors required for destabilization of reactivated contextual fear memories. *Learning and Memory, 15*, 426–433.

Tay, K. R., Flavell, C. R., Cassini, L., Wimber, M., and Lee, J. L. (2019). Postretrieval relearning strengthens hippocampal memories via destabilization and reconsolidation. *Journal of Neuroscience, 39*, 1109–1118.

Tulving, E. and Thomson, D. (1973). Encoding specificity and retrieval processes in episodic memory. *Psychological Review, 86*, 739–748.

PART 3
Neural Systems and Memory

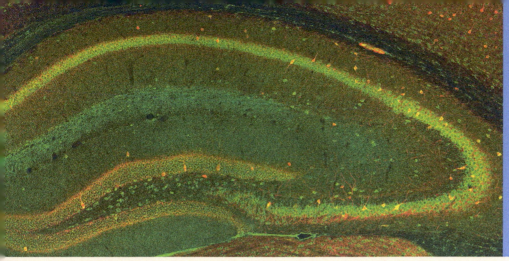

Memory Systems and the Hippocampus

We are our memories. Without a record of our experiences we would be disconnected from our past, have no recognition of our relatives and friends, possess no knowledge of the world, and would always be completely lost. We could not anticipate dangerous situations or locate the food and water we need to survive. We would be unable to acquire even the most rudimentary of skills, let alone learn to drive a car or become an expert violinist or tennis player. We could not be left alone.

The activities and functions that our memories support are remarkably varied and should make us ask, *how can the brain do all of this?* A part of the answer is that the brain contains specialized systems that are designed to store and utilize the different kinds of information contained in our experiences. Neurobiologists have achieved some basic understanding of how these systems are organized to support different types of memory.

The purpose of this chapter and the remaining ones is to introduce some of what is now known about these different systems. It begins with a quick overview of the multiple memory systems perspective, one of the important achievements of modern memory research (see Squire, 2004 for a historical overview).

The Multiple Memory Systems Perspective

The content of our experience matters to the brain. It sorts content and assigns its storage to different regions of the brain. This idea is the essence of what is called the **multiple memory systems** perspective (McDonald and White, 1993; Squire, 2004; White and McDonald, 2002). Some examples will help to explain this concept.

Example 1: Personal Facts and Emotions

Suppose you were in a minor automobile accident and no one was injured. As a consequence of that experience, you would very likely remember many of the details leading up to the accident—whom you were with, where it happened, who you thought was at fault, and so on. Now imagine that you were in a much more serious accident, you suffered facial lacerations and multiple fractures in one leg, and you were pinned in the car for some time. It was bad. This second case contains additional content. The experience was quite aversive and frightening. In addition to recording the details of the accident, your brain would record the aversive aspects of the experience in ways that might later alter your behavior. Not only would you be able to recall the cold facts of the experience, you might be afraid to drive or even get into an automobile.

The details that make up an episode and the impact of the experience are stored in different brain regions. Memory researchers have been aware of this possibility for a long time. For example, Édouard Claparède (1951), a French psychologist, reported on a test he performed on an amnesic patient with a brain pathology. He concealed a pin in his hand and then shook hands with the patient, who quickly withdrew her hand in pain. A few minutes later Claparède offered his hand to the patient again. The patient resisted shaking it. When asked why, the patient replied, "Doesn't one have a right to withdraw her hand?" Claparède then insisted on further explanation and the patient said, "Is there, perhaps, a pin hidden in your hand?" However, the patient could not give any reason why she had this suspicion.

Consider how you would react to such an experience. You also would be reluctant to shake hands, but you would be able to recall the content of the experience as an explanation of your behavior. Although Claparède's patient's brain pathology produced amnesia for the episode, it is reasonable to conclude that this pathology spared the system in the brain that was modified to produce a reluctance to shake hands. This example suggests that some aspect of the aversive content of the experience, as well as associations with the cues of the doctor, were stored outside of the region of the brain that supported recollection of the experience.

Example 2: Personal Facts and Skills

We ride bikes, drive cars, play musical instruments, ride skateboards, and do many other things quite well. The level of accomplishment obtained by individuals such as concert violinists or professional skateboarders is truly amazing. Obviously, to achieve even a functional level of performance, such as needed to safely drive a car, requires an enormous amount of practice. Once a skill is acquired, it can be performed without having any sense of awareness. The many hours of practice have left an enduring impression in the brain that now supports the skill. In addition to acquiring a skill, however, you will also remember much about the practice sessions, where they occurred, who your instructors were, and how difficult it was initially to perform. Nevertheless, these aspects of your memory have absolutely nothing to do with your ability to perform the skill. We know this because people who are amnesic in the sense of having no recollection of their training episodes can still perform (Bayley et al., 2005). The inescapable conclusion is that the memory system that supports skillful behaviors is outside of the region of the brain that supports our ability to recollect the training episodes.

Such examples and brain research have led memory researchers to believe that: (1) a complete understanding of memory can only be achieved by recognizing that the content of experience is important; and (2) memories are segregated into different brain regions according to their content. The remainder of this chapter explores the episodic memory system, how memory researchers learned that episodic memory depends on a neural system that involves the hippocampus (Figure 16.1), and different models researchers have used to study this system. The story begins with patient H.M.

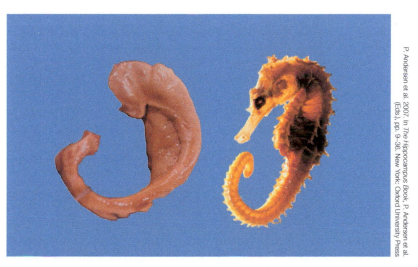

P. Andersen et al. 2007. In *The Hippocampus Book*, P. Andersen et al. (Eds.), pp. 9–36. New York: Oxford University Press

FIGURE 16.1 A hippocampus dissected from a human brain (left) and the tropical fish *hippocampus* or seahorse (right). The striking similarity in shape is undoubtedly why the Bolognese anatomist Giulio Cesare Aranzi named this brain region the hippocampus.

The Case of Henry Molaison

The two previous examples made the point that brain insults can result in the loss of the ability to recall personal experiences, while sparing memories such as those that support emotional responses, skills, and habits. It was not until Brenda Milner (Scoville and Milner, 1957) reported her analysis of the then anonymous amnesic, Henry Molaison (previously known only as H.M.), that memory researchers first gained insight into the regions of the brain that are responsible for the ability to remember experiences.

Henry Molaison is the most famous and important amnesic in the history of memory research. His personal tragedy revolutionized how we think about the relationship between memory and the brain. The seeds of Henry's tragedy were sown when, at the age of nine, he sustained a head injury that eventually led to epilepsy. Over the years his seizures became more frequent, and by the age of 27 they were so disturbing that he was no longer able to function. Because Henry's seizures were thought to originate in the temporal lobes, the decision was made to bilaterally remove these regions. This was the first time these regions had been bilaterally removed. The surgery was successful in reducing his epilepsy. Moreover, Henry's cognitive abilities were left intact; his IQ actually increased. Unfortunately, however, shortly after the surgery it was discovered that the surgery profoundly and permanently affected his memory.

Henry was brought to the attention of Milner, who then tested him in a variety of ways and described her results to the scientific community (Milner, 1965; Milner, 1970; Scoville and Milner, 1957). The essence of her analysis was that Henry had severe anterograde amnesia; he could not acquire some types of new memories. For example, he never recognized Milner even though they interacted many times. Soon after eating he could not remember what he ate or that he had eaten. His experiences registered initially and could be maintained for a short period of time. However, the memory vanished if he was distracted. Thus, although H.M.'s short-term memory was intact, his long-term memory was severely disturbed.

Although Henry had some preserved childhood memories, he had extensive retrograde amnesia that disconnected him with most of his personal past. Thus, even though other intellectual capacities remained intact, Henry could not acquire enduring new memories or remember a significant part of his past.

In spite of these severe memory impairments, formal tests revealed that some of his memory capacities were spared. For example, he was able to learn and remember the skill of mirror tracing (Figure 16.2), which requires coordinating hand movement with an inverted image of the object being traced, and a rotary-pursuit task (Corkin, 1968), which requires acquiring a new motor skill. Remarkably, even though Henry's performance improved on these tasks, he never recalled the training experiences that established the skills.

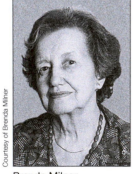

Courtesy of Brenda Milner

Brenda Milner

(A) The mirror-tracing task

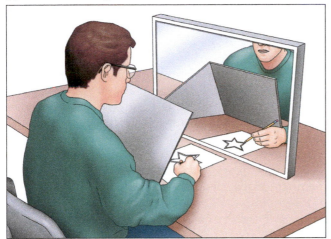

FIGURE 16.2 (A) The mirror-tracing task. (B) H.M.'s performance improved with training. (After B. Milner. 1965. In *Cognitive Processes and the Brain: An Enduring Problem for Psychology,* P. M. Milner and S. Glickman (Eds.), pp. 97–111. Princeton, NJ: Van Nostrand.)

(B) Performance of H.M. on mirror-tracing task

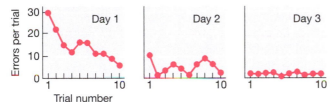

Although Henry was severely amnesic, he had some understanding of his state. Milner (1970, p. 37) reported that between tests he would suddenly look up and say rather anxiously: "Right now, I'm wondering. Have I done or said anything amiss. You see at this moment everything looks clear to me, but what happened just before? That's what worries me. It's like waking from a dream; I just don't remember."

It is difficult to overestimate how important Henry's tragedy was for memory research. He wasn't the first patient to display amnesia for certain types of information. What was unique was that the location of the brain damage was known because the surgeon, William Scoville, had made a careful record of the surgery. This meant that for the first time, researchers had a testable hypothesis about just what regions of the brain may be critical for memory. In addition, that Henry's intellectual capacities were intact meant that memory functions could be separated from other cognitive abilities. That his anterograde and retrograde amnesia were restricted to certain kinds of content also provided a foundation for the multiple memory systems view.

The Episodic Memory System

Today many researchers believe that the removal of Henry's medial temporal lobes disrupted what is called the **episodic memory system**. This is the system that supports what most of us mean when we use the term memory. It extracts and stores the content from our experiences (episodes), which allows us to answer questions such as: What did you have for lunch? Where did you park your car? Who went with you to the movies? Thus, it supports the ability to consciously recollect and report on facts and events that we have experienced. We can declare that we have a memory. The episodic memory system has other properties that are discussed in more detail in Chapter 17.

It is important to emphasize that Henry had some spared memory capacities. He could learn and retain the skills needed to perform the mirror-tracing and rotary-pursuit tasks. These abilities and others are supported by memory systems that depend on different regions of the brain. Some of these other systems are discussed in later chapters.

Henry's tragedy revealed that there are regions in the brain that are essential to the episodic memory system. At the time of surgery, Scoville estimated that a large part of what is called the medial temporal lobe was bilaterally removed, including much of the hippocampus, amygdala, and some of the surrounding regions of the underlying neocortex (Figure 16.3). Modern neuroimaging techniques largely confirmed Scoville's estimates. However, it is notable that more of the posterior part of the hippocampus was spared than was originally estimated. Portions of the ventral perirhinal cortex were spared and the parahippocampal cortex was largely intact (Corkin et al., 1997).

Given the extent of Henry's brain damage, it is difficult to know if one region was more critical to the episodic memory system than any other. It is interesting, however, that based on her analysis of patients with different combinations of brain damage, Milner (1970) speculated that the hippocampus might have been a critical region of the medial temporal lobes that supported the recall of the memories lost by Henry. Much research has been directed at trying to define critical regions of the brain responsible for Henry's memory impairment.

There are two ways that one can determine the critical brain regions that support episodic memory. One is by using laboratory animals (rodents and primates) to answer the question. The other is by studying patients that have selective damage to a particular medial temporal lobe structure or structures. Let's first consider the animal model strategy, including a memory testing procedure developed to determine what part of the brain supports episodic memory, before discussing humans with hippocampal damage.

The Animal Model Strategy

The animal model strategy has the advantage that the researcher has some control over the location of the brain damage and can selectively target different regions. However, there is a fundamental problem with this approach that

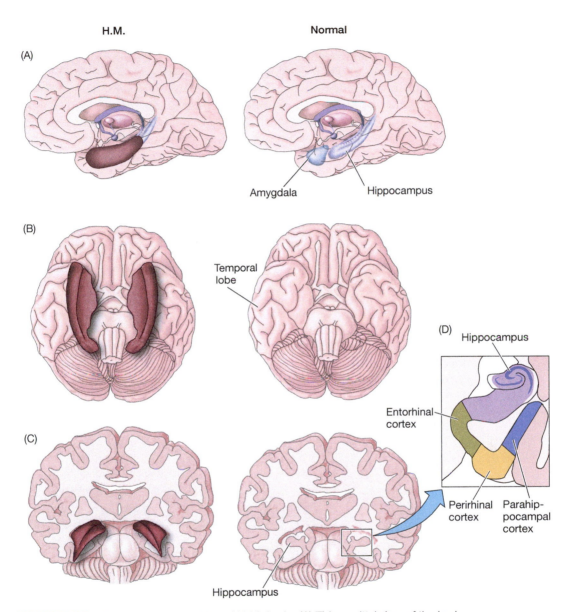

H.M.   **Normal**

(A)

Amygdala   Hippocampus

(B)

Temporal
lobe

(D) Hippocampus

Entorhinal
cortex

(C)

Perirhinal   Parahip-
cortex   pocampal
              cortex

Hippocampus

FIGURE 16.3 The tissue removed from H.M.'s brain. (A) This sagittal view of the brain shows that most of the amygdala and hippocampus were removed. (B) This view shows the extent to which underlying cortical tissue was removed. (C) This coronal section illustrates the combined loss of the cortical regions and hippocampus. (D) Another coronal view shows the cortical regions (entorhinal cortex, perirhinal cortex, parahippocampal cortex) and hippocampus in more detail. (C, D after W. B. Scoville and B. Milner. 1957. *J Neurol Neurosurg Psychiatry* 20: 11–21.)

has never been completely solved. Specifically, the most important and easily demonstrated property of the episodic memory system is that it supports our ability to consciously recall our experiences. When I ask my wife what she had for lunch and she tells me she had a salad, unless she lied I can be confident that she consciously recalled the experience, and that her response depended on her episodic memory system. In contrast, my cat also might remember what she had for breakfast, but I have no way of knowing if she can consciously recollect this experience. Thus, researchers who use the animal model approach are faced with the problem of trying to convince themselves, and the rest of the scientific community, that the particular task they use measures episodic memory.

Milner's analysis of H.M. provides a related problem for animal models of episodic memory. H.M.'s primary impairment was relatively selective. He lost the ability to acquire memories that could be consciously recollected. However, some of his other memory capacities, such as his ability to improve on the rotary-pursuit task, were spared. Since we cannot ask animals to consciously recollect their daily events, it is likely that many of the tasks used to study memory in animals may not depend on the hippocampus because the memory-based performance can be supported by other neural systems that do not include the hippocampus. Given these problems, it is not surprising that it is difficult to develop a consensus on an animal model of episodic memory.

The primate brain is anatomically similar to our brain, so in the late 1970s Mortimer Mishkin (1978, 1982) decided to use primates to determine what brain regions contributed to Henry's memory loss. To do this he developed a memory testing procedure called **delayed nonmatching to sample (DNMS)**, which is illustrated in Figure 16.4. In the DNMS task each trial consists of two components. First, the monkey is shown a three-dimensional object. It is called the sample. Some time later he is presented with a choice between the sample

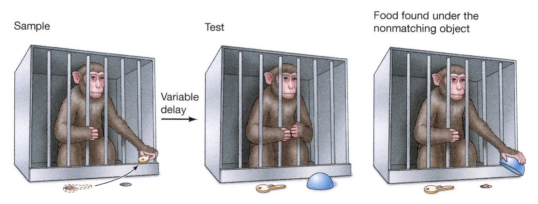

FIGURE 16.4   The delayed nonmatching-to-sample task was invented to study episodic memory in monkeys. The animal's task is to remember the object it sampled and to choose the novel object on the choice trial.

object and a new object. This is called the choice component. If the monkey chooses the new object, he will find a reward such as a grape or a peanut. The task is called nonmatching to sample because the correct object on the choice test does not match the sample. There are two important features of this task: (1) new objects are used on every trial; and (2) the experimenter can vary the interval between the sample and the choice trial.

To make the correct choice the monkey must retain information about the sampled object. It is the to-be-remembered episode. Implicit in the use of the DNMS task is the assumption that when the monkey chooses the correct object, it is telling the experimenter, "I remember seeing the old object at a particular time and in this particular place." If this assumption is true, then this task depends on the episodic memory system. If one believes that the DNMS task exclusively measures episodic memory, then evaluating monkeys with selective damage to medial temporal lobes should reveal which of these regions were responsible for Henry's amnesia.

Mishkin initially used this task to determine if damage to the hippocampus and/or amygdala caused Henry's amnesia. Viewed against Milner's hypothesis, the results of his experiments and others were somewhat surprising. They revealed that damage to either the hippocampus or the amygdala had very little effect on DNMS performance; however, damage to both regions dramatically impaired performance. Moreover, monkeys with damage to both of these regions were able to acquire motor skills (Squire, 1987). This outcome initially encouraged the belief that it was the combined damage to both the hippocampus and the amygdala that produced Henry's amnesia.

Larry Squire, however, pointed out that the surgical approaches used to remove both the hippocampus and amygdala produced extensive damage to the immediate surrounding cortical tissue compared to when only the hippocampus was surgically removed (Squire, 1987). Subsequent research led to the conclusion that it was the damage to the rhinal cortex, not damage to either the amygdala or hippocampus, which drastically impaired performance on the DNMS task (Meunier et al., 1993; Murray and Mishkin, 1998; Zola-Morgan et al., 1989). An example of these results is presented in Figure 16.5. Thus, researchers agree that this medial temporal lobe region is critical for performance on the DNMS, and that neither the hippocampus nor the amygdala is critical.

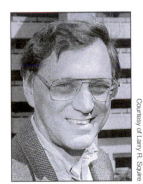

Larry Squire

Studies of Patients with Selective Hippocampal Damage

The above discussion illustrates the difficulties one encounters using the DNMS animal model to define a neural circuit for episodic memory. We don't know when nonverbal animals are actually recollecting events from their past. Thus, ultimately conclusions about the critical contribution the hippocampus makes to the episodic memory system must be derived from people with brain damage limited to the hippocampus. A number of patients with relatively selective damage to the hippocampus have been identified. Although there is

(A)

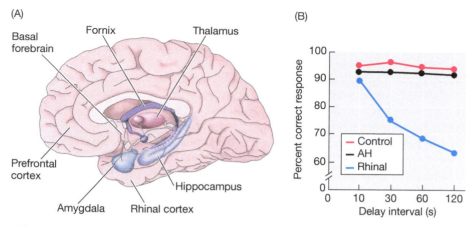

(B)

FIGURE 16.5 (A) A sagittal view of the human brain. (B) The performance on the delayed nonmatching-to-sample task. Primates with damage to both the amygdala and hippocampus (AH) performed normally. However, removal of the rhinal cortical regions profoundly disrupted performance. (B after E. A. Murray and M. Mishkin. 1998. *J Neurosci* 18: 6568–6582. © 1998 Society for Neuroscience; M. Meunier et al. 1993. *J Neurosci* 13: 5418–5432. © 1993 Society for Neuroscience.)

debate about the recognition memory capacity of these patients, no one doubts that they all are impaired in acquiring new episodic memories.

Stuart Zola-Morgan et al. (1986) described patient R.B. The onset of R.B.'s amnesia was associated with complications of a second artery bypass surgery. Zola-Morgan and his colleagues tested R.B.'s memory and, at his death, conducted an extensive neuropathological evaluation of R.B.'s brain. Formal memory tests indicated that he had difficulty acquiring new information. For example, after a story was read to him, R.B. could recall only a small fraction of the material. He also could recall only a small percentage of words that were read to him twice. Informally R.B. reported that he had severe memory problems. He reported that if he had talked to his children on the phone he did not remember doing so the next day. Thus, R.B. had significant anterograde amnesia. However, formal tests found no evidence of retrograde amnesia, that is, loss of memory for events that occurred prior to the cardiac episode. There was some speculation based on informal observations that he may have had loss of memory for some events that occurred a few years prior to the cardiac episode.

Remarkably, the neuropathological assessment of R.B.'s brain indicated that the pathology was restricted to the CA1 region of the hippocampus (Figure 16.6). Bilaterally, there was a complete loss of neurons from the CA1 field. The CA1 field is a final stage whereby information processed by other regions is sent out via the subiculum and entorhinal cortex. Thus, although the damage was restricted, it was in a location that would be expected to significantly diminish the ability of the hippocampus to make its normal contribution to memory.

Cipolotti et al. (2001) described the case of V.C., who became profoundly amnesic at the age of 67, apparently after experiencing an epileptic seizure. Assessment of his brain damage by magnetic resonance imaging indicated that

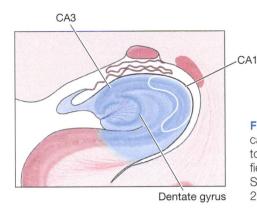

CA3

CA1

Dentate gyrus

FIGURE 16.6 Damage to the hippocampus of patient R.B. was restricted
to a massive loss of neurons in the CA1
field, outlined in white in the figure. (After
S. Zola-Morgan et al. 1986. *J Neurosci* 6:
2950–2967.)

there was significant loss of volume over the entire rostral–caudal length of the
hippocampus. However, critical surrounding cortical regions—the entorhinal
and parahippocampal cortices—were normal, as were the adjacent temporal
lobes. Thus, V.C.'s damage was restricted primarily to the hippocampus. Formal
tests revealed that V.C. had profound anterograde amnesia. He was severely
impaired on all measures of recall, such as the recall of a story and word associations. V.C. also had extensive retrograde amnesia.

Thus, studies of patients with much more selective damage to the hippocampus support Brenda Milner's original conjecture that the hippocampus is
critically involved in episodic memory.

The DNMS Paradox Resolved

The results generated by the DNMS task—that monkeys with damage to the hippocampus are not impaired on this task—are both surprising and disconcerting
as they imply that the hippocampus is not part of the episodic memory system.
And that conclusion runs counter to Milner's hypothesis that it was damage to
the hippocampus that was responsible for H.M.'s selective memory impairments.

Baxter and Murray (2001) reviewed all of the relevant studies and concluded
that extensive damage to the hippocampus has a smaller effect on DNMS than
does limited damage (but see Zola and Squire, 2001). Based on this review, one
would have to conclude that either (a) the hippocampus is not part of the episodic
memory system or (b) the DNMS task has a solution that does not depend on
episodic memory. Given that it is now generally agreed that the hippocampus *is*
a central component of the episodic memory system, the latter hypothesis is the
more likely explanation and there are theoretical reasons for favoring it.

The DNMS task belongs to a category of tasks called **recognition memory
tasks**. Such tasks require the subject to make a judgment about whether something has previously occurred. Today many theorists believe that two different
processes can support recognition. One type is called **familiarity** and the other
is called **recollection** (Brown and Aggleton, 2001; Rugg and Yonelinas, 2003;
Sutherland and Rudy, 1989). To appreciate this distinction, you need only to
reflect on how often you have recognized a person as familiar without being able

to recall information about the place and time you met her. This would be an example of recognition without recall. It would be based on familiarity and not recollection. Recollection would also include the information about such things as where and when you met the person and her name, content that is supported by the episodic memory system, as described in the next chapter. Often you will get a sense of familiarity before you recollect the details of past encounters.

Contemporary theorists have proposed that recognition based on recollection depends on the hippocampus, whereas recognition based on familiarity depends on surrounding cortices (Brown and Aggleton, 2001). If two processes can support recognition memory, it is possible to explain why extensive damage to the hippocampus can have little or no effect on DNMS performance. The monkeys in the DNMS task were using the familiarity process to make their correct choice (Sutherland and Rudy, 1989) and this does not depend on the episodic memory system that supports recollection.

The MTH System: Episodic Memory and Semantic Memory

Some memory researchers believe the episodic memory belongs to a broader, long-term memory category called **declarative memory**, which includes not only episodic memory but also **semantic memory**. Semantic memory is believed to support memory for facts and the ability to extract generalizations from multiple experiences. For example, past experiences allow us to answer questions like, is a violin a musical instrument or an automobile? We can also answer factual questions such as, what day was your mother born? Note that to answer these questions requires intentional retrieval and explicit recollection. Thus, semantic memory and episodic memory are similar in that we can intentionally retrieve information from them and in some sense declare we have the memory. The content of semantic memory, however, is not tied to the place or context where it was acquired. It is sometimes said to be context free. This means that we can know the facts about something without remembering when or where we learned them.

The inclusion of both episodic and semantic memory into a more general category—declarative memory—implies that they are supported by the same neural system. Indeed, some researchers (Manns, Hopkins, Reed et al., 2003; Squire and Zola, 1996, 1998; Squire and Zola-Morgan, 1991) have argued that the **medial temporal hippocampal (MTH) system** (which is composed of the parahippocampal cortex, perirhinal cortex, entorhinal cortex, hippocampus, and subiculum) provides support for both types of memory. This is called the **unitary view** (Figure 16.7A). It suggests that damage to any component of this system will produce the same degree of impairment in tests of episodic and semantic memory.

Other researchers, however, believe that only episodic memory requires the entire MTH system. This is called the **modular view**. Researchers who support this view believe that (a) semantic memories can be acquired even when the hippocampus is selectively removed, and (b) while episodic and semantic memory may share some components of the MTH system, the overlap is not complete and episodic and semantic memory are not part of a single declarative memory system (Figure 16.7B). This position suggests that the MTH system has a modular organization—that is, components of the system are relatively dedicated to specific functions.

(A) Unitary view

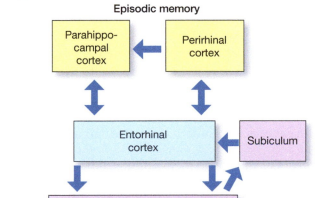

(B) Modular view

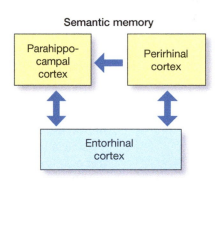

FIGURE 16.7   (A) The unitary view of the medial temporal hippocampal (MTH) system. Supporters of this view believe that the system is needed to support both episodic and semantic memory. (B) The modular view. Supporters of this view believe that the entire system, including the hippocampal formation, is required for episodic memory but that semantic memory does not require the hippocampus.

A Modular MTH System

The components of the MTH system are highly interconnected, so one might imagine that it would be difficult to assign particular functions to them. Nevertheless, several lines of research suggest that a modular view of the MTH system is useful. Two sources of evidence are considered. One comes from the discovery of individuals who grew up with a compromised hippocampus, while the other comes from studies of recognition memory.

Growing Up without the Hippocampus

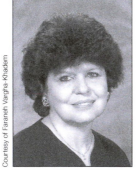

Faraneh Vargha-Khadem

The modular view emerged when Faraneh Vargha-Khadem and her colleagues (Vargha-Khadem et al., 1997) reported the results for three patients with amnesia caused by relatively selective damage to the hippocampus sustained very early in life. Each of these patients developed pronounced memory impairments as a result of an anoxic–ischemic episode, that is, they experienced a reduction in oxygen supply (hypoxia) combined with reduced blood flow (ischemia) to the brain.

As revealed by quantitative magnetic resonance imaging, these patients had bilateral damage to approximately 50% of their hippocampus and very little damage to the surrounding cortices. The insult producing the pathology occurred at birth or when the patient was 4 or 9 years old. These children thus grew up without a functioning hippocampus.

These patients were 13, 16, and 19 years old when they received their first neuropsychological examination. The IQ of one of the patients was 109, which is well within the average range, whereas the IQs of the other two were in the low average range (82 and 86). Their memory for everyday experiences was so poor that none of them could be left alone for any extended period of time. Formal tests of their memory confirmed that they were profoundly amnesic.

The surprising aspect of these patients is that even though they had no episodic memory, they all developed normal language and social skills. Moreover, they were all educated in mainstream schools. They learned to read and write and acquired new factual information at levels consistent with their verbal

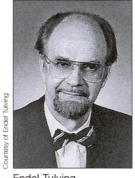

Endel Tulving

IQs. In fact, all three patients had fully normal scores on the vocabulary, information, and comprehension subtests of the Wechsler Intelligence Scale. Given these findings, Vargha-Khadem and her colleagues concluded that there was a disproportionate sparing of semantic memory compared to episodic memory in these patients who suffered selective damage to their hippocampus early in life.

The strong implication of the Vargha-Khadem findings is that the MTH system is not a homogeneous system (Mishkin et al., 1997; Vargha-Khadem et al., 1997) and that semantic memory may be supported by components of the MTH system that remain after the hippocampus has been removed. This view is consistent with the position proposed by Endel Tulving, who was first to strongly argue for the distinction between episodic and semantic memory (Tulving, 1972). He argued that episodic memory should be considered as separate from declarative memory (Tulving and Markowitsch, 1998).

Subsequent reports have provided additional support for the modular view of the MTH system (Bindschaedler et al., 2010; Gadian et al., 2000). For example, Bindschaedler and his colleagues reported on patient V.J., who had severe atrophy of the hippocampus but otherwise had a normal perirhinal cortex. His hippocampus loss was believed to be the result of a neurological episode experienced a few hours after birth. When V.J. was 8 years old, his parents became concerned that he might have memory disturbances. This was confirmed and researchers tested him on a regular basis from that age to his teenage years. Based on this extensive testing, Bindschaedler and his colleagues concluded that V.J. had persistent impairments related to his episodic memory. Remarkably, at 8 years of age, his general world knowledge and understanding of the meaning of words was spared. Moreover, V.J.'s memory progression to teenage years was normal. Bindschaedler and his colleagues concluded that V.J.'s case adds support to the view that episodic and semantic memory are partially independent.

The organization of the MTH system may be modular but it should be appreciated that the absence of the hippocampus, which interacts with the other components of the MTH system, will compromise acquisition of semantic information. For example, Holdstock et al. (2002) suggested that the hippocampal formation is critical for rapid acquisition of new semantic information, whereas semantic information via the adjacent cortices is acquired slowly over multiple trials.

Recognition Memory and MTH Modularity

It was noted that Mishkin (1978) developed the DNMS task to determine the contribution of medial temporal brain regions to episodic memory. Research during his era, however, revealed that the hippocampus was not needed to recognize previously experienced objects. In discussing this outcome, it was noted that this type of recognition memory task could be based on either a familiarity signal or recollection process. In the current context, the familiarity signal does not contain information about the context of the experience, whereas recollection-based recognition contains such information (see Sutherland and Rudy, 1989). Based on this analysis, damage to the hippocampus spared performance because the surrounding perirhinal cortex was able to support familiarity-based recognition.

If this conclusion is correct, then studies of recognition memory should provide additional support for a modular view of the MTH system. Additional evidence is provided by functional neuroimaging studies of both normal and brain-damaged patients. The general conclusion from this work is that recollection-based recognition is associated with the hippocampus, whereas familiarity is supported by perirhinal cortex (Aggleton et al., 2005; Vilberg and Rugg, 2007; Yonelinas et al., 2002). It is worth mentioning that V.J., who grew up without the hippocampus, displayed relatively spared recognition compared to recall and that "overall pattern of performance … is consistent with the hypothesis that spared recognition was based on familiarity processes" (Bindschaedler et al., 2010, p. 941).

Research with rodents also supports the modular view. Rats with damage to the hippocampus recognize previously experienced objects. However, as described earlier in Figure 16.6, they cannot remember the context where an object was experienced (Mumby et al., 2002; Mumby et al., 2005). These results are consistent with the idea that the hippocampus is not required to support familiarity-based recognition but is required to place the recognized item into the surrounding context and thus provide an episodic quality to the memory.

Although there is strong support for the modular view, it is not universally accepted (see Manns, Hopkins, Reed et al., 2003; Manns, Hopkins, and Squire, 2003). Manns and his colleagues, for example, presented data from patients thought to have bilateral damage primarily to the hippocampal region and claimed that their ability to acquire factual knowledge was just as impaired as their memory for episodes. They suggested that the division of labor among the medial structures might not be absolute and that it may not be possible to map psychological categories like episodic and semantic memory precisely onto the hippocampal formation and its adjacent cortical regions because these regions are so interconnected. This is a difficult argument to reject, in part because when damage is inflicted on the hippocampus it is difficult to know the extent to which it spreads and causes damage to the surrounding cortices. Moreover, it is difficult to know exactly how to compare the extent to which semantic memory for facts is impaired relative to episodic memory.

Summary

The content of experience matters to the brain. Different attributes are assigned to different regions of the brain for storage. The idea that the brain has multiple memory systems is now central to the neurobiology of memory.

The perspective that different brain regions support different memory systems gained support when Brenda Milner's analysis of patient H.M. revealed that the removal of the medial temporal lobes left him with no long-term episodic memory but did not influence his ability to learn complex motor tasks or perceptual motor adjustments. Milner proposed that it was the damage to the hippocampus that was critical to H.M.'s profound episodic memory impairment.

The DNMS recognition memory task was invented in an attempt to develop an animal model aimed at determining which regions of the medial temporal lobes are critical for episodic memory. This research revealed that the hippocampus is not necessary for animals to perform this task but that the cortical areas surrounding the hippocampus are. However, studies of human patients with more selective damage to the hippocampus support Milner's hypothesis that the hippocampus is critical for episodic memory.

Most researchers believe that recognition is based on both a familiarity process that depends on the cortical areas surrounding the hippocampus and a recollection process that contains information about where and when the event happens, which depends on the hippocampus. Just how the hippocampus supports episodic memory is the topic of the next chapter.

The relationship between the medial temporal hippocampal neural system and episodic and semantic memories also was explored. Studies of patients with selective hippocampus pathology that developed at a young age suggest that episodic memories require the entire MTH system, but semantic memories can be acquired when the hippocampal formation is removed. Such findings support the idea that the organization of the MTH system is modular. The modular view is also supported by studies that show that recollection-based recognition memory requires the entire MTH system but familiarity-based recognition does not require the hippocampus.

References

Aggleton, J. P., Vann, S. D., Denby, C., Dix, S., Mayes, A. R., Roberts, N., and Yonelinas, A. P. (2005). Sparing of the familiarity component of recognition memory in a patient with hippocampal pathology. *Neuropsychologia, 43*, 1810–1843.

Andersen, P., Morris, R., Amaral, D., Bliss, T., and O'Keefe, J. (2007). Historical perspective: proposed functions, biological characteristics, and neurobiological models of the hippocampus. In P. Andersen, R. Morris, D. Amaral, T. Bliss, and J. O'Keefe (Eds.), *The Hippocampus Book* (pp. 9–36). New York: Oxford University Press.

Baxter, M. G. and Murray, E. A. (2001). Opposite relationship of hippocampal and rhinal cortex damage to delayed nonmatching-to-sample deficits in monkeys. *Hippocampus, 11*, 61–71.

Bayley, P. J., Frascino, J. C., and Squire, L. R. (2005). Robust habit learning in the absence of awareness and independent of the medial temporal lobe. *Nature, 436*, 550–553.

Bindschaedler, C., Peter-Favre, C., Maeder, P., Hirsbrunner, T., and Clarke, S. (2010). Growing up with bilateral hippocampal atrophy: from childhood to teenage. *Cortex, 47*, 931–944.

Brown, M. W. and Aggleton, J. P. (2001). Recognition memory: what are the roles of the perirhinal cortex and hippocampus? *Nature Reviews Neuroscience, 2*, 51–61.

Cipolotti, L., Shallice, T., Chan, D., Fox, N., Scahill, R., Harrison, G., Stevens, J., and Rudge, P. (2001). Long-term retrograde amnesia...the crucial role of the hippocampus. *Neuropsychologia, 39*, 151–172.

Claparède, É. (1951). Recognition and me-ness. In D. Rapaport (Ed.), *Organization and Pathology of Thought* (pp. 58–75). New York: Columbia University Press.

Corkin, S. (1968). Acquisition of a motor skill after bilateral medial temporal lobe excision. *Neuropsychologia, 6*, 255–265.

Corkin, S., Amaral, D. G., Gonzalez, R. G., Johnson, K. A., and Hyman, B. T. (1997). H.M.'s medial temporal lobe lesion: findings from magnetic resonance imaging. *Journal of Neuroscience, 17*, 3964–3979.

Gadian, D. G., Aicardi, J., Watkins, K. E., Porter, D. A., Mishkin, M., and Vargha-Khadem, F. (2000). Developmental amnesia associated with early hypoxic-ischaemic injury. *Brain, 123*, 499–507.

Holdstock, J. S., Mayes, A. R., Isaac, C. L., Gong, Q., and Roberts, N. (2002). Differential involvement of the hippocampus and temporal lobes cortices in rapid and slow learning of new semantic information. *Neuropsychologia, 40*, 748–768.

Manns, J. R., Hopkins, R. O., Reed, J. M., Kitchener, E. G., and Squire, L. R. (2003). Recognition memory and the human hippocampus. *Neuron, 7*, 171–180.

Manns, J. R., Hopkins, R. O., and Squire, L. R. (2003). Semantic memory and the human hippocampus. *Neuron, 38*, 127–133.

McDonald, R. J. and White, N. M. (1993). A triple dissociation of memory systems: hippocampus, amygdala, and dorsal striatum. *Behavioral Neuroscience, 107*, 3–22.

Meunier, M., Bachevalier, J., Mishkin, M., and Murray, E. A. (1993). Effects on visual recognition of combined and separate ablations of the entorhinal and perirhinal cortex in rhesus monkeys. *Journal of Neuroscience, 13*, 5418–5432.

Milner, B. (1965). Memory disturbances after bilateral hippocampal damage. In P. M. Milner and S. Glickman (Eds.), *Cognitive Processes and the Brain: An Enduring Problem for Psychology* (pp. 97–113). Princeton, NJ: Van Nostrand.

Milner, B. (1970). Memory and the medial temporal lobe regions of the brain. In K. H. Pribram and D. E. Broadbent (Eds.), *Biology of Memory* (pp. 29–50). New York: Academic Press.

Mishkin, M. (1978). Memory in monkeys severely impaired by combined but not by separate removal of amygdala and hippocampus. *Nature, 273*, 297–298.

Mishkin, M. (1982). A memory system in the monkey. *Philosophical Transactions of the Royal Society London, 298*, 83–95.

Mishkin, M., Suzuki, W. A., Gadian, D. G., and Vargha-Khadem, F. (1997). Hierarchical organization of cognitive memory. *Philosophical Transactions of the Royal Society of London B, 352*, 1461–1467.

Mumby, D. G., Gaskin, S., Glenn, M. J., Schramek, T. E., and Lehmann, H. (2002). Hippocampal damage and exploratory preferences in rats: memory for objects, places, and contexts. *Learning and Memory, 9*, 49–57.

Mumby, D. G., Tremblay, A., Lecluse, V., and Lehmann, H. (2005). Hippocampal damage and anterograde object-recognition in rats after long retention intervals. *Hippocampus, 15*, 1050–1056.

Murray, E. A. and Mishkin, M. (1998). Object recognition and location memory in monkeys with excitotoxic lesions of the amygdala and hippocampus. *Journal of Neuroscience, 18*, 6568–6582.

Rugg, M. D. and Yonelinas, A. P. (2003). Human recognition memory: a cognitive neuroscience perspective. *Trends in Cognitive Sciences, 7*, 313–319.

Scoville, W. B. and Milner, B. (1957). Loss of recent memory after bilateral hippocampal lesions. *Journal of Neurology, Neurosurgery, and Psychiatry, 20*, 11–12.

Squire, L. R. (1987). *Memory and Brain*. New York: Oxford University Press.

Squire, L. R. (2004). Memory systems of the brain: a brief history and current perspective. *Neurobiology of Learning and Memory, 82*, 171–177.

Squire, L. R. and Zola, S. M. (1996). Structure and function of declarative and nondeclarative memory systems. *Proceedings of the National Academy of Sciences USA, 93*, 13515–13522.

Squire, L. R. and Zola, S. M. (1998). Episodic memory, semantic memory, and amnesia. *Hippocampus, 8*, 205–211.

Squire, L. R. and Zola-Morgan, S. (1991). The medial temporal lobe memory system. *Science, 253*, 1380–1386.

Sutherland, R. J. and Rudy, J. W. (1989). Configural association theory: the role of the hippocampal formation in learning, memory, and amnesia. *Psychobiology, 17*, 129–144.

Tulving, E. (1972). Episodic and semantic memory. In E. Tulving and W. Donaldson (Eds.), *Organization of Memory* (pp. 381–403). New York: Academic Press.

Tulving, E. and Markowitsch, H. J. (1998). Episodic and declarative memory: role of the hippocampus. *Hippocampus, 8*, 198–204.

Vargha-Khadem, F., Gadian, D. G., Watkins, K. E., Connelly, A., Van Paesschen, W., and Mishkin, M. (1997). Differential effects of early hippocampal pathology on episodic and semantic memory. *Science, 277*, 376–380.

Vilberg, K. L. and Rugg, M. D. (2007). Dissociation of the neural correlates of recognition memory according to familiarity, recollection, and amount of recollected information. *Neuropsychologia, 45*, 2216–2225.

White, N. M. and McDonald, R. J. (2002). Multiple parallel memory systems in the brain of the rat. *Neurobiology of Learning and Memory, 77*, 125–184.

Yonelinas, A. P., Kroll, N. E. A., Quamme, J. R., Lazzara, M. M., Sauve, M. J., and Widaman, K. F. (2002). Effects of extensive temporal lobe damage or mild hypoxia on recollection and familiarity. *Nature Neuroscience, 5*, 1236–1241.

Zola, S. M. and Squire, L. R. (2001). Relationship between magnitude of damage to the hippocampus and impaired recognition memory in monkeys. *Hippocampus, 11*, 92–98.

Zola-Morgan, S., Squire, L. R., and Amaral, D. G. (1986). Human amnesia and the medial temporal region: enduring memory impairment following a bilateral lesion limited to field CA1 of the hippocampus. *Journal of Neuroscience, 6*, 2950–2967.

Zola-Morgan, S., Squire, L. R., Amaral, D. G., and Suzuki, W. A. (1989). Lesions of perirhinal and parahippocampal cortex that spare the amygdala and hippocampal formation produce severe memory impairment. *Journal of Neuroscience, 9*, 4355–4370.

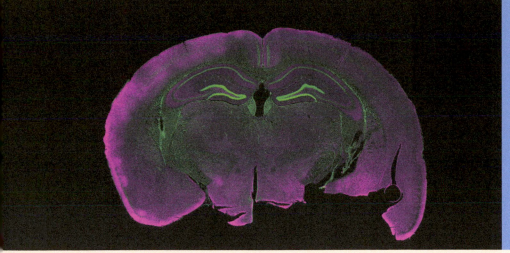

The Hippocampus Index and Episodic Memory

As learned in the previous chapter, the episodic memory system captures the content of our experiences in a form that permits us to recollect or replay them. When the hippocampus is significantly damaged, this capacity is lost and we become disconnected from our past. Thus, there is something special about the hippocampus and its connections with other brain regions that is fundamental to the episodic memory system. How do the hippocampus and its related cortical structures store the content of our personal experiences so that it can be recollected or recalled? The goal of this chapter is to answer this question, by describing:

- properties of the episodic memory system;
- the neural system in which the hippocampus is situated;
- the indexing theory of episodic memory; and
- current evidence supporting the indexing theory.

Properties of Episodic Memory

Episodic memory has several important properties or attributes, including (1) its support of conscious recollection and storage of temporal–spatial contextual information for later retrieval, (2) its ability to automatically capture episodic and incidental information, and (3) its ability to acquire information about an event that occurs only once, yet protect the representations it stores from interfering with each other.

Conscious Recollection and Contextual Information Storage

The episodic system is most often described as supporting memories that can be consciously recollected or recalled. The term **conscious recollection** has two meanings (Schacter, 1989).

1. It means that you intentionally initiated a search of your memory. This meaning refers to the manner in which retrieval is initiated.
2. It also means that you have an awareness of remembering—a sense that a memory trace has been successfully activated. This meaning refers to a subjective feeling that is a product of the retrieval process.

Our personal experience is consistent with the idea that we can be aware that we have retrieved a memory or had a remembering experience. It also is the case that we can intentionally initiate a memory search that leads to recalling a memory. However, this does not mean that memories retrieved from the episodic system have to evoke a state of conscious awareness to influence behavior. Nor does it mean that our episodic memory system can only be accessed if we intentionally initiate a search.

To appreciate this last point, we also can draw on personal experiences such as encountering a friend whom we haven't seen in a while or visiting an old neighborhood. Such experiences often initiate the recall of many events associated with the friend or neighborhood without any intention on our part to retrieve these memories. Moreover, it is likely that we became aware of having a remembering experience.

The subjective state of conscious awareness that can occur when we have successfully remembered some event may be associated with the content of the memory trace. A number of researchers agree that the feeling of remembering emerges when a retrieved memory trace contains information about the time, place, or context of the experience that established the memory (Nadel and Moscovitch, 1997; Squire and Kandel, 1999; Squire and Zola-Morgan, 1991). Being able to retrieve this contextual information enables a replay of the experience and allows us to declare that we remember. In describing the importance of contextual information for recollection, for example, Squire and Kandel (1999, p. 69) wrote, "Once the context is reconstructed, it may seem surprising how easy it is to recall the scene and what took place. In this way, one can become immersed in sustained recollection, sometimes accompanied by strong emotions and by a compelling sense of personal familiarity with what is remembered."

Obviously, information about the spatial and temporal context of the experience must be stored if conscious recollection depends on its retrieval. Thus, the episodic memory system must be critically involved in both the storage and retrieval of contextual information.

Automatic Capture of Episodic and Incidental Information

Many theorists believe that the episodic memory system automatically captures information simply as a consequence of our exploring and experiencing the environment (O'Keefe and Nadel, 1978; O'Reilly and Rudy, 2001; Teyler and DiScenna, 1986; Teyler and Rudy, 2007). The term automatic is used to note that the information is captured without intention on our part to do so. You can prove this is true by recalling your experiences of the past several days. You will undoubtedly remember a surprising amount of information. Now ask yourself if you intentionally attempted to store any of this information. Your likely answer will be no.

To be sure, you may be able to co-opt this system by instructing yourself to remember a phone number or an address. However, the basic point is that the hippocampus does not need to be driven by our intentions or goals to capture information. It contributes to the episodic memory system by automatically capturing the information it receives as we attend to and explore the world. For this reason, some researchers also say that the episodic memory system captures incidental information. This means that it will capture information that is incidental to the task at hand. Thus, when you deliberately remember a phone number, it is unlikely that you intend to remember the episode of memorizing the number, but it is likely that you will. Or, if you are trying to learn a new tune on the piano, you do not instruct yourself to remember the practice session. Nevertheless, the episodic memory system likely captures a great deal of this incidental information so that you can later recall much about the practice session.

Single Episode Capture with Protection from Interference

The term episodic memory means that the system captures information about single episodes of our lives. What constitutes the duration of an episode is vague. However, the gist of this idea is that the episodic memory system can acquire information about an event that occurs only once. It has been suggested that from the viewpoint of the episodic system, every episode of our lives is unique, even if it contains highly overlapping information (Nadel and Moscovitch, 1997). Thus, we can remember many different instances of practicing the piano or driving our car to the same parking lot.

If the episodic memory system is constantly capturing information about our daily events, then it must be able to store highly similar episodes, such as where you parked your car today versus where you parked it yesterday, so that these memories do not interfere with each other. Our success in keeping memories of similar events separate suggests that an important property of the episodic system is that the representations it stores are somehow protected from interference (O'Keefe and Nadel, 1978; O'Reilly and McClelland, 1994; O'Reilly and Rudy, 2001).

Properties Summary

In summary, many researchers agree about the fundamental attributes of the episodic memory system. It automatically captures information about the single episodes of our lives. The memory trace includes information about the spatial and temporal context of the episode and it is when this contextual information is retrieved that we are consciously aware of the memory and can declare that we remembered some event. The next sections describe how the hippocampus contributes to these properties and supports memories.

A Neural System that Supports Episodic Memory

The hippocampus can support episodic memories because (a) it is embedded in a neural system in which it interacts with other regions of the brain and (b) both its intrinsic organization and the properties of its synaptic connections are unique. The work of a number of neuroanatomists has led to an understanding of the connectivity of these regions of the brain (Amaral and Lavenex, 2007; Lavenex and Amaral, 2000; Van Hoesen and Pandya, 1975).

The Hierarchy and the Loop

The neural system that supports episodic memory can be organized around two principles (Lavenex and Amaral, 2000) that are illustrated in Figure 17.1.

1. The organization is hierarchical. The level of integration or abstraction of information increases as it flows from the neocortex to the perirhinal and parahippocampal cortices to the entorhinal cortex and through the hippocampus.

2. The circuit is a loop. This means that information carried forward to the hippocampus also is then projected back to the sites lower in the hierarchy that initially brought the information to the hippocampus.

The flow of information to the medial temporal lobes begins when sensory information (for example, visual, auditory, somatosensory) arrives at different regions of the neocortex (called unimodal associative and polymodal associative areas). Information at this level is not well integrated. However, these regions project to what Lavenex and Amaral call the first level of integration—the perirhinal and parahippocampal cortices. Information from these regions projects forward to the second level of integration in the entorhinal cortex that projects to the highest level of integration—the hippocampus. At each stage the information becomes more compressed or abstract.

(A)

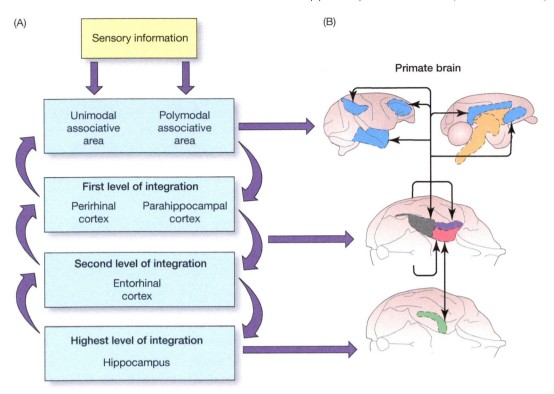

(B)

Primate brain

FIGURE 17.1   (A) A schematic representation of the flow of information from the neocortical unimodal and polymodal associative areas to the medial temporal lobe regions. Information flows to the highest level of integration and then loops back to the neocortical areas. (B) The location of these regions in the primate brain. (A after P. Lavenex and D. G. Amaral. 2000. *Hippocampus* 10: 420–430; B after H. Eichenbaum. 2000. *Nature Rev Neurosci* 1: 41–50.)

Information is processed through the hippocampus and then projects back to the entorhinal cortex. The entorhinal cortex also projects back to the perirhinal and parahippocampal cortices that in turn project back to the neocortical regions. Figure 17.2 provides a more complete representation of the flow of information into and out of the hippocampus. It shows that the entorhinal cortex projects into two regions of the hippocampus, the dentate gyrus and the CA1 region, and that information projects out of the hippocampus to the entorhinal cortex via

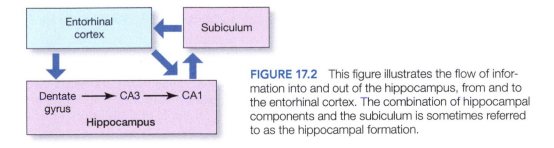

FIGURE 17.2   This figure illustrates the flow of information into and out of the hippocampus, from and to the entorhinal cortex. The combination of hippocampal components and the subiculum is sometimes referred to as the hippocampal formation.

a region called the **subiculum**. This combination of hippocampal components and the subiculum is sometimes called the **hippocampal formation**.

The MTH System

Most researchers agree that the critical components of this hierarchical system are located in the medial temporal lobes. As described in the previous chapter, this system is sometimes referred to as the medial temporal hippocampal (MTH) system, consisting of the perirhinal, parahippocampal, and entorhinal cortices and the hippocampal formation (see Figure 17.2). This MTH system has the following functional implications.

1. Because the hippocampus sits at the top of a hierarchically organized system, it is in a position to receive convergent information from a wide range of cortical regions. In a sense, it sees what is going on in other regions of the brain.

2. The information is so highly processed by the time it reaches the hippocampus that it is described as amodal (Lavenex and Amaral, 2000). This means that hippocampal neurons do not know whether they are receiving auditory, visual, or somatosensory information.

3. The perirhinal, parahippocampal, and entorhinal cortices also have to be considered as part of the episodic memory system because without them the hippocampus receives no information. They are the last stage of information processing before information enters the hippocampus. Thus, whether or not these regions can support other memory functions, such as familiarity-based recognition, they are critical to episodic memory.

Now consider a theory of just what the hippocampus contributes to episodic memory.

The Indexing Theory of Episodic Memory

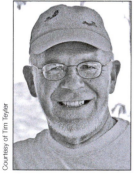

Courtesy of Tim Teyler

Tim Teyler

Any theoretical account of how the hippocampus supports episodic memory must be consistent with the anatomy and physiology of the system. Tim Teyler and Pascal DiScenna (1986) provided one such account and called it the hippocampal memory indexing theory (see also Marr, 1971). This theory has been supported by a wealth of data (Teyler and Rudy, 2007) and its basic ideas are shared by a number of theorists (Marr, 1971; McNaughton, 1991; McNaughton and Morris, 1987; O'Reilly and Rudy, 2001; Squire, 1992).

Indexing theory was designed to provide an in-principle account of how the neural system in which the hippocampus is embedded (see Figures 17.1 and 17.2) can naturally explain episodic memory. It explored three fundamental areas: (1) the role of the hippocampus in the formation of the engram; (2) the nature of the engram; and (3) the role of the hippocampus in memory retrieval.

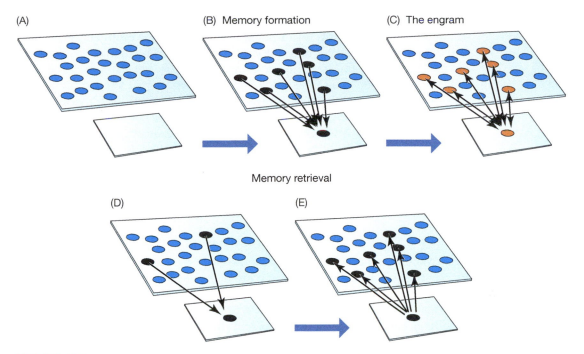

(A)

(B) Memory formation

(C) The engram

Memory retrieval

(D)

(E)

FIGURE 17.3 This figure illustrates the important ideas contained in the hippocampal indexing theory of episodic memory. (A) Here the top layer represents potential patterns of neocortical activity (blue dots), while the bottom layer represents the hippocampus. (B) Memory formation begins when a set of neocortical patterns (black dots) activated by a particular experience is projected to the hippocampus and activates a unique set of synapses that will become the index. (C) The resulting *engram* consists of those patterns of neocortical activity conjoined by the indexing neurons in the hippocampus (orange dots). (D) During memory retrieval, when a subset of the initial input pattern activates the hippocampal index, output from the hippocampus projects back to the neocortex to activate the original neocortical pattern. (After T. J. Teyler and J. W. Rudy. 2007. *Hippocampus* 17: 1158–1169, based on T. Teyler and P. DiScenna. 1986. *Behav Neurosci* 100: 147–152.)

The resulting conclusions can be understood by referring to Figure 17.3. Memory *formation* begins when the individual features of an episode activate a pattern of neocortical activity, which then projects to the hippocampus (see Figure 17.3B). As a consequence, synapses in the hippocampus responding to the neocortical inputs are strengthened by mechanisms that support long-term potentiation (see Chapters 2 through 7). The resulting *engram* consists of those patterns of neocortical activity conjoined by the indexing neurons in the hippocampus (see Figure 17.3C). Memory *retrieval* occurs when a subset of the original neocortical pattern is experienced and activates the indexing neurons above the threshold needed to project back to the neocortex to activate the neocortical pattern representing the entire experience (see Figure 17.3D,E).

The index concept can be understood in relationship to a library. A library often contains thousands of books. This creates an obvious problem—how do you find the one you want? Librarians solved the retrieval problem by creating an indexing system that contains information about the location of the book. So you go to the index and find the book's address. Note that the content you are looking for is in the book. The index has no content; it just tells you where to find the book that contains the desired information. Likewise, indexing theory assumes the rich content of our experience is stored in neocortical regions of the brain and all that the hippocampus stores is information about how to retrieve the memories stored in the neocortex. It provides an index to the content represented in the neocortex. In this context there are two important related concepts that need to be further discussed in relationship to indexing theory—**pattern completion** and **pattern separation**. Understanding these concepts is central to understanding how the index retrieves an episodic memory.

Pattern Completion and Pattern Separation

When a subset or portion of the experience that originally established the memory trace is encountered, it can activate or replay the entire experience (see Figure 17.3D,E). The process by which this happens is called pattern completion. It is the most fundamental process provided by the index. This process is possible because synapses on neurons in the hippocampus that represent the patterns of activity in the neocortex have been strengthened (this is the index) and because neurons in the hippocampus project back to the same neocortical regions (for example, entorhinal cortex) that projected to it (see Figures 17.1 and 17.2). Note that this could not happen if there were no return projections back from the hippocampus to the neocortex.

As noted previously, one of the remarkable aspects of the episodic memory system is that it has the capacity to maintain distinct representations of similar, but separately occurring, episodes. Many theorists believe that this property of episodic memory derives from the architecture of the hippocampus and its relationship to the neocortex. The basic idea is that outputs from widespread patterns of activity in the neocortex will randomly converge onto and activate a much smaller set of neurons in the hippocampus (O'Reilly and McClelland, 1994; O'Reilly and Rudy, 2001). Because the similar (but different) inputs are likely to converge onto different neurons in the hippocampus, the two similar patterns are likely to create different indices. Thus, the hippocampus is said to support a process called pattern separation that keeps representations of similar experiences segregated (Figure 17.4).

Why Not Just Store the Memory in the Neocortex?

The way in which the engram is built by the indexing system might seem overly complex. Why should the brain need an elaborate hierarchical system in which neocortical regions project to the hippocampus and then loop back to the neocortex to store a memory? Why not just directly strengthen the connections between those patterns of activity in the neocortex? There are at least two reasons why a hierarchical system has evolved. The first has to do with

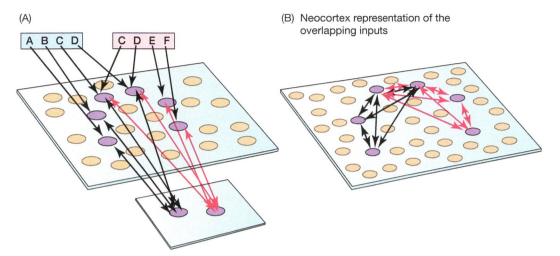

FIGURE 17.4 The hippocampus keeps memories of similar episodes separated. (A) Two similar input patterns (ABCD and CDEF) activate their respective patterns of neocortical activity. Projections from these similar neocortical patterns converge onto different neurons in the hippocampus. The synaptic connections from the cortical projections to and among the hippocampus neurons are strengthened. Thus, the hippocampus provides a separate index for the two similar memories that keeps them separated. Presenting the AC combination selectively activates the ABCD pattern, and the CE combination activates the CDEF pattern. (B) In contrast, the neocortex has difficulty keeping the memories for similar episodes separated. Because the patterns share common features (CD), they are interconnected and the memories for the different episodes lose their identity. Any combination of inputs (for example, AC, CE, or BD) activates the entire blended network.

the associative connectivity problem, while the second is related to the interference problem.

The associative connectivity problem relates to the potential connections among neurons in the different neocortical regions that support representations of experience. There may not be enough of these connections to support the rapid changes needed to associate patterns of activation distributed widely across the neocortex (Rolls and Treves, 1998). Thus, although there may be on the order of 10^{10} principal neurons in the cortex, they are not richly interconnected. This makes it difficult to strengthen associative connections among the patterns of activity produced by experience. Without these patterns being strongly connected, pattern completion (the activation of the entire pattern by a subset of the original experience) would be difficult.

In contrast, two regions in the hippocampus, the dentate gyrus and CA3, have high internal connectivity and modifiable synapses. In CA3, in particular, interconnectivity is so high that most of the pyramidal cells are connected within two to three synaptic steps (Rolls and Treves, 1998). Thus, unlike the neocortex, the hippocampus is well designed to associate arbitrary input patterns. Moreover, these synapses are easily modified, and mechanisms of synaptic plasticity revealed by studies of LTP (see Chapters 2 through 7) may very well support the changes in synaptic strength needed to maintain new associative connections.

The second reason why the hierarchical organization may be favored is related to the interference problem. Many of the episodes that make up our daily experiences occur in similar situations. For these individual episodes to be kept separate, they must be stored so that two similar episodes are not confused. Memory traces composed of directly connected patterns of neocortical activity may not be well suited to solve this problem. Consider what might happen if you have two related experiences such as lunch in the same place with two different friends. As described earlier, the hippocampus index supports pattern separation and thus would keep these two related but different experiences separate (illustrated in Figure 17.4A as ABCD and CDEF). In the neocortex, however, these two similar experiences would be integrated into a common representation. The key difference, shown in Figure 17.4B, is that in the neocortex any combination of inputs (AC, CE, or BD) would activate the integrated representation.

Indexing Theory and Properties of Episodic Memory

Indexing theory was developed with the intent of explaining how the neural system in which the hippocampus is situated can support the fundamental features of episodic memory. The properties of episodic memory emerge quite naturally from this theory.

- Conscious recollection and awareness emerge when pattern completion processes activate a representation of the entire event, including the context in which it occurs, sufficiently to replay the memory.

- The automatic or incidental storage property emerges because the synapses that support the memory are automatically strengthened just by the fact that experience generates new patterns of neural activity in the neocortex that project into the hippocampus. Such a mechanism captures the contextual information in which experience occurs because it binds the cortical representations of the entire experience.

- The episodic nature of the memory trace is due to single experiences, each generating unique patterns of neural activity in the neocortex that are captured by the hippocampus index.

- Interference among similar memory traces is reduced because the hippocampus supports pattern separation.

Evidence for the Indexing Theory

In this section some of the literature that provides support for indexing theory is presented. The experiments were chosen because they comment on some component of the theoretical ideas that have been presented. Two sources of the data include studies of amnesic people with damage to the hippocampus and studies of animals.

As described in Chapter 16, people with significant damage to the hippocampus are selectively impaired in their ability to consciously recall episodes of their personal experiences and events that occurred at specific times and places. Recall that H.M. improved his performance on motor and perceptual reorganization tasks, yet he had no recollection of ever participating in these tasks. Formal tests of other patients with much more selective damage to the hippocampus (such as patients R.B. and V.C.) also revealed that their recall of recent experiences was severely impaired (Cipolotti et al., 2001; Zola-Morgan et al., 1986).

Animal Studies

As previously noted, an advantage of studying memory in animals (primarily rodents) other than people is that the experimenter can precisely damage a particular region of the brain, including the hippocampus or its surrounding cortical regions. The disadvantage of this approach is that nonhuman animals cannot consciously recollect. Nevertheless, Howard Eichenbaum (2000) has made the point that the anatomical organization of the neural system that contains the hippocampus in primates and rodents is remarkably similar to that system in humans (see Figure 17.1). Thus, even though conscious recollection can be demonstrated only in people, given the anatomy of the rodent brain one should expect that it could support a rudimentary episodic memory system.

Indexing theory makes several claims about the role of the hippocampus in episodic memory that can be evaluated even in animals that cannot consciously recollect. These claims are that the hippocampus:

- is critical to forming context representations;
- provides a basis for conscious awareness and recollection;
- automatically captures context (incidental) information;
- captures single episodes;
- supports cued recall through pattern completion; and
- keeps separate episodes distinct.

Evidence supporting these basic claims is presented below. In addition, evidence based on the modern methods of neurobiology are discussed.

Context Representations Depend on the Hippocampus

A large number of studies with rodents support the idea that the hippocampus is critical to forming a representation of the context in which events are experienced. The context preexposure paradigm developed by Michael Fanselow (1990) provides a powerful tool to study context representations. It is based on a phenomenon called the immediate shock effect. If a rat is placed into a fear conditioning chamber and shocked immediately (within 6 seconds), it will later show little or

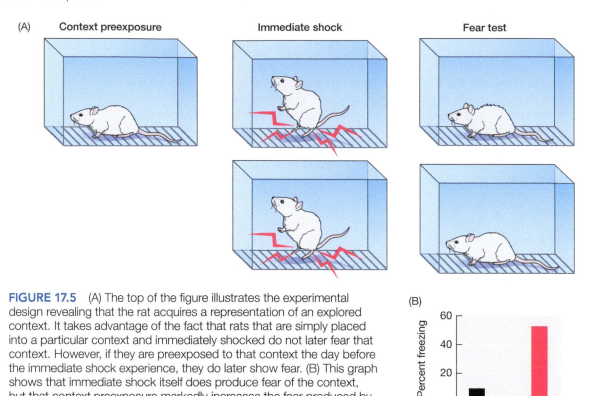

(A) Context preexposure   Immediate shock   Fear test

FIGURE 17.5 (A) The top of the figure illustrates the experimental design revealing that the rat acquires a representation of an explored context. It takes advantage of the fact that rats that are simply placed into a particular context and immediately shocked do not later fear that context. However, if they are preexposed to that context the day before the immediate shock experience, they do later show fear. (B) This graph shows that immediate shock itself does produce fear of the context, but that context preexposure markedly increases the fear produced by immediate shock. This result, called the context preexposure effect, indicates that the rat acquires a representation of the explored context. (After M. S. Fanselow. 1990. *Anim Learn Behav* 18: 264–270.)

(B)

Percent freezing

Immediate shock | Context preexposure + Immediate shock

no fear of the conditioning chamber. However, if the rat is allowed to explore the conditioning chamber for a couple of minutes the day before it receives immediate shock, it will subsequently show substantial fear to that context (Figure 17.5).

This result is called the **context preexposure facilitation effect**. It is believed to demonstrate that the rat acquired a representation of the context during the preexposure phase. If this is true then damage to the hippocampus should prevent the context preexposure effect. This result has been obtained many times. In fact, temporarily inactivating the hippocampus before either of the three phases of the context preexposure experiment eliminates the context preexposure facilitation effect (Barrientos et al., 2002; Matus-Amat et al., 2004, 2007; Rudy et al., 2002, 2004).

However, the important theoretical question is, how does the memory acquired during context preexposure result in immediate shock producing fear to the context? Index theory explains this result as being due to the cues associated with the preexposure procedure activating pattern completion processes to retrieve the context memory just prior to the immediate shock. The implication is that the animal is conditioning to the memory representation of the preexposed context and not to the place where the immediate shock occurs (Figure 17.6). This explanation makes two predictions. First, following immediate shock, during the fear test, the animal will display more fear to the preexposed context than to the place where it was actually shocked. Second, damage to the hippocampus will eliminate the context preexposure. Rudy et al.

(A)

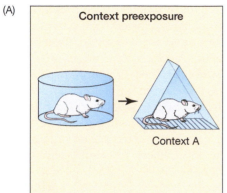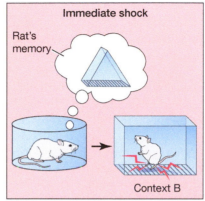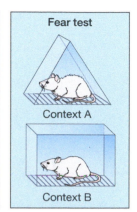

(B)

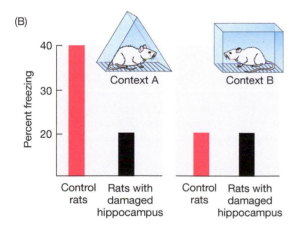

FIGURE 17.6 (A) An experiment demonstrating that rats can retrieve a memory of an explored context. During the context preexposure phase, the rats were transported in a bucket several times to a novel context (context A) and allowed to explore that context. The purpose of this procedure was to allow the transport bucket to become a cue that could retrieve the rat's memory of the explored context. In the immediate-shock phase of the experiment, the rats were transported in the same bucket to a shock chamber (context B), where they received an immediate shock. Note that the shock chamber was quite different from the previously explored context. The rats were then tested in either context A or context B. (B) The control rats displayed no fear in context B, where they were actually shocked, but displayed fear in context A, where they had been allowed to explore and had received no shock. This means that during the immediate-shock phase the control rats recalled the memory of context A (where they thought they were being transported to) and associated it with the shock. This created a false memory. Rats with damage to the hippocampus, however, did not show fear to either context A or context B, which means they were not able to acquire or retrieve the memory representation of the preexposed context. (After J. W. Rudy et al. 2002. *Behav Neurosci* 116: 530–538.)

(2002) confirmed both of these predictions. In effect, the preexposure facilitation effect is the result of the training procedure creating a **false memory**. The animals were never shocked in the preexposed context but displayed fear to it because its memory representation was present when it was shocked.

Conscious Awareness and Recollection

Indexing theory assumes that conscious recollection derives, in part, from the index representation that binds components of the episode into a representation of the context. Thus, encountering some component of the episode activates the index that in turn projects back to the neocortex and activates the cortical representation of the context. Strong activation of this representation might provide a basis for conscious awareness (see Eichenbaum et al., 2007 for a similar analysis).

Animals other than people cannot express their subjective feelings. However, it is possible to tell if they have the kind of representation just described. Studies of object recognition indicate that they do. For example, when given a choice between exploring a novel object and one previously experienced (a familiar object), rats spend more time exploring the novel object. Rats with damage to the hippocampus also explore a novel object more than a familiar one. However, what they apparently can't do is remember the context in which a particular object was experienced. This point is illustrated in Figure 17.7. A normal rat is first allowed to explore the cube in context A and the cylinder in context B. In the test phase, the rat is presented with each object in context A and in context B. A normal rat will explore the object presented in the different context as if it were novel. This means the representation of the object was bound together with features of the context in which it was explored. This kind of representation should require an index and be dependent on the hippocampus. In fact, rats with damage to the hippocampus treat explored objects as familiar, whether they are tested in their training context or the other context (Eacott and Norman, 2004; Mumby et al., 2002; see Eichenbaum et al., 2007 for a review).

Automatic Capture of Single Episodes

As noted earlier, the episodic memory system is always online, automatically capturing the events that make up our daily experiences. The studies just described make the case that this property also depends on the hippocampus. To appreciate this point, reconsider the context dependency of the object-recognition study illustrated in Figure 17.7. There are no explicit demands embedded in an object-recognition task. Nothing forces the animal to remember that the cube occurred in context A and the cylinder occurred in context B, any more than a normal person must remember where he or she had breakfast. However, this happens and it depends on an intact hippocampus. For that matter nothing forces the animals to acquire a representation of the context in the context preexposure experiments (see Figures 17.5 and 17.6). Note also that in these examples the memory representations are captured in a single experience.

(A) Exploration

(B) Test

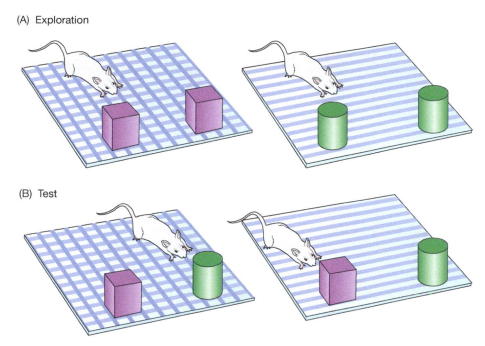

FIGURE 17.7   (A) Rats were allowed to explore two objects, a cube and a cylinder. Each object was explored in a different context. (B) The rats were then tested twice. Both objects were presented in each context. Control rats spent more time exploring the object that had not previously been experienced in the test context. In contrast, rats with damage to the hippocampus explored the objects equally. This means that control animals had a memory of the object and the context in which it occurred, but rats with damage to the hippocampus did not.

Pattern Separation

One of the important properties of the episodic memory system is that it keeps similar episodes somewhat distinct. As noted, an index in the hippocampus provides an advantage over a straight neocortical memory system. There is evidence that pattern separation is better when the hippocampus is intact. One source of such evidence is the study of what is called generalized contextual fear conditioning. In such studies, rats are shocked in one context (context A) and then tested in either that context or a similar but not identical context (context B). To the extent that they show fear to the similar context, they are said to generalize their fear to another context.

Imagine that you were in an automobile accident. You might display fear of being in the specific car involved in the accident and/or generalized fear to other, similar cars. Rats lacking a hippocampus display more generalized fear than normal rats (Antoniadis and McDonald, 2000; Frankland et al., 1998). This result suggests that the hippocampus provides processes that enable the rat to discriminate the context paired with shock from a similar one that was not paired with shock.

Gilbert and Kesner (2006) have provided another source of evidence that the hippocampus is necessary for pattern separation. They reported that rats with selective neurotoxic damage to the dentate gyrus could discriminate the location of two identical objects (a covered food well, for example) when the physical distance between them (their spatial separation) was great, but they performed poorly as the distance decreased. In contrast, normal rats were unaffected by the degree of spatial separation. Thus, the hippocampus was necessary for the rats to remember separate, similar spatial locations.

Modern Tests

In Chapter 14 a number of methods were introduced that enable researchers to identify and manipulate so-called engram cells. These methods have permitted strong tests of the indexing theory. Three examples are described below.

1. Direct activation of the indexing neurons can produce false memories.
2. Silencing identified indexing neurons prevents memory retrieval.
3. Engram cells in the neocortex are controlled by the hippocampal index.

FALSE MEMORIES   In the discussion of the context preexposure facilitation effect presented in Figure 17.6, it was noted that during the immediate shock phase the rats were conditioning to the memory representation of the preexposed context and this in effect produced a false memory because the rats were never shocked there. According to indexing theory it should also be possible to create a false memory if one could identify and directly activate neurons in the hippocampus that index the preexposed context.

Steve Ramirez and Xu Liu (Ramirez et al., 2013) used optogenetic methods to test and confirm this prediction (Figure 17.8). In their experiments they used a viral vector system to deliver channelrhodopsin-2 (ChR2) to a small set of neurons in the dentate gyrus. ChR2 would not be expressed as long as doxycycline was in the diet.

When doxycycline was removed from the diet they exposed mice to context A. Thus, during this period indexing neurons that were active in the dentate gyrus would express ChR2. Mice were put back on doxycycline (to prevent further expression of ChR2) and then placed in context B where they experienced shock. However, before shock was presented blue light was delivered to the dentate gyrus to activate the hippocampal cells theoretically indexing context A, so that this representation could become associated with the shock. If it did, even though they were never shocked there, the mice should display freezing when tested in context A. As predicted by indexing theory mice indeed displayed freezing behavior in context A—revealing a false memory (see Figure 17.8E).

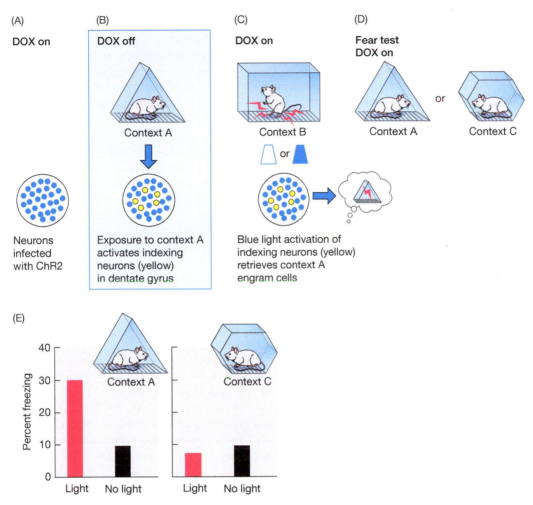

FIGURE 17.8 In this experiment, optogenetic methods were used to create a false memory. (A) When on doxycycline (DOX on), neurons in the dentate gyrus did not express channelrhodopsin-2 (ChR2). (B) Doxycycline was removed from the diet (DOX off) and the mice were allowed to explore context A, thus allowing active neurons in the dentate gyrus to express ChR2. (C) In the DOX-on state the mice were placed in context B and shocked. Blue light stimulation was delivered to the dentate gyrus of some animals to activate indexing neurons (the light condition). Theoretically, this should activate the memory of context A so that it could be associated with shock. Blue light was not delivered to mice in the control (no light) condition. (D) Mice were tested for fear in context A or context C. (E) Mice in the light-on condition displayed freezing in context A but not in context C. These results support the hypothesis that activating the index to the context A representation when the animals were shocked in context B established a false memory. (After S. Ramirez et al. 2013. *Science* 341: 387–391.)

SILENCING INDEXING NEURONS PREVENTS RETRIEVAL   If neurons in the hippocampus are indeed indexing the context memory, it should be possible to prevent memory retrieval by silencing them during the fear test. Using optogenetic methods, other researchers have demonstrated that silencing neurons can prevent retrieval of a conditioned fear memory. Silencing indexing neurons in either the dentate gyrus or CA3 (Denny et al., 2014) or in CA1 (Tanaka et al., 2014) prevents the retrieval of a contextual fear memory (Figure 17.9).

THE INDEX CONTROLS ACTIVATION OF CORTICAL ENGRAM NEURONS
According to the indexing theory, memories are retrieved when a subset of the original episode activates the relevant indexing neurons sufficiently to project back to the neocortex to activate the neocortical pattern representing the entire experience. Thus, indexing theory predicts that (a) engram neurons controlled by the index will be widely distributed over the neocortex and (b) silencing indexing neurons during retrieval will prevent the activation of the engram cells.

In order to test the first prediction, the researcher has to tag neurons all over the brain that are activated by the memory-producing event for later identification and then determine if some of these same neurons are in fact engram cells. If this is true they will also be activated at the time of retrieval. To test the second prediction, the researcher has to determine if silencing indexing neurons in the hippocampus prevents the activation of neocortical engram cells.

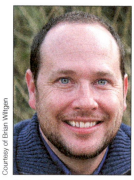

Brian Wiltgen

Brian Wiltgen's laboratory developed what is called the H2B-GFP Tet-Tag mouse to address these predictions (Tanaka et al., 2014; Tayler et al., 2013). This transgenic mouse was genetically engineered so that activated neurons all over the brain would express a **green fluorescent protein (GFP)** tag. The expression of the gene, however, was controlled by doxycycline. GFP would only be expressed when doxycycline was not in the diet and this tag would endure for over two weeks. Contextual fear conditioning was used as the memory-producing procedure.

To determine which neurons activated by the conditioning procedure were engram cells, doxycycline was reintroduced into the diet and the mice were tested for their fear response. To qualify as an engram cell, a neuron had to express both GFP and the immediate early gene *c-Fos*, another marker of neuronal activity. Thus, in any particular brain region, there would be cells that express only GFP, only *c-Fos*, or both. Note that the logic of the experiment is similar to that introduced by Mark Mayford's group (Reijmers et al., 2007) who were the first to identify engram cells (see Figure 14.4).

Using this logic, Tayler et al. (2013) discovered that a large number of neurons in the hippocampus and throughout the neocortex and amygdala expressed GFP. However, only a small percentage of these cells expressed both GFP and *c-Fos*

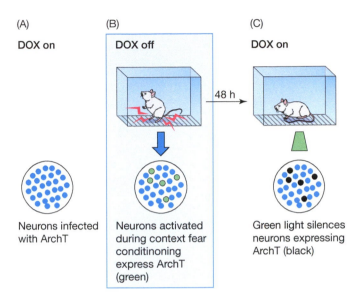

(A)
DOX on

(B)
DOX off

(C)
DOX on

48 h

Neurons infected
with ArchT

Neurons activated
during context fear
conditinoning
express ArchT
(green)

Green light silences
neurons expressing
ArchT (black)

(D)

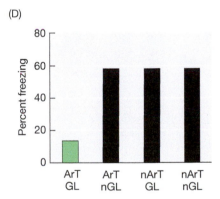

FIGURE 17.9 In this experiment, optogenetic methods were used to silence neurons to prevent retrieval of a context fear memory. (A) When on doxycycline (DOX on), neurons in the CA1 did not express the neuron silencer, ArchT (abbreviated in the graph as ArT). (B) Doxycycline was removed from the diet (DOX off) and the mice experienced a fear condition, thus allowing active neurons in CA1 to express ArchT. (C) During the test for fear conditioning, green light (GL) was delivered to the CA1 region to silence the indexing neurons that express ArchT. (D) Mice expressing ArchT and stimulated with the green light did not freeze during the test but did freeze if not stimulated (nGL), as did mice in the control conditions that did not express ArchT (nArT). Thus, silencing indexing neurons in CA1 prevented retrieval of the context fear memory. (After K. Z. Tanaka et al. 2014. *Neuron* 84: 347–354.)

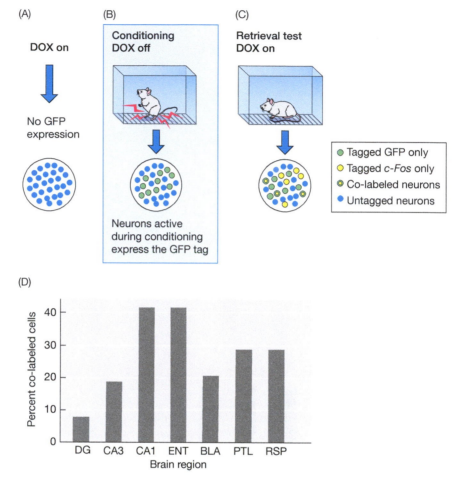

FIGURE 17.10 The H2B-GFP TetTag mouse was genetically engineered so activated neurons express a green fluorescent protein (GFP), but only when doxycycline (DOX) was removed from its diet. (A) When doxycycline was in the diet, GFP was not expressed. (B) When doxycycline was removed from the diet, all neurons activated by the fear conditioning experience expressed GFP. (C) Following the retrieval test, the experimenter would expect to see neurons expressing only GFP, expressing only *c-Fos*, or expressing both GFP and *c-Fos*. Only the neurons that co-express both GFP and *c-Fos* would count as engram cells because they would be cells that were active during both memory formation and retrieval. (D) A small percentage of co-labeled cells (engram cells) were found throughout the brain. Key: DG = dentate gyrus; ENT = entorhinal cortex; BLA = basolateral amygdala; PTL = posterior parietal association; RSP = retrosplenial cortex. (After K. K. Tayler et al. 2013. *Cur Biol* 23: 99–106.)

(Figure 17.10), which is consistent with studies discussed in Chapter 14. Tanaka et al. (2014) then determined the effect of optogenetically silencing indexing

(A)

(B)

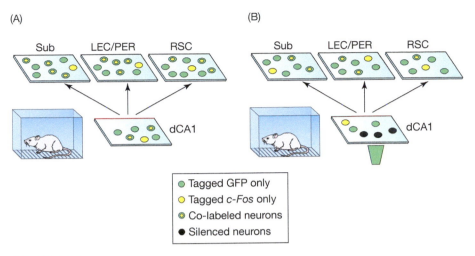

- ◉ Tagged GFP only
- ○ Tagged c-Fos only
- ◎ Co-labeled neurons
- ● Silenced neurons

FIGURE 17.11 (A) Illustrates that retrieval of a contextual fear memory activates co-labeled neurons throughout the dorsal hippocampus and neocortex. (B) Optogenetically silencing neurons in the dorsal hippocampus CA1 (dCA1) expressing ArchT dramatically reduces the number of co-labeled neurons in these regions. Key: Sub = subiculum; LEC = lateral entorhinal cortex; PER = perirhinal cortex; RSC = retrosplenial cortex. (After K. Z. Tanaka et al. 2014. *Neuron* 84: 347–354.)

neurons in CA1 upon the activation of engram cells in the neocortex. As illustrated in Figure 17.11, silencing indexing neurons reduced the number of co-labeled neurons obtained in neocortal regions produced by retrieval.

In summary, consistent with the predictions of indexing theory, the work from Wiltgen's group has demonstrated that (a) engram cells controlled by indexing neurons are distributed throughout the neocortex, and (b) silencing indexing neurons in the hippocampus prevents their activation during retrieval and prevents the expression of contextual fear.

Summary

The episodic memory system supports our ability to consciously recollect the daily episodes of our lives. The hippocampus is a critical component of the neural system that supports the storage and retrieval of episodic memories. Information flows from the neocortical regions to the hippocampus and then returns to the neocortical projection sites.

The hippocampal indexing theory was developed to provide an in-principle account of how the neural system in which the hippocampus is embedded contributes to memory formation, the resulting engram, and memory retrieval. It assumes that the content of experience is stored in the neocortex and that the hippocampus creates indices to memories for different episodes. It does this by binding the inputs it receives from different regions of the neocortex into a neural ensemble that represents the conjunction of their co-occurrence. Because the hippocampus projects back to the neocortical areas (see Figure 17.1A), when this index is activated it can activate or replay the activity patterns that are the memory of the episode.

The hippocampus supports pattern completion, whereby a subset of the original episode can activate the whole pattern. It also supports pattern separation by creating different indices for similar episodes and thus segregating them. The neocortex is not well suited to rapidly acquire memories for single episodes because potential associative connectivity across neocortical regions is low and patterns of neocortical activity produced by separate but similar experiences may become blended and thus lose their episodic nature. Studies with both people and rodents support this view of the role of the hippocampus in episodic memory. Activating indexing neurons can retrieve context memories. Silencing these neurons can prevent both the activation of neocortical engram neurons and memory retrieval.

References

Amaral, D. and Lavenex, P. (2007). Hippocampal anatomy. In P. Andersen, R. Morris, D. Amaral, T. Bliss, and J. O'Keefe (Eds.), *The Hippocampus Book* (pp. 37–114). New York: Oxford University Press.

Antoniadis, E. A. and McDonald, R. J. (2000). Amygdala, hippocampus, and discrimination fear conditioning to context. *Behavioural Brain Research, 108*, 1–19.

Barrientos, R. M., O'Reilly, R. C., and Rudy, J. W. (2002). Memory for context is impaired by injecting anisomycin into dorsal hippocampus following context exploration. *Behavioural Brain Research, 134*, 291–298.

Cipolotti, L., Shallice, T., Chan, D., Fox, N., Scahill, R., Harrison, G. J., Stevens, J., and Rudge, P. (2001). Long-term retrograde amnesia: the crucial role of the hippocampus. *Neuropsychologia, 39*, 151–172.

Denny, C. A., Kheirbek, M. A., Alba, E. L., Tanaka, K. F., Brachman, R. A., Laughman, K. B., Tomm, N. K., Turi, G. F., Losonczy, A., and Hen, R. (2014). Hippocampal memory traces are differentially modulated by experience, time, and adult neurogenesis. *Neuron, 83*, 189–201.

Eacott, M. J. and Norman, G. (2004). Integrated memory for object, place, and context in rats: a possible model of episodic-like memory? *Journal of Neuroscience, 24*, 1948–1953.

Eichenbaum, H. (2000). A cortical-hippocampal system for declarative memory. *Nature Reviews Neuroscience, 1*, 41–50.

Eichenbaum, H., Yonelinas, A. R., and Ranganath, C. (2007). The medial temporal lobe and recognition memory. *Annual Reviews of Neuroscience, 30*, 123–152.

Fanselow, M. S. (1990). Factors governing one-trial contextual conditioning. *Animal Learning and Behavior, 18*, 264–270.

Frankland, P. W., Cestari, V., Filipkowski, R. K., McDonald, R. J., and Silva, A. J. (1998). The dorsal hippocampus is essential for context discrimination but not for contextual conditioning. *Behavioral Neuroscience, 112*, 863–874.

Gilbert, P. E. and Kesner, R. P. (2006). The role of dorsal CA3 hippocampal subregion in spatial working memory and pattern separation. *Behavioural Brain Research, 169*, 142–149.

Lavenex, P. and Amaral, D. G. (2000). Hippocampal–neocortical interaction: a hierarchy of associativity. *Hippocampus, 10*, 420–430.

Marr, D. (1971). Simple memory: a theory for archicortex. *Proceedings of the Royal Society of London B Biological Sciences, 262*, 23–81.

Matus-Amat, P., Higgins, E. A., Barrientos, R. M., and Rudy, J. W. (2004). The role of the dorsal hippocampus in the acquisition and retrieval of context memory representations. *Journal of Neuroscience, 24*, 2431–2439.

Matus-Amat, P., Higgins, E. A., Sprunger, D., Wright-Hardesty, K., and Rudy, J. W. (2007). The role of dorsal hippocampus and basolateral amygdala NMDA receptors in the acquisition and retrieval of context and context fear memories. *Behavioral Neuroscience, 121*(4), 721–731.

McNaughton, B. L. (1991). Associative pattern completion in hippocampal circuits: new evidence and new questions. *Brain Research Review, 16*, 193–220.

McNaughton, B. L. and Morris, R. G. M. (1987). Hippocampal synaptic enhancement and information storage within a distributed memory system. *Trends in Neurosciences, 10*, 408–415.

Mumby, D. G., Gaskin, S., Glenn, M. J., Schramek, T. E., and Lehmann, H. (2002). Hippocampal damage and exploratory preferences in rats: memory for objects, places, and contexts. *Learning and Memory, 9*, 49–57.

Nadel, L. and Moscovitch, M. (1997). Memory consolidation, retrograde amnesia and the hippocampal complex. *Current Opinion in Neurobiology, 17*, 217–227.

O'Keefe, J. and Nadel, L. (1978). *The Hippocampus as a Cognitive Map*. Oxford: Clarendon Press.

O'Reilly, R. C. and McClelland, J. L. (1994). Hippocampal conjunctive encoding, storage, and recall: avoiding a trade-off. *Hippocampus, 4*, 661–682.

O'Reilly, R. C. and Rudy, J. W. (2001). Conjunctive representations in learning and memory: principles of cortical and hippocampal function. *Psychological Review, 108*, 311–345.

Ramirez, S., Liu, X., Lin, P. A., Suh, J., Pignatelli, M., Redondo, R. L., Ryan, T. J., and Tonegawa, S. (2013). Creating a false memory in the hippocampus. *Science, 341*, 387–391.

Reijmers, L. G., Perkins, B. L., Matsuo, N., and Mayford, M. (2007). Localization of a stable neural correlate of associative memory. *Science, 317*, 1230–1233.

Rolls, E. T. and Treves, A. (1998). *Neural Networks and Brain Function*. Oxford: Oxford University Press.

Rudy, J. W., Barrientos, R. M., and O'Reilly, R. C. (2002). The hippocampal formation supports conditioning to memory of a context. *Behavioral Neuroscience, 116,* 530–538.

Rudy, J. W., Huff, N., and Matus-Amat, P. (2004). Understanding contextual fear conditioning: insights from a two-process model. *Neuroscience Biobehavioral Review, 28,* 675–686.

Schacter, D. L. (1989). On the relation between memory and consciousness: dissociable interactions and conscious experience. In H. L. Roediger, III, and F. I. M. Craik (Eds.), *Varieties of Memory and Consciousness: Essays in Honor of Endel Tulving* (pp. 355–389). Hillsdale, NJ: Erlbaum Associates.

Squire, L. R. (1992). Memory and the hippocampus: a synthesis from findings with rats, monkeys and humans. *Psychology Review, 99,* 195–231.

Squire, L. R. and Kandel, E. R. (1999). *Memory: From Mind to Molecules.* New York: W. H. Freeman and Company.

Squire, L. R. and Zola-Morgan, S. (1991). The medial temporal lobe memory system. *Science, 253,* 1380–1386.

Tanaka, K. Z., Pevzner, A., Hamidi, A. B., Nakazawa, Y., Graham, J., and Wiltgen, B. J. (2014). Cortical representations are reinstated by the hippocampus during memory retrieval. *Neuron, 84,* 347–354.

Tayler, K. K., Tanaka, K. Z., Reijmers, L. G., and Wiltgen, B. J. (2013). Reactivation of neural ensembles during the retrieval of recent and remote memory. *Current Biology, 23,* 99–106.

Teyler, T. J. and DiScenna, P. (1986). The hippocampal memory indexing theory. *Behavioral Neuroscience, 100,* 147–152.

Teyler, T. J. and Rudy, J. W. (2007). The hippocampus indexing theory of episodic memory: updating the index. *Hippocampus, 17,* 1158–1169.

Van Hoesen, G. and Pandya, D. N. (1975). Some connections of the entorhinal (area 28) and perirhinal (area 35) cortices of the rhesus monkey. I. Temporal lobe afferents. *Brain Research, 95,* 1–24.

Zola-Morgan, S., Squire, L. R., and Amaral, D. G. (1986). Human amnesia and the medial temporal region: enduring memory impairment following a bilateral lesion limited to field CA1 of the hippocampus. *Journal of Neuroscience, 6,* 2950–2967.

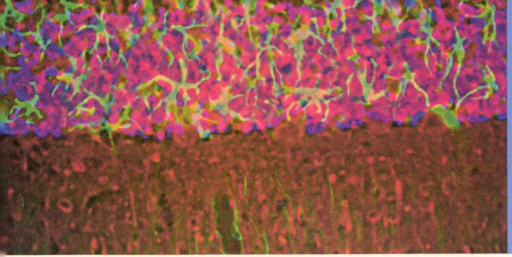

Courtesy of Heidi E. W. Day

When Memories Age

Episodic memories are supported by the medial temporal hippocampal (MTH) system. What happens to these memories as they age? The most likely outcome is that they will be forgotten either due to interference produced by similar experiences or because the underlying supporting synapses will degrade (see Chapter 13). For example, in an experiment designed to study memory for real life episodes, Misra et al. (2018) had participants spend an hour walking a novel route with a GoPro camera attached to their foreheads to record where they gazed. The striking result was that, when tested the next day, participants could barely distinguish between scenes recorded from their own personal episodic experience from those of other participants that followed the same route. Such forgetting is of little consequence because much of what is experienced on a daily basis is of no lasting significance—such as what we had for breakfast, whom we encountered at the grocery store, or some conversation that we had about the weather.

Most everyday uneventful memories established in the MTH system likely will be lost. Recall, however, that Ribot's Law suggests that as some memories age they become resistant to disruption (see Chapter 1). By itself this claim is not surprising because (a) the experience that produced the initial memory is more likely to be repeated and (b) older memories, compared to new memories, are more likely to have been recalled a few times. Both of these factors would increase the strength of the memory.

However, in the modern era Ribot's Law has been nuanced to give an explicit role for the MTH system in protecting old memories from disruption and in reorganizing and strengthening memories in the neocortex. This chapter discusses some of the theoretical claims and empirical issues associated with Ribot's Law. It introduces and evaluates what is called the standard model of systems consolidation and ends with a discussion of another view, called competitive trace theory.

The Standard Model of Systems Consolidation

When the memory impairments associated with H.M. were first reported it was believed that his retrograde amnesia was temporally graded—meaning that it was limited to a 2–3 year period just prior to the surgical removal of his medial temporal lobes. Based largely on this observation, Larry Squire, Neal Cohen, and Lynn Nadel (1984) proposed that Ribot's Law could be related to the MTH system. Their position is called the **standard model of systems consolidation**. They proposed that experience initially lays down a memory trace that depends, for both storage and retrieval, on interactions between the neocortical areas and the MTH system, described in Figure 18.1. There are two other important assumptions associated with this position (Squire et al., 1984).

First, the critical interaction between the MTH system and other cortical sites is required for only a limited time after learning. When a memory is originally formed, the MTH system maintains its coherence—it holds together the components of the trace that are distributed over various regions of the brain. Processes intrinsic to the neocortical storage sites are responsible for consolidating the memory in the brain regions outside of the MTH system. During this period the integrity of the MTH system is also necessary to retrieve the memory. Once this process is sufficiently complete, however, the MTH system is no longer needed for retrieval of that memory. Squire and his colleagues never specified what constitutes a limited amount of time. However, based on their discussion of H.M. and other literature, it appears that they assumed consolidation requires about 3 years.

Second, the MTH system–neocortical interaction is needed only to consolidate declarative memory (episodic and semantic memories). It is not involved in what is sometimes called **procedural memory**—memories that support learned skills such as bike riding or skiing.

In summary, the standard model explains Ribot's Law by assuming that:

- disruptive events primarily impact the MTH system;
- new memories require the hippocampus for ongoing systems consolidation and retrieval; and
- old memories are more resistant to disruption than new memories because they have been consolidated in the neocortex and no longer depend on the MTH system for retrieval (Squire et al., 1984).

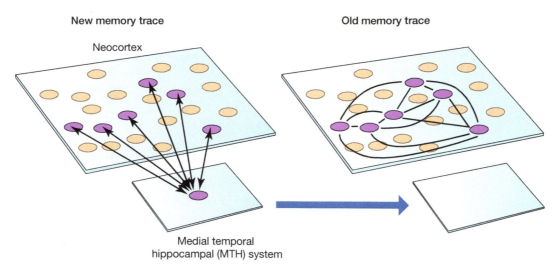

New memory trace

Old memory trace

Neocortex

Medial temporal
hippocampal (MTH) system

FIGURE 18.1   A schematic representation of the standard model of systems consolidation. Initially the memory trace consists of weakly connected neocortical representations of the features (purple circles) of the experience held together by their temporary connections with the medial temporal hippocampal (MTH) system. New memories require the MTH system for retrieval. As the memory ages, intrinsic processes result in the consolidation or strengthening of the connections among the neocortical representations. Because of the strengthened connections the memory can now be retrieved without the hippocampus. (After L. Squire et al. 1984. In *Memory Consolidation: Psychobiology of Cognition*, H. Weingartner and E. Parker (Eds.), pp. 185–210. Hillsdale, NJ: Erlbaum and Associates.)

It should be noted that the concept of systems consolidation is quite different from the concept of **cellular consolidation**. Cellular consolidation refers to the biochemical and molecular events that take place immediately following the behavioral experience that initially forms the memory trace. Several hours may be required for these processes, which are discussed extensively in previous chapters, to consolidate the trace. Systems consolidation refers to changes in the strength of the memory trace brought about by interactions between brain regions (the MTH system and neocortex) that take place after the memory is initially established. Systems consolidation begins after the trace is initially stored and operates over a much longer time frame—days, months, or years (Figure 18.2).

Two other points about systems consolidation need to be considered. First, there is no mention of a role for recall or repetition within this framework. So experience lays down the trace and for months thereafter intrinsic processes operate to consolidate the memory in the cortex, while the hippocampus in some way maintains the coherence of the neural patterns in the cortex that represent the memory. Thus, in principle this intrinsic activity requires no additional input from experience (recall or repetition) to carry out its function.

FIGURE 18.2 Two types of processes are thought to contribute to the consolidation of long-term stability of memories.

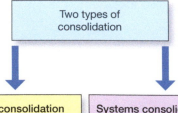

Two types of consolidation

Cellular consolidation

- Consequence of synaptic biochemical events initiated by the original experience

- Time frame of hours

Systems consolidation

- Consequence of an interaction between the medial temporal hippo- campal system and neocortex

- Time frame largely unspecified—days, weeks, months, years

More recent versions of the theory assign the intrinsic activity to neural processes occurring during sleep (see Klinzing et al., 2019; Skelin et al., 2019). Second, the standard model assumes that this process consolidates declarative memories (both episodic and semantic).

Evaluating the Standard Model

The standard model makes a strong prediction: damage to the hippocampal formation will spare old episodic and semantic memories, but new episodic and semantic memories will be lost—a temporally graded retrograde amnesia. This prediction is illustrated in Figure 18.3A. However, if damage to the MTH system produces a flat gradient (Figure 18.3B), this would be a problem for the model.

Clinical Evidence

Case studies of individuals who are known to have damage to regions in the medial temporal lobes provide an important source of data for evaluating this prediction. For many years, H.M. was the only patient available with known bilateral damage to the medial temporal lobes. Over the years, however, a number of patients with damage to the MTH system have been identified and evaluated. When Lynn Nadel and Morris Moscovitch (1997) reviewed this literature, they reached a surprising conclusion: the evidence does not support the standard model. They concluded that when damage to the MTH system is complete there is no sparing of either new or old episodic memories. Spared old episodic memories are only found when damage to the MTH system is incomplete. Thus, they asserted that the MTH system continues to be critical to retrieval throughout the life

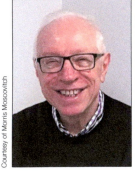

Courtesy of Morris Moscovitch

Morris Moscovitch

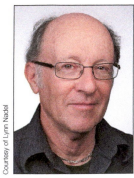

Courtesy of Lynn Nadel

Lynn Nadel

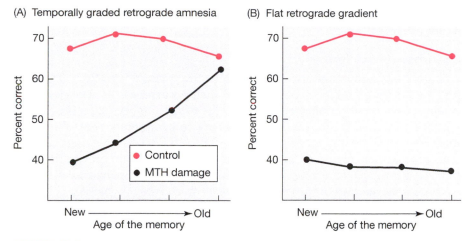

FIGURE 18.3 These graphs illustrate patterns of results that would either support or be evidence against the standard model of systems consolidation. (A) This pattern would support the model because it shows that damage to the hippocampus results in temporally graded retrograde amnesia. (B) This pattern would be evidence against the standard model because it shows that damage to the hippocampus produces a flat retrograde amnesia.

of an episodic memory. Their conclusion regarding the fate of old semantic memories was less clear. They suggested that retrograde damage for general semantic memories is more variable but less severe.

The relevant literature reviewed by Nadel and Moscovitch is complex and controversial; not everyone agrees with their conclusion. For example, some researchers argue that the loss of old memories reflects the fact that the brain injury extends beyond the MTH system into neocortical areas that would be the storage sites of old memories (Bayley et al., 2003; Bayley et al., 2005; Reed and Squire, 1998). It is interesting to note that Suzanne Corkin, who knew and worked with H.M. for over 40 years, reevaluated him to determine the extent of his retrograde amnesia, using modern methods that discriminated between episodic and semantic memories (Corkin, 2002; Steinvorth et al., 2005). Her review concluded that H.M.'s episodic memory was severely impaired and that there was no sparing of old memories. Moreover, his semantic memory was very much in the range of control subjects matched for age, IQ, and level of education. It is interesting that H.M.'s episodic memory impairment was much more severe than was initially believed (Corkin, 1984; Milner et al., 1968).

Based on the new clinical data, a number of contemporary researchers believe that damage to the MTH system or perhaps even just to the hippocampal formation produces a profound retrograde amnesia for both new and old episodic memories. If this is true, then the human clinical literature provides little or no support for the standard model of systems consolidation and its view that, for the retrieval of episodic memories, the MTH system is needed only for a limited time.

Experimental Evidence

There are many problems associated with testing people who have damage to the medial temporal lobes produced by such occurrences as strokes or encephalitis. Two main problems are that (1) the brain damage extends beyond the regions of interest and (2) there is no way to completely control for the initial strength of the memory. For these reasons researchers have used laboratory animals, primarily rodents, to experimentally assess the contribution the hippocampus makes to new and old memories. This strategy has the obvious advantage that one can (a) provide animals with a known behavioral experience, (b) vary the exact time between the experience and the occurrence of the brain damage, and (c) vary the extent of the brain damage. One can also hold constant the length of time between when the brain is damaged and when the animals are tested.

As noted in Chapter 17, there is an inherent difficulty in studying episodic memory in rodents and nonhuman primates—for the simple reason that they cannot directly tell the experimenter about their past experiences. They cannot tell us what they had for lunch, let alone who was with them and where it happened. Thus, the choice of how to study systems consolidation in animals has boiled down to finding tasks in which a memory can be established in a single episode and persist for a long time.

In 1992, Jeansok Kim and Michael Fanselow reported that contextual fear conditioning would be a good choice. They found that a single conditioning session produced a memory (as expressed by the animal freezing in the conditioning context) that lasted for at least 28 days. Moreover, with time the memory became resistant to disruption produced by damage to the dorsal hippocampus. This result was in line with the prediction of the standard model. Thereafter, the contextual fear conditioning task became the dominant animal model for evaluating the standard model of systems consolidation, so most of the narrative that follows focuses on results obtained with this methodology.

Damage to the Hippocampus Disrupts Old and New Memories

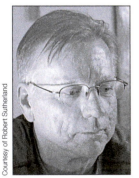

Courtesy of Robert Sutherland

Robert Sutherland

Unfortunately, Kim and Fanselow's result did not hold up. More systematic explorations of this paradigm have revealed that both partial and complete damage to the hippocampus equally disrupt old and new contextual fear memories. For example, Robert Sutherland and his colleagues (Lehmann et al., 2007) have compared the effects of partial and complete lesions of the hippocampus on the rat's contextual fear memory. They damaged the hippocampus either 1 week, 3 months, or 6 months following the conditioning session. Partial damage to the hippocampus produced less amnesia than large lesions, but the age of the memory at the time of the lesion did not

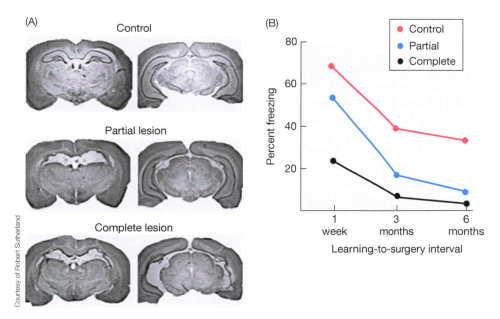

FIGURE 18.4   (A) These images illustrate the extent of the damage to the hippocampus. (B) These data show that over the 6-month retention interval, control rats showed evidence of forgetting. Note, however, that there was no evidence that the 3-month and 6-month-old memories were protected from damage to the hippocampus. (B after H. Lehmann et al. 2007. *Eur J Neurosci* 25: 1278–1286.)

matter (Figure 18.4). Furthermore, Broadbent and Clark (2013) explored a range of parameters, including the type of lesion, extent of the damage to the hippocampus, and number of conditioning trials. No matter what the condition, old contextual fear memories were not protected from disruption by hippocampal damage. They concluded that the preponderance of available evidence indicates that context fear memory remains hippocampus dependent indefinitely (see also Lehmann et al., 2007; Sparks et al, 2013; Sutherland et al., 2001). More recently, Ocampo et al. (2017) reported that selective lesioning of CA1, the output region of the hippocampus, equally impaired new and old contextual fear memories. These results obviously provide no support for the standard model.

Learning the spatial locations of the type required by the place-learning version of the Morris water-escape task (see Chapter 9) requires that animals acquire what is sometimes called a cognitive map (see O'Keefe and Nadel, 1978)—a representation that links together the various features of the environment into a coherent framework which can then be used to guide behavior. This representation is similar to that formed in a contextual fear conditioning experiment. Moreover, animals with damage to the hippocampus cannot learn the location of a hidden platform. Thus, researchers have also asked if old memories for place location are protected from damage to the hippocampus.

A variety of tasks have been used to address this question and in every case the answer is no—old memories are just as disrupted by damage to the hippocampus as new ones (Clark et al., 2005a, 2005b; Martin et al., 2005; Ocampo et al., 2017; Sutherland et al., 2001).

The surgical removal of a brain region is often used to gain insight into the role of that structure in memory. However, interpretation of the lesion data is complicated. For example, it is possible that a resulting impairment is due to unintended damage to other nearby regions. In principle, optogenetics methodology provides a much more precise means of identifying the contribution of specific sets of neurons to a particular behavioral outcome and eliminates many issues that are associated with lesions or other methodologies (see Chapter 9). Thus, it has been used to address the contribution of hippocampal neurons to the retrieval of new and old contextual fear memories. To do this, Inbal Goshen and her colleagues (Goshen et al., 2011) used a viral vector system to deliver a gene for inhibitory channels to CA1 neurons. When activated by light, neurons expressing these channels are inhibited. To the researchers' surprise, inhibiting these neurons during the retrieval test equally impaired the expression of both new (1-day old) and old (4–12 weeks old) contextual fear memories. This experiment provides no support for the standard model prediction—that retrieval of a contextual fear memory becomes independent of the hippocampus as the memory ages.

Goshen et al. (2011) provided an additional interesting observation. In the initial experiments the neurons were inactivated only during the few minutes of the retrieval test. In a subsequent experiment, however, they inhibited these neurons for 30 minutes prior to and during the retrieval test. Under these conditions, the old memory was retrieved. The authors suggested that this 30-minute period allowed time for the neocortical sites to adapt to the removal of the hippocampal input. This result indicates that it is possible to retrieve a contextual fear memory when a small set of CA1 neurons is inhibited. However, it is difficult to know what if any implications these results have for systems consolidation. This is because these researchers did not examine the effect of this long-lasting inhibition on retrieval of a new fear memory. So it is very possible this same treatment would also allow the retrieval of a new memory.

Memory without the Hippocampus

This review of the human and animal literature provides *very little support for the standard model's explanation of Ribot's Law*—that old memories are more resistant to disruption than new ones because they are liberated from the hippocampus. However, there is a second claim embedded in the standard model, specifically: *the hippocampus participates in a time-dependent manner in reorganizing and increasing the contribution of neocortical regions to the retrieval of old memories*. This claim predicts that the hippocampus is necessary to establish long-lasting memories that reside in the neocortex. The evidence relevant to this prediction is presented below. First, however, the concept of an extrahippocampal system needs to be introduced.

A number of neocortical regions have been identified as contributors to retrieval of contextual fear memories. They include prefrontal, anterior cingulate, perirhinal, postrhinal, and retrosplenial cortex (Burwell et al., 2004; Coelho et al., 2018; Frankland and Bontempi, 2005; Keene and Bucci, 2008; Takehara-Nishiuchi, 2014; Todd et al., 2017; Zelikowsky et al., 2013). Hereafter, these regions collectively are referred to as the **extrahippocampal system**, a neural system that does not include the hippocampus. Evidence discussed below reveals that this system is able to acquire and retrieve the contextual fear memory independent of the hippocampus.

RETROGRADE BUT NOT ANTEROGRADE DAMAGE PRODUCES AMNESIA Over 20 years ago, Steve Maren and colleagues (Maren et al., 1997; see also Coelho et al., 2018; Wiltgen et al., 2006) reported that damage to the hippocampus *shortly after* contextual fear conditioning produced a profound retrograde amnesia. Yet, damage to the hippocampus *prior to* conditioning had no effect on retrieval of the memory; these rats displayed as much freezing as the control animals (Figure 18.5A).

As just noted, newly acquired contextual fear memories created when the hippocampus is intact often cannot be retrieved if the hippocampus is subsequently damaged. Under some circumstances, however, even when the hippocampus is present, a newly acquired contextual fear memory can be established that survives subsequent damage to the hippocampus. This happens if animals receive several conditioning sessions, distributed over several days prior to the lesion (Lehmann et al., 2009; Figure 18.5B).

THE EXTRAHIPPOCAMPAL SYSTEM SUPPORTS LONG-LASTING FEAR MEMORIES A contextual fear memory can be established in the extrahippocampal system when the hippocampus is not present. It is also important to ask if this memory will persist as it ages. The standard model would predict that it should not last. Zelikowsky et al. (2012) first addressed this question and reported that retrieval of the context memory systematically decreased over a 30-day retention interval. However, Darryl

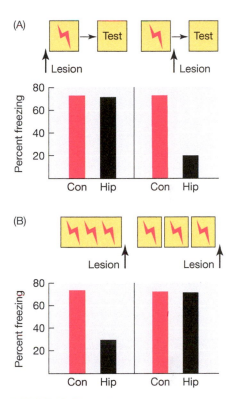

FIGURE 18.5 (A) Damage to the hippocampus prior to contextual fear conditioning does not impair retrieval of the memory, but damage to the hippocampus after conditioning prevents subsequent retrieval of the memory. (B) Contextual fear conditioning produced by several shocks delivered in the same session is impaired by subsequent damage to the hippocampus, but contextual fear produced by the same number of shocks delivered in separate sessions is not affected by subsequent damage to the hippocampus. Lightning bolt symbol represents the delivery of shock. Key: Con = control; Hip = hippocampus. (A after S. Maren et al. 1997. *Behav Brain Res* 88: 261–274; B after H. Lehmann et al. 2009. *Learn Mem* 16: 417–420.)

Gidyk, a Ph.D student in Robert Sutherland's laboratory, provided a more systematic investigation of this question (Gidyk, 2019; Gidyk et al., 2016). In these experiments the extent of the damage to the hippocampus was either complete or restricted to the dorsal hippocampus prior to conditioning. In neither case did damage to the hippocampus impair retention of the contextual fear memory, even when there was a 30-day retention interval. Moreover, even at the longest retention interval, there was no evidence that the quality of the memory representation diminished because animals with damage to the hippocampus did not generalize their fear to a similar context any more than the nonlesioned controls. Consistent with this finding, Wang et al. (2009) reported that extrahippocampal brain regions can maintain a precise representation of a conditioning context. These results indicated that the hippocampus is not required for the extrahippocampal system to maintain a long-lasting context fear memory.

THE EXTRAHIPPOCAMPAL SYSTEM ACQUIRES THE MEMORY WHEN THE HIPPOCAMPUS IS PRESENT   Nevertheless, under some conditions damage to the hippocampus after conditioning equally disrupts retrieval of both new and old contextual fear memories (Broadbent and Clark, 2013; Maren et al., 1997; Sutherland et al., 2008). This result suggests that the presence of the hippocampus might interfere with the acquisition of the fear memory by the extrahippocampal system. Recall, however, that Goshen et al. (2011) reported that optogenetic silencing of the hippocampus for about 30 minutes prior to the retrieval test allowed an old contextual fear memory to be retrieved, which indicated that the old memory was available in the extrahippocampal system. But Goshen and her colleagues did not determine if this procedure would also uncover the existence of a new memory.

However, Sparks et al. (2011; see also Holt and Maren, 1999) uncovered the existence of a newly established contextual fear memory when they silenced the hippocampus by pharmacological treatments that inhibit its function (muscimol or bupivacaine). In their experiment the hippocampus was functioning normally at the time of conditioning but silenced prior to the retrieval test by infusing the drug into the dorsal and ventral hippocampus (Figure 18.6).

More recently Brian Wiltgen and his colleagues (Krueger et al., 2019) confirmed Sparks et al.'s findings using modern optogenetic and chemogenetic methods, specifically the DREADD methodology (see Chapter 9), to silence the CA1 region of the hippocampus during the retrieval test. An important difference between the optogenetic and DREADD methodologies is their time frame of action. The optogenetic

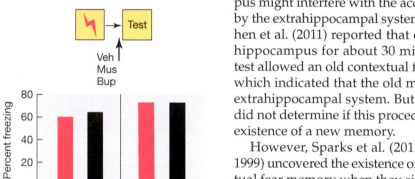

FIGURE 18.6 Silencing the hippocampus with either muscimol or bupivacaine prior to the retrieval test has no effect on retrieval of a contextual fear memory acquired when the hippocampus was functioning normally. This result indicates that the presence of the hippocampus does not prevent the extrahippocampal system from acquiring the contextual fear memory. Key: Veh = vehicle; Mus = muscimol; Bup = bupivacaine. (After F. T. Sparks et al. 2011. *Eur J Neurosci* 34: 780–786.)

method immediately shuts down the hippocampus, whereas the DREADD method does so very gradually over about an hour. The time course of the DREADD methodology corresponds more closely to that of the pharmacological methods than optogenetics. Both the DREADD and pharmacological treatments give the extrahippocampal system time to adjust to the absence of the hippocampal input, whereas silencing with optogenetics does not. Wiltgen's group found that silencing with the DREADD method prior to retrieval revealed the presence of a context fear memory acquired when the hippocampus was present, whereas optogenetic silencing prevented retrieval of the memory.

Summary and Implications

It is clear that there is a robust extrahippocampal system that can acquire a contextual fear memory that will persist as the memory ages. Moreover, this system will acquire the memory even when the hippocampus is present and retrieve it when the hippocampus is removed. Collectively, the animal studies provide no support for the primary predictions of the standard model of systems consolidation that (a) as memories age they become independent of the hippocampus and (b) in order to persist in the cortex, memories require an interaction with the hippocampus for some period of time.

Given these results it is tempting to conclude that the standard model is wrong. However, this conclusion is not justified. It is likely, in retrospect, that the use of the contextual fear conditioning preparation as an animal model to study systems consolidation was a bad choice. There are several reasons why this is so.

As assumed by the indexing theory (see Chapter 17), the hippocampus is critical to episodic memories because it supports pattern completion processes, that is, a subset of the original experiences can retrieve the entire episode. Pattern completion afforded by the indexing properties of the hippocampus provide a continuous representation of the current context and a place to store the episodes of our lives (Nadel and Willner, 1980; Nadel et al., 1985; Rudy, 2009). A fundamental problem with the contextual fear conditioning paradigm is that it does not depend on pattern completion processes. *There is no need for the animal to pattern complete because all the features of the context are present as the animal continuously explores the context.* This allows the extrahippocampal system to capture representations of these features and associate them with the shock.

Moreover, a central feature of the contextual fear conditioning paradigm is the aversive experience produced by shock, which dramatically changes the emotional state of the animal and recruits a behavior system designed to protect us from danger (see Chapter 20). Such a system likely evolved to support long-lasting memories of aversive experiences. While the contextual fear conditioning procedure produces a long-lasting memory, it does not model the kinds of everyday experiences that are rich in contextual detail, such as celebrations, news events, or routine social interactions. To finalize this last point, consider a result reported by Antonio Damasio's laboratory about 25 years ago (Bechara et al., 1995). They conditioned a patient who had bilateral hippocampal damage but no damage to the amygdala. This patient displayed the conditioned response as strongly as control subjects. However, the patient could not remember any of the contextual details surrounding the experience. Rodents with damage to the hippocampus acquire and display a contextual fear memory. However, if they could talk it is unlikely that they would be able to recollect the experience, and therein lies the problem. In the absence of the hippocampus they lack the essential pattern completion–separation processes needed to acquire or retrieve episodic memories.

Systems Consolidation: Another Look

The animal studies provide no support for the standard model but they also provide no basis for rejecting it. They tell us what the brain can do without a hippocampus but say nothing about its normal contribution. The results are interesting but may be irrelevant to evaluating the model. Thus, any new insights into systems consolidating will likely come from thinking about how our (human) memories change with age.

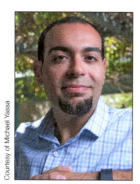

Courtesy of Michael Yassa

Michael Yassa

Michael Yassa (Yassa and Reagh, 2013) proposed a more sophisticated model of systems consolidation called **competitive trace theory** (**CTT**). It offers a different perspective on how the hippocampus and neocortex interact to change memories as they age. To understand this model, recall that episodic and semantic memory can be distinguished by the level of contextual detail present when a memory is retrieved; episodic memories are rich in contextual details, whereas retrieved semantic memories are lacking in such details. A major claim of the CTT model is that memories are more episodic and more veridical (more accurate) when first acquired. With each subsequent reactivation or retrieval of the memory that occurs as it ages, the memory becomes less veridical (less accurate) and either devoid of contextual detail or contaminated with false details. However, the representation of the core content of the memory contained in the neocortical units becomes strongly consolidated and very accurate. In effect, reactivation either by retrieval or through intrinsic processes operating during sleep will move the memory along a continuum from containing detailed episodic content to becoming semantic and lacking contextual detail.

To make this discussion less abstract, consider the first time you learned your mother's birthdate. Shortly thereafter, if you were asked when your mother was born, you could give the correct answer and recall the contextual details (about where the memory was established). With the passage of time you would still recall the correct date but the incidental contextual details would diminish and you also might falsely recall some of the details—you might mistakenly recall that you acquired the memory while at home with your sister but in reality you acquired it when visiting your grandmother. Nevertheless, suppose a day or so after you last recalled the birthdate you were asked when your mother was born and where you last recalled your mother's birthdate. You would give the correct date and a detailed, accurate account of when and where you last recalled it. In effect the most recent reactivation would have recontextualized the core memory. With enough time, however, this new contextual information also would be degraded, but the core would remain.

According to CTT, memory changes that occur over time are the product of interactions between the hippocampus and neocortical units provided by the principles of indexing theory (Teyler and DiScenna, 1986; see Chapter 17). Each replay through the hippocampal index will activate neocortical units that overlap with those activated when the memory was established (the core), but might add or subtract contextual detail to the core memory. These interactions will consolidate connections among the content-holding neocortical units to the point at which *the core is semantic and can be retrieved in the absence of the hippocampus*. The core memory will lose its episodic nature because the nonoverlapping contextual features embedded in the replay cannot successfully be retrieved.

As predicted by CTT, the quality of recollections changes dramatically as the memory ages. For example, Heyworth and Squire (2019) had participants encounter 11 planned events while on a guided tour. They were tested for their recollection of the events directly after the walk, after 1 month, or 2.6 years later. The subjects' recall did not change significantly between the first and second test but fell off significantly by the third test, as did the accuracy of recall. The quality of their recollections, as measured by the richness of contextual details, also decreased significantly from the first to the third test 2.6 years later.

CTT also predicts that over time memories for significant events can become distorted. Schmolck et al.'s study (2000) supports this prediction. Three days following the announcement of the verdict of the famous O. J. Simpson murder trial they asked college students how they heard the news. When asked the same question 32 months later, compared to their initial responses, there were major distortions in their recollections. For example, a student might initially report learning the verdict while watching television at school with other students but later report learning the verdict at home with family members.

To summarize this discussion of CTT, the indexing properties of the hippocampus allow for the rapid acquisition of an episodic memory that is both accurate and rich in contextual detail. Ironically, however, as the memory ages, these properties also permit the fidelity of the memory to be eroded and distorted because it has been subject to bouts of retrieval or intrinsic reactivation that obscure or erase the original contextual detail. Yet, at the same time, these retrieval–replay events establish a semantic memory that is devoid of the contextual detail surrounding its origin and might be recalled in the absence of the hippocampus. The bottom line is that episodic memories that are rich in contextual detail (accurate or inaccurate) will always depend on an intact hippocampus, whereas semantic memories may not.

Summary

This chapter examines the contribution of the MTH system to the fate of old memories. A primary role of the MTH system is to provide support for episodic memories—the everyday events that make up our lives. Much of daily life is uneventful and need not be remembered for any appreciable period of time. In contrast to forgetting that occurs with time, Ribot proposed that memories can become more resistant to disruption as they age. This standard model of systems consolidation proposed that the MTH system was fundamental to Ribot's Law. Old memories are resistant to disruption because they have become consolidated in the neocortical regions that are more immune to disrupting influences.

This idea has proven controversial and unsupported by a large body of human clinical data and animal research. Research centered on the contextual fear conditioning procedure indicated that both new and old memories are lost if the hippocampus is damaged following conditioning. However, research with this procedure also revealed that there is a robust extrahippocampal system that can acquire a contextual fear memory whether the hippocampus is present or absent, and the memory acquired in its absence can persist for weeks.

Although these data provide no support for the standard model of systems consolidation they do not rule it out. Instead, it is more likely that the contextual fear conditioning task is not appropriate for evaluating the model because the acquisition and retrieval of the memory does not depend on the pattern completion properties of the hippocampus, and the use of aversive shock engages a powerful behavioral system designed to protect us from danger.

Competitive trace theory provides another way of thinking about how memories are altered by hippocampal–neocortical interactions as they age. When memories are initially acquired they are veridical and the rich contextual detail in which they are embedded can be recalled. As memories age, however, retrieval or intrinsic replay can both degrade and add false contextual detail to the memory. Moreover, this repetition and replay consolidates connections among the core overlapping elements of neocortical units to create a semantic memory that may be recalled in the absence of the hippocampus. In short, retrieval of memories with episodic contextual detail will always require the hippocampus, but the recall of memories lacking contextual detail may become independent of the hippocampus. It is interesting that when H.M. was reevaluated, his semantic memory was in the normal range for age-matched controls but he had no episodic memory (Steinvorth et al., 2005).

References

Bayley, P. J., Gold, J. J., Hopkins, R. O., and Squire, L. R. (2005). The neuroanatomy of remote memory. *Neuron, 46,* 799–810.

Bayley, P. J., Hopkins, R. O., and Squire, L. R. (2003). Successful recollection of remote autobiographical memories by amnesic patients with medial temporal lobe lesions. *Neuron, 38,* 135–144.

Bechara, A., Tranel, D., Damasio, H., Adolphs, R., Rockland, C., and Damasio, A. R. (1995). Double dissociation of conditioning and declarative knowledge relative to the amygdala and hippocampus in humans. *Science, 269,* 1115–1118.

Broadbent, N. J. and Clark, R. E. (2013). Remote context fear conditioning remains hippocampus-dependent irrespective of training protocol, training-surgery interval, lesion size, and lesion method. *Neurobiology of Learning and Memory, 106,* 300–308.

Burwell, R. D., Bucci, D. J., Sanborn, M. R., and Jutras, M. J. (2004). Perirhinal and postrhinal contributions to remote memory for context. *Journal of Neuroscience, 24,* 11023–11028.

Clark, R. E., Broadbent, N. J., and Squire L. R. (2005a). Hippocampus and remote spatial memory in rats. *Hippocampus, 15,* 260–272.

Clark, R. E., Broadbent, N. J, and Squire, L. R. (2005b). Impaired remote spatial memory after hippocampal lesions despite extensive training beginning early in life. *Hippocampus, 15,* 340–346.

Corkin, S. (1984). Lasting consequences of bilateral medial temporal lobectomy: clinical course and experimental findings in H.M. *Seminars in Neurology, 4,* 249–259.

Corkin, S. (2002). What's new with the amnesic patient H.M.? *Nature Reviews Neuroscience, 2,* 153–160.

Frankland, P. W. and Bontempi, B. (2005). The organization of recent and remote memories. *Nature Reviews Neuroscience, 6,* 119–130.

Gidyk, D. C. (2019). Maintenance and behavioral expression of long-term memories acquired in the absence of the hippocampus. Unpublished PhD dissertation, University of Lethbridge.

Gidyk, D. C., McDonald, R. J., and Sutherland, R. J. (2016). Persistence of long-term contextual fear and visual discrimination memory in the absence of the hippocampus. In *Society for Neuroscience Abstracts.* San Diego, CA. Online.

Goshen, I., Brodsky, M., Prakash, R., Wallace, J., Gradinaru, V., Ramakrishnan, C., and Deisseroth, K. (2011). Dynamics of retrieval strategies for remote memories. *Cell, 147,* 678–689.

Heyworth, N. C. and Squire, L. R. (2019). The nature of recollection across months and years and after medial temporal lobe damage. *Proceedings of the National Academy of Sciences USA, 116,* 4619–4624.

Holt, W. and Maren, S. (1999). Muscimol inactivation of the dorsal hippocampus impairs contextual retrieval of fear memory. *Journal of Neuroscience, 19,* 9054–9062.

Keene, C. S. and Bucci, D. J. (2008). Contributions of the retrosplenial and posterior parietal cortices to cue-specific and contextual fear conditioning. *Behavioral Neuroscience, 122,* 89–97.

Kim, J. J. and Fanselow, M. S. (1992). Modality-specific retrograde amnesia of fear. *Science, 256,* 675–677.

Klinzing, J. G., Neithard, N., and Born, J. (2019). Mechanisms of systems memory consolidation during sleep. *Nature Neuroscience, 22,* 1598–1610.

Krueger, J. N., Wilmot, J. H., Teratani-Ota, Y., Puhger, K. R., Nemes, S. E., Lafreniere, M., and Wiltgen, B. J. (2019). Recently formed context fear memories can be retrieved without the hippocampus. *bioRxiv* 843342; DOI: 10.1101/bioRxiv.843342.

Lehmann, H., Lacanilao, S., and Sutherland, R. J. (2007). Complete or partial hippocampal damage produces equivalent retrograde amnesia for remote contextual fear memories. *European Journal of Neuroscience, 25,* 1278–1286.

Lehmann, H., Sparks, F. T., Spanswick, S. C., Hadikin, C., McDonald, R. J., and Sutherland R. J. (2009). Making context memories independent of the hippocampus. *Learning and Memory, 16,* 417–420.

Maren, S., Aharonov, G., and Fanselow, M. S. (1997). Neurotoxic lesions of the dorsal hippocampus and Pavlovian fear conditioning in rats. *Behavioural Brain Research, 88,* 261–274.

Martin, S. J., de Hoz, L., and Morris, R. G. (2005). Retrograde amnesia: neither partial nor complete hippocampal lesions in rats result in preferential sparing of remote spatial memory, even after reminding. *Neuropsychologia, 43,* 609–624.

Milner, B., Corkin, S., and Teuber, H. L. (1968). Further analysis of the hippocampal amnesic syndrome: 14-year follow-up study of H.M. *Neuropsychologia, 6,* 215–234.

Misra, P., Marconi, A., Peterson, M., and Kreiman, G. (2018). Minimal memory for details in real life events. *Scientific Reports, 8,* 16701–16711.

Nadel, L. and Moscovitch, M. (1997). Memory consolidation, retrograde amnesia and the hippocampal complex. *Current Opinion in Neurobiology, 7,* 217–227.

Nadel, L. and Willner, J. (1980). Context and conditioning: a place for space. *Physiology and Behavior, 8,* 218–228.

Nadel, L., Willner, J., and Kurz, E. M. (1985). Cognitive maps and environmental context. In P. Balsam and A. Tomie (Eds.), *Context and Learning* (pp. 385–406). Hillsdale, NJ: Erlbaum and Associates.

Ocampo, A.C., Squire, L. R., and Clark, R. E. (2017). Hippocampal area CA1 and remote memory in rats. *Learning and Memory, 24,* 563–568.

O'Keefe, J. and Nadel, L. (1978). *The Hippocampus as a Cognitive Map*. Oxford: Clarendon Press.

Reed, J. M. and Squire, L. R. (1998). Retrograde amnesia for facts and events: findings from four new cases. *Journal of Neuroscience, 18*, 3943–3954.

Rudy, J. W. (2009). Context representations, context functions, and the parahippocampal-hippocampal system. *Learning and Memory, 16*, 573–589.

Schmolck, H., Buffalo, E. A., and Squire, L. R. (2000). Memory distortions develop over time: recollections of the O.J. Simpson trial verdict after 15 and 32 months. *Psychological Science, 11*, 39–45.

Skelin, I., Kilianske, S., and McNaughton, B. L. (2019). Hippocampal coupling with cortical and subcortical structures in the context of memory consolidation. *Neurobiology of Learning and Memory, 160*, 21–31.

Sparks, F. T., Lehmann, H., and Sutherland, R. J. (2011). Between-systems memory interference during retrieval. *The European Journal of Neuroscience, 34*, 780–786.

Sparks, F. T., Spanswick, S. C., Lehmann, H., and Sutherland, R. J. (2013). Neither time nor number of context-shock pairings affect long-term dependence of memory on hippocampus. *Neurobiology of Learning and Memory, 106*, 309–313.

Squire, L. R., Cohen, N. J., and Nadel, L. (1984). The medial temporal region and memory consolidation: a new hypothesis. In H. Weingartner and E. Parker (Eds.), *Memory Consolidation* (pp. 185–210). Hillsdale, NJ: Erlbaum and Associates.

Steinvorth, S., Levine, B., and Corkin, S. (2005). Medial temporal lobe structures are needed to re-experience remote autobiographical memories: evidence from H.M. and W.R. *Neuropsychologia, 43*, 479–496.

Sutherland, R. J., O'Brien, J., and Lehmann, H. (2008). Absence of systems consolidation of fear memories after dorsal, ventral, or complete hippocampal damage. *Hippocampus, 18*, 710–718.

Sutherland, R. J., Weisend, M. P., Mumby, D., Astur, R. S., Hanlon, F. M., Koerner, A., Thomas, M. J., Wu, Y., Moses, S. N., and Cole, C. (2001). Retrograde amnesia after hippocampal damage: recent vs. remote memories in two tasks. *Hippocampus, 11*, 27–42.

Takehara-Nishiuchi, K. (2014). Entorhinal cortex and consolidated memory. *Neuroscience Research, 84*, 27–33.

Teyler, T. J. and DiScenna, P. (1986). The hippocampal memory indexing theory. *Behavioral Neuroscience, 100*, 147–152.

Todd, T. P., DeAngeli, N. E., Jiang, M. Y., and Bucci, D. J. (2017). Retrograde amnesia of contextual fear conditioning: evidence for retrosplenial cortex involvement in configural processing. *Behavioral Neuroscience, 131*, 46–54.

Wang, S. H., Teixeira, C. M., Wheeler, A. L., and Frankland, P. W. (2009). The precision of remote context memories does not require the hippocampus. *Nature Neuroscience, 12*, 253–255.

Wiltgen, B, J., Sanders, M. J., Anagnostaras, S. G., Sage, J. R., and Fanselow, M. S. (2006). Context fear learning in the absence of the hippocampus. *Journal of Neuroscience, 26*, 5484–5491.

Yassa, M. A. and Reagh, Z. (2013). Competitive trace theory: a role for the hippocampus in contextual interference during retrieval. *Frontiers in Behavioral Neuroscience, 7*, Article 107.

Zelikowsky, M., Bissiere, S., and Fanselow, M. S. (2012). Contextual fear memories formed in the absence of the dorsal hippocampus decay across time. *Journal of Neuroscience, 32*, 3393–3397.

Zelikowsky, M., Bissiere, S., Hast, T. A., Bennett, R. Z., Abdipranoto, A., Vissel, B., and Fanselow, M. S. (2013). Prefrontal microcircuit underlies contextual learning after hippocampal loss. *Proceedings of the National Academy of Sciences USA, 110*, 9938–9943.

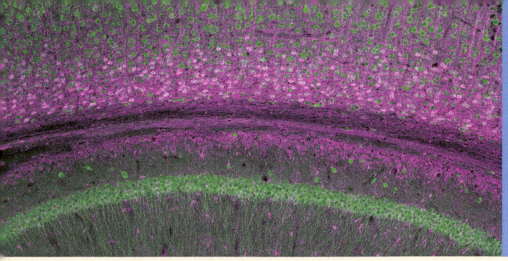

19

© Alexandros A Lavdas/Shutterstock.com

Actions, Habits, and the Cortico-Striatal System

Our brains are sensitive to the outcomes produced by our behaviors. Consequently, we can rapidly adjust our behaviors in response to a changing world and acquire complex behavioral skills. Psychologists have been concerned with how this happens for more than 120 years, and in the last 30 years neurobiologists have also weighed in on this topic. We now understand some of the basic psychological principles that govern the acquisition of new behaviors and how those principles might relate to systems in the brain. This chapter explores this complex relationship, first discussing the concept and two theories of instrumental behavior and then describing two categories of such behavior— **actions** and **habits**—and the cortico-striatal neural system of the brain that supports them.

To appreciate the basic problems addressed in this chapter, you might think back to when you initially learned to drive a car. In order to competently drive you had to learn and coordinate many complex behaviors, such as:

- insert the ignition key;
- turn on the ignition key;
- release the handbrake;

- put the car in gear;
- put your foot on the accelerator;
- generate just the right amount of gas;
- adjust the steering wheel to maintain or change the trajectory; and
- apply just the amount of pressure on the brake to stop.

Remarkably, once these skills are learned, a competent driver can execute them in a seamless manner and at the same time carry on a conversation and sometimes drive for miles while unaware of even being on the road. However, this was certainly not the case when you were learning to drive. The initial execution of each of these behaviors was an intentional, goal-driven act that was motivated by your knowledge or expectancy that it would produce a particular outcome. Only with extensive practice did you acquire and integrate into a well-coordinated process the individual behaviors that comprise the collection of skills needed to drive a car. The initial crude actions you performed while learning to drive later became highly refined motor patterns, liberated from your intentions and conscious control. Driving then became a habit.

The Concept of Instrumental Behavior

Most psychologists use the term **instrumental learning** or **instrumental behavior** when referring to the study of how behavior is modified by the outcome it produces. These terms recognize that our behaviors can be viewed as instruments that can change or modify our environments. For example, when you turn the ignition key, the engine starts.

The experimental study of instrumental learning emerged when, as a graduate student, E. L. Thorndike (1898) wanted to gain some insight into the "mind" of animals. He was unhappy with the speculation of his contemporaries about what kinds of representations of the world existed in the minds of dogs and cats and how these representations were acquired. This was because the speculation was made on the basis of anecdotal accounts of the behavior of animals and, when explaining behavior, psychologists of his era tended to anthropomorphize, that is, attribute human characteristics to animals. So, as described in Chapter 1, Thorndike developed a novel methodology, called the Thorndike puzzle box, to study how animals solve problems and represent the solution (Figure 19.1A). A cat, dog, or chicken was placed into the box and it had to learn a particular behavior to escape—for example, to pull the ring attached by a rope to the door.

The important feature of this methodology was that it arranged an explicit contingency between the animal's behavior and a change in the environment. Specifically, the opening of the escape door was contingent or dependent upon the animal generating a particular behavior—pulling the ring. If the specified response was not made, the door did not open.

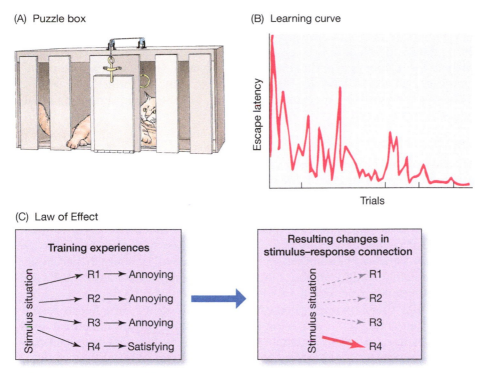

FIGURE 19.1   (A) Thorndike contributed the puzzle box and learning curves to the study of instrumental learning. (B) These learning curves represented escape latency as a function of trials. (C) He also proposed a theory of instrumental learning known as the Law of Effect. Training experiences: When the animal is placed in the puzzle box, the stimulus situation (S) initiates many responses (R1, R2, R3, R4). The S–R connections linking S to wrong responses (R1, R2, R3) are followed by annoying consequences. The connection linking S to the correct response (R4, ring pull) is followed by a satisfying consequence (the door opens). Resulting changes: Over trials the incorrect S–R connections are weakened (as indicated by dashed arrows) and the correct connection is strengthened, as represented by the red arrow.

More importantly, the animal's behavior was modified by the behavioral contingency Thorndike arranged. In attempting to escape from the box, the animal initially engaged in a wide range of behaviors that had no influence on its situation. However, it gradually learned the behavior that opened the door. Thorndike documented this change in behavior by presenting what may have been the first example of "learning curves." These learning curves represented escape latency as a function of trials (Figure 19.1B). He found that escape latency gradually decreased as a function of those trials, indicating that the animal had learned to escape.

Two Theories of Instrumental Behavior

Two general ideas about how outcomes change our behavior emerged quite early in the history of experimental psychology and continue to be influential. One idea, called the Law of Effect, originated with Thorndike. The second idea, called **cognitive expectancy theory**, is associated with Edward C. Tolman (1948, 1949).

Thorndike's Law of Effect

The essence of Thorndike's theory is that outcomes produced by behavior ultimately adapt the animal to the situation by strengthening and weakening existing stimulus–response (S–R) connections. Outcomes that are rewarding strengthen S–R connections, while nonrewarding outcomes weaken connections. His Law of Effect, illustrated in Figure 19.1C, can be stated as follows: If in the presence of a stimulus a response is followed by a satisfying state of affairs, the connection between the stimulus and the response will be strengthened. If the response is followed by an annoying state of affairs, the connection between the stimulus and response will be weakened (Thorndike, 1905).

Note that Thorndike described outcomes produced by behavior as resulting in either annoying or satisfying events. The term **reward** or **reinforcer** is often used to represent an outcome that strengthens stimulus–response connections and the term **nonreward** is used to designate an event that weakens such connections.

It is useful to highlight some of the implications of Thorndike's theory. A strengthened S–R connection can produce the appropriate response, but it contains no information about either the behavioral contingency (that is, that the outcome depended on the response) or the nature of the outcome (a reward or nonreward). More generally stated, the instrumental behavior itself should not be considered purposeful or goal directed. Thus, if you asked Thorndike's cat why it pulled the ring every time it was placed in the box, if it could answer it would say something like, "I don't know. It's very strange but when I am placed into the box I get an irresistible urge to pull the ring." A behavior supported by S–R connections is a habit, acquired through frequent repetition.

Tolman's Cognitive Expectancy Theory

No one believes that Thorndike's theory provides a complete description of the processes that control our behavior or how we represent our past experiences. Tolman certainly did not accept this theory. He believed that instrumental behaviors are purposeful and organized around goals. He would say that when the cat solves Thorndike's puzzle box it would learn the relationship between its behavior and the outcome that it produced. The cat acquired an expectancy about the relationship between its actions and the outcomes they produced. More generally speaking, Tolman believed that our brains detect and store information about relationships among all the events provided by a particular

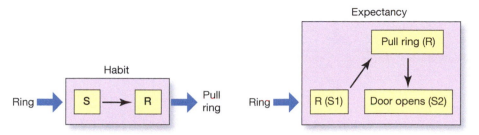

FIGURE 19.2 This figure provides a comparison of the S–R habit versus an expectancy representation of the cat's solution to the puzzle box. Note that the sight of the ring directly evokes a strengthened S–R connection to produce the pull-ring response. In contrast, according to expectancy theory, the sight of the ring activates the representation of the pull-ring response and the consequence it produces—the door opening. Activating the expectancy does not necessarily result in the response. Thus, the expectancy contains information about what would happen, but it does not force a response. This depends on the value of the outcome.

experience. An expectancy is a three-term association (S1–R–S2) that includes a representation of the stimulus situation (S1) that preceded the response, a representation of the response (R), and a representation of the outcome (S2) produced by the response. The expectancy concept is illustrated in Figure 19.2 in relation to Thorndike's S–R habit.

Tolman's cognitive expectancy–goal-directed theory of behavior placed a heavy emphasis on the value of the outcome produced by an instrumental behavior. The associations that make up an expectancy contain information about relationships between stimuli and relationships between behavior and stimulus outcomes. Whether or not you act, however, depends on the value of the outcome you expect the behavior to produce. So even though the cat "knows" how to escape from the box, it does not have to automatically initiate the escape response. It does so only if the outcome has value—if the cat has some motivation to escape. Similarly, you may know a friend's telephone number, but seeing a telephone does not always result in your dialing the number. You only do so when you want to speak to your friend, that is, when the outcome has value.

Action and Habit Systems

Together, the theories of Thorndike and Tolman imply that there are two categories of instrumental behavior (Figure 19.3). Hereafter they will be called actions and habits. They differ on four dimensions.

1. *Purpose.* The action system is goal directed and purposeful and motivated by an anticipated outcome. Habits are not goal directed or purposeful.

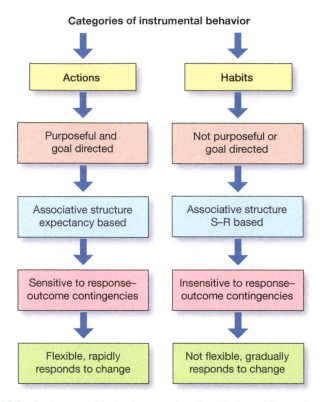

Categories of instrumental behavior

Actions	Habits
Purposeful and goal directed	Not purposeful or goal directed
Associative structure expectancy based	Associative structure S–R based
Sensitive to response–outcome contingencies	Insensitive to response–outcome contingencies
Flexible, rapidly responds to change	Not flexible, gradually responds to change

FIGURE 19.3 Instrumental behaviors can be classified as either actions or habits.

2. *Sensitivity to outcomes.* The action system is sensitive to the response–reward contingencies. It rapidly detects outcomes associated with behavior and assesses the causal relationship—did the response actually produce the outcome? The habit system is not sensitive to response–reward contingencies.

3. *Associative structure.* The action system acquires expectancies, whereas the habit system acquires stimulus–response associations.

4. *Flexibility.* The action system is flexible and designed to rapidly respond to changes in response contingencies. The habit system has to unlearn or overcome existing S–R associations by slowly acquiring new ones.

Under normal circumstances if you were watching a cat escape from the puzzle box or someone opened a door, you would have difficulty determining if the behavior was an action or a habit. However, researchers can use two strategies to determine if a particular instrumental behavior is supported by the action system or the habit system: the reward devaluation strategy and the discrimination reversal learning strategy.

The **reward devaluation** strategy is used to determine if the instrumental behavior is purposeful and goal directed. This strategy centers on changing the value of the outcome after the animal has solved the problem. The logic of the strategy, which has been used with both primates and rodents, is described as follows.

Since actions are purposeful and generated to produce a specific outcome, when the outcome has value, the animal should produce the appropriate response. But when the outcome has no value, the animal may not produce the response. In contrast, since habits are not goal directed, they should be produced regardless of the value of the outcome or reward. Thus, by changing the value of the reward–outcome after an instrumental response has been learned, one can determine if the response is an action or a habit. If the response is controlled by the action system, devaluing the outcome should reduce the likelihood that the response will occur. If it is a habit, then reward devaluation will not influence the behavior.

An example of the devaluation strategy is illustrated in Figure 19.4. A monkey is trained to solve two discriminations. In the first problem the reward is a grape. If the monkey chooses the pyramid it will find the grape, but it will receive nothing if it chooses the cylinder. In the second problem the reward is a peanut. If it chooses the cube it will find the peanut, but if it chooses the cone it will find nothing (Baxter and Murray, 2002). Monkeys easily solve such problems. How can you tell whether the correct response is an action supported by an expectancy or a habit supported by an S–R connection? The answer is, *by changing the value of the reward*.

This can easily be done. After the problems have been solved the monkey receives a test in which the two correct stimuli from each discrimination problem—the pyramid (with the grape) and the cube (with the peanut)—are presented several times. Before the test, however, the monkey is satiated with one of the rewards. It is allowed to eat either all the peanuts or all the grapes it wants. This treatment reduces the value of one of the rewards. No reward is given on the test. If the monkey's response is an action, it will choose the object associated with the reward that still has "value." However, if the monkey's choice is random this means that the choice response was a habit.

The action system is said to be more flexible than the habit system. This means that the action system is more sensitive to changes in the contingencies associated with behavior than the habit system and it can use new information to rapidly adapt to changes in the environment. For example, someone raised in the United States who visits England faces a potentially lethal situation. In the United States when a pedestrian prepares to cross a street the dominant response is to look to the left before crossing. This is because cars in the closest lane will be coming from the left. However, in England if you look left and then step into the street you have a good chance of being hit by a car because in England traffic in the inside lane is coming from the pedestrian's right. Thus, to survive in England, one has to rapidly adjust to the new response

Training

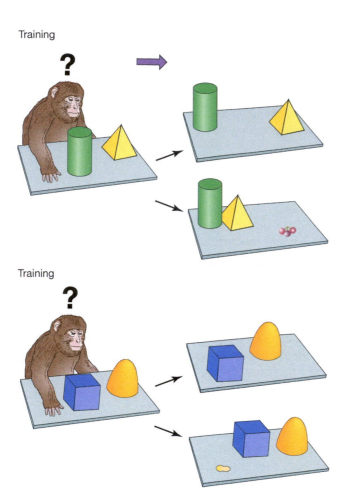

FIGURE 19.4 The figure illustrates the satiation method for devaluing a reward. A monkey is trained to solve two discrimination problems. In the first problem the pyramid is the correct choice and the reward is a grape. In the second problem the correct choice is the cube and the reward is a peanut. After solving the two problems, the monkey is given a choice between the two correct objects (cube and pyramid). Before the test, however, the monkey is allowed to have either all the grapes or all the peanuts it wants, thus reducing the value of one of the outcomes. Typically, monkeys choose the object that contains the reward that it was not fed prior to the test. (After M. G. Baxter and E. A. Murray. 2002. *Nature Rev Neurosci* 3: 563–573.)

Training

Tests

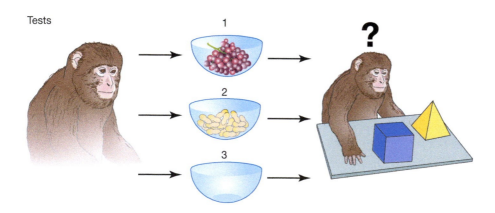

contingencies and learn to look to the right before crossing. The action system is thought to provide the basis for this rapid adjustment and to override the habit system, which is thought to respond to change by incrementally changing S–R connections.

The **discrimination reversal learning** strategy is commonly used to assess the flexibility of the system supporting the instrumental response. For example, after the monkey initially solves the cylinder (reward) versus pyramid (no reward) problem, the solution would be reversed and it would have to learn that the pyramid is now the correct choice. The idea behind this strategy is that the action system would facilitate learning these reversals but the habit system would interfere with reversal learning because it is slow to change.

With Practice, Actions Become Habits

The devaluation methodology has provided evidence for the existence of both actions and habits. In addition, research with animals has revealed a dominance principle. With limited training instrumental behaviors are goal-directed actions, but with practice, instrumental behaviors tend to shift from actions to habits, meaning they become insensitive to reward devaluation.

This point is illustrated in Figure 19.5, which presents the results of an experiment in which rats were trained to press a lever to receive food. Thus, lever pressing was the instrumental response and food was the outcome–reward. In one condition the rats were given only a limited amount of lever-press training, while in the other they were given extended training. Prior to the test phase, the outcome–reward was devalued for one set of rats. During the test phase, food was no longer delivered in response to lever pressing. Rats that had limited training were sensitive to the value of the reward, making fewer lever-pressing responses than the control rats. In this case, the lever press was

(A)

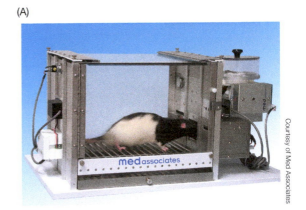

Courtesy of Med Associates

(B)

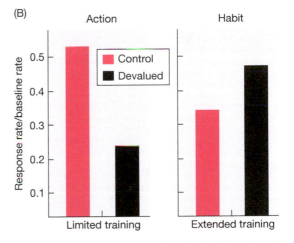

FIGURE 19.5 (A) A rat is collecting food produced by pressing a lever. In this experiment, in one condition the rats were given only a limited amount of lever-press training, while in the other they were given extended training. Prior to the test phase, the food reward was devalued for one set of rats. (B) Rats that had limited training were sensitive to the value of the reward, pressing the lever less than control rats. In this case, the lever press was considered an action. In contrast, rats that had experienced extended training were insensitive to the value of the reward, pressing the lever as often as the control rats. In this case the lever press was considered a habit. (B after C. D. Adams. 1982. *Q J Exp Psychol [B]* 34: 77-98.)

considered an action. In contrast, rats that had experienced extended training were insensitive to the value of the reward, pressing the lever as often as the control rats (Adams, 1982). In this case the lever press was considered a habit.

With repetition, an action can become a habit. However, one should not conclude that the expectancy representation of an action is replaced by an S–R representation of a habit. Instead, once established, the two representations co-exist. As the next section explains, what changes with practice is which representation controls behavior (Killcross and Coutureau, 2003).

A Conceptual Model for Actions and Habits

Behavioral neuroscientists have begun to uncover regions in the brain that contribute to the support of actions and habits. The unfolding story is complex and incomplete, so to facilitate understanding of the concepts, a conceptual model is provided in Figure 19.6 to illustrate the general idea that instrumental behaviors can be generated by either an action system or a habit system.

In this simple model a stimulus–response–outcome experience is represented at two levels in the brain (see Figure 19.6A). The representations of the experience activated in level I are fed forward to level II. The processes operating in level II are responsible for assembling these representations into a goal-directed action, but ultimately processes in level I that associate the stimulus representation and response representation produce habits. The action and habit systems both generate the instrumental behavior (IB) by activating the representation of the response in level I.

More specifically, the associations that support actions form in level II after limited training. They link (a) the stimulus representation to both the outcome representation and the response representation, (b) the response representation to the outcome representation, and (c) the outcome representation to the response representation. If the outcome representation has value (+), this association will contribute to activating the response representation in level II. If the response representation in level II is sufficiently activated, its output will project back to the response representation in level I and produce the instrumental behavior. However, if the outcome has no value (–), then the response representation in level II will not be sufficiently activated to stimulate the response representation in level I, and the instrumental behavior will not occur (see Figure 19.6B).

With extended training an S–R habit can emerge in level I (see Figure 19.6C). This happens because with repetition the action system repeatedly produces the same response in the presence of the antecedent stimulus, thereby creating the opportunity for it to be directly associated with a representation of the response. After extended training, both the action system and the habit system can produce the instrumental behavior, but the habit system tends to dominate.

Action and Habit Systems Compete

Under normal circumstance the action and habit systems cooperate to allow us to adapt to our environment. The action system initially assembles the relevant task information to generate the correct instrumental response. Then, as the correct response is repeated it becomes controlled by the habit system. *But what happens when the response contingencies are changed?* For example, suppose a rat has learned to respond to two levers. However, pressing lever 1 is more likely to produce a reward than pressing lever 2. Thus, the animal learns to press lever 1 more often than lever 2. After this pattern is established, the contingencies are reversed (using the discrimination reversal learning strategy described above), so that pressing lever 2 is more likely to produce a reward than pressing lever 1,

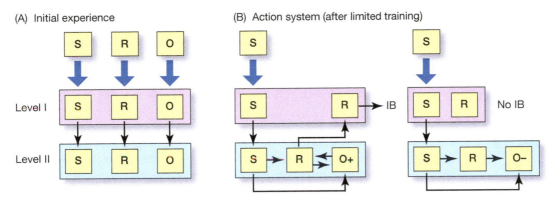

FIGURE 19.6 (A) An animal has an initial experience composed of a sequence of an antecedent stimulus (S), a response (R), and an outcome (O) produced by the response. This experience is represented in two levels of the brain, I and II. (B) With limited training, the representations in level II are associated with and can support an action. The diagram on the left shows that the action system generates an instrumental behavior (IB) if the outcome has value (+). In this case, when S occurs the level II associations are activated and the output of the action system projects back to the response representation in level I to generate the instrumental behavior. The diagram on the right illustrates the case when the outcome has been devalued (–). In this case the outcome representation does not strongly project onto the response representation in level II. Thus, the response representation in level I is not activated and the instrumental behavior is not produced. (C) With extended training, a habit is formed, that is, connections between the stimulus and response representations in level I become strong enough to support the generation of an instrumental behavior, without projections back from level II.

and the animal now has to acquire this conflicting information and learn to respond more to lever 2 than lever 1.

The action system is designed to acquire the new information and provide a basis for a rapid shift to the lever that produces more rewards. However, the habit system is slow to adjust and its output may interfere with adjusting to the new contingencies. The animal must unlearn or suppress the old habit. This description suggests that information contained in the habit system will interfere with the rat learning to shift to the better lever. Wolfgang Pauli and his colleagues (Pauli et al., 2012) reasoned that if the action system were removed (by inactivating the region of the brain that supports the action system), rats would learn more slowly to make this adjustment. In contrast, if the habit system were removed (by inactivating the region of the brain that supports the habit system), rats would more rapidly learn to shift to the more favorable lever. (Note: these brain regions are described in great detail in the section below on the cortico-striatal system.) To test these predictions these regions were inactivated immediately prior to the test session when the response–reward contingencies reversed. The researchers' predictions were confirmed and the results of their experiment also support the hypothesis that the action and habit systems initially compete for control of instrumental behaviors when the requirements of a situation are reversed.

Action Systems Are Vulnerable

Development of an instrumental response occurs in a temporally overlapping sequence in which the action system initially acquires the information needed to generate the response. However, once the appropriate response occurs reliably, the habit system takes over. These ideas now play a prominent role in guiding research in other areas (see Graybiel, 2008). One principle that has emerged is that the action system is more vulnerable to disruption than the habit system. For example, there is evidence that exposure to psychostimulants such as amphetamines can unduly favor control of instrumental behaviors by the habit system (Nelson and Killcross, 2006).

Jane Taylor and her colleagues (Gourly et al., 2013) reported that an injection of cocaine following training prevents the consolidation of the memory supporting the action system's ability to store the memory of the response–reward contingency—the instrumental response of animals treated with cocaine was controlled by the habit system. Moreover, this group found that this happens because cocaine selectively interferes with actin reorganization in spines located on neurons in the region of the brain that supports the action system.

In another domain, it has been found that chronic stress dramatically alters components of the action system and this results in the habit system controlling instrumental behaviors (Dias-Ferreira et al., 2009). Graybiel (2008) has discussed the implications of the action–habit analysis for a number of domains, such as obsessive–compulsive disorder and Tourette syndrome.

A Cortico-Striatal System
Supports Instrumental Behavior

The conceptual model for actions and habits described above is complex, but even so it is an oversimplification. The reality is that many components of the brain make a contribution to the learning of instrumental behavior, and no one has yet provided a theory that shows how all the relevant components are integrated to produce such behavior. Nevertheless, important components of the neural system that supports the acquisition and production of instrumental behavior have been identified.

One important component of this system, located deep in the center of the brain, is the **basal ganglia**. This region of the brain consists of a number of subcortical nuclei including the caudate nucleus, putamen, globus pallidus, subthalamic nucleus, nucleus accumbens, and substantia nigra. Together, the caudate nucleus, putamen, and nucleus accumbens components of the basal ganglia form a region of the brain called the **striatum**.

The striatum is the basic input segment of the basal ganglia. It receives input from many cortical regions of the brain and projects out through the globus pallidus and substantia nigra to the thalamus and ultimately back to areas of the cortex from which it received input. Thus, the striatum is at the center of what is sometimes called the **cortico-striatal system**. Because the striatum projects back to some of the cortical regions that project to it, the cortico-striatal system has the same sort of return-loop organization that characterizes the medial temporal hippocampal (MTH) system that supports episodic memory, discussed in Chapters 16 and 17. Note in particular that the striatum projects back to the motor cortex. This is important because motor cortices are critical for the generation of behaviors. Many researchers believe that the striatum is the key anatomical region for creating instrumental behaviors (Divac et al., 1967; Shiflett and Balleine, 2011; White and McDonald, 2002).

An experiment by Raymond Kesner (Cook and Kesner, 1988) used a radial maze with eight arms to illustrate this point (Figure 19.7). Each rat was placed randomly into one of these arms and then released. Normally, when released the rat will move out into the arena and enter some distant arm. However, in what is called the adjacent-arm task, no matter which arm it was placed into to start a trial, the rat was only rewarded if its first choice upon release was to enter one of the two adjacent arms. Normal rats learned this task, but rats with damage to the striatum were quite impaired. Thus, these animals had difficulty learning what would appear to be the simple task of turning left or right.

Figure 19.8 illustrates the rat's striatum and some of the cortical and other regions in the brain that it interacts with to produce instrumental behavior. This figure provides a framework for discussing some of the key components of the neural system that contribute to assembling and performing action patterns. It

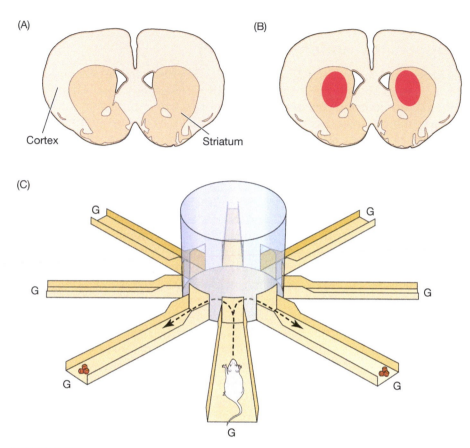

FIGURE 19.7 (A) This illustration of a normal rat brain shows the cortex and striatum. (B) This illustration shows the location of the experimentally induced lesion in the dorsal striatum. (C) An illustration of a rat in the eight-arm radial maze task. On each trial the rat is started randomly from one arm of the maze. In order to receive a reward the rat must leave the start arm and enter an adjacent arm. Rats with damage to the dorsal striatum are greatly impaired on this instrumental learning task. (C after D. Cook and R. P. Kesner. 1988. *Behav Neural Biol* 49: 332–343.)

is useful to think of the cortico-striatal system as performing the functions of level II in the conceptual model of instrumental behavior described previously and illustrated in Figure 19.6.

Neural Support for Actions

Much of what is known about the contribution different regions of the brain make to support instrumental behavior comes from the combined use of neurobiological methods to influence the brain and devaluation techniques to determine if the instrumental response is an action or a habit. Researchers use

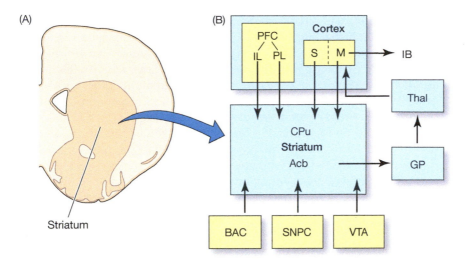

FIGURE 19.8   (A) The rodent striatum and surrounding cortex. (B) A highly schematic representation of the rat striatum and some of the important regions of the brain that project to it. Note that information processed by the striatum projects back to the motor (M) cortex via the thalamus (Thal). The striatum of the rat is composed of the caudate putamen (CPu) and the nucleus accumbens (Acb). Key: S = sensory cortex; PFC = prefrontal cortex; PL = prelimbic cortex; IL = infralimbic cortex; BAC = basal amygdala complex; VTA = ventral tegmental area; SNPC = substantia nigra pars compacta; IB = instrumental behavior; GP = globus pallidus.

lesions to permanently remove a particular component of the neural system and use inactivation methods to temporarily but reversibly prevent a region from contributing to the behavioral outcome. In addition, drugs that influence synaptic plasticity, such as the NMDA receptor antagonist APV, are employed to determine if synapses in a particular region of the brain are modified by experience.

As noted earlier, actions are said to be goal directed and purposeful. Thus, the reward devaluation strategy is used to determine regions of the brain that are part of the action system. If a reward devaluation procedure reduces the production of the instrumental behavior, that behavior is said to be a goal-directed action. Consequently, if the function of a brain region is impaired and the reward devaluation procedure has no effect on instrumental responding (does not reduce responding), one might conclude that the brain region is part of the action system. In contrast, if the function of a brain region is impaired and the devaluation reduces instrumental responding, then one would conclude that this brain region is not part of the action system. Based on this logic, three brain regions have been linked to the action system: (1) the **dorsomedial striatum (DMS)**, (2) the **basolateral amygdala**, and (3) the **prelimbic prefrontal cortex**.

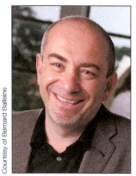

Bernard Balleine

DORSOMEDIAL STRIATUM   Bernard Balleine and his colleagues reported several findings that suggest that the DMS plays an important role in goal-directed actions. In one study, they damaged this region of the brain either before or after training rats on a two-lever pressing task (Yin, Ostlund, et al., 2005). Pressing each lever produced a different outcome: a food pellet or a sip of a sucrose solution. Prior to the test, they satiated the animals on one or the other of the rewards. During the test no reward was given. When satiated on food pellets, control rats were sensitive to the devaluation treatment and pressed the lever that in the past produced the sucrose. Rats with damage to the DMS, however, were not sensitive to the devaluation; they pressed the lever as much when the reward was devalued as they did when it was not, and they pressed each lever equally as often. These results (Figure 19.9) suggest that the control rats' behavior was produced by the action system and that the DMS is part of this system.

A different set of experiments, in which the NMDA-receptor antagonist APV was injected into the DMS, resulted in similar findings, further supporting the idea that neurons in the DMS are important in action learning (Yin, Knowlton, et al., 2005).

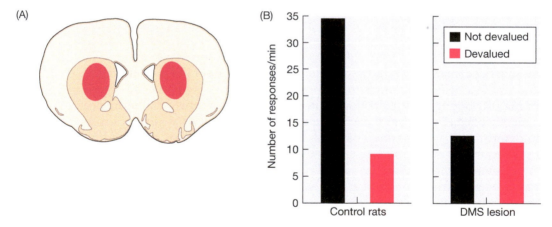

FIGURE 19.9   (A) This illustration shows the location of damage to the dorsomedial striatum (DMS) in rats. In this experiment, the rats were trained to press two levers that each produced a different reward. Following training, one of the rewards was devalued. (B) During the test, when no rewards were delivered, control rats pressed the lever that was associated with the now devalued reward far less than they pressed the other lever. This result indicates that their instrumental behavior was controlled by the action system. In contrast, rats with damage to the DMS pressed the two levers equally often. This result suggests that the DMS is part of the neural system that supports actions. (B after H. H. Yin et al. 2005. *Eur J Neurosci* 22: 513–523.)

BASOLATERAL AMYGDALA   The production of an action depends on the value of the outcome it produces; however, outcomes have particular sensory qualities—steak does not taste like oatmeal and peanuts do not taste like raisins. When a particular food is experienced, a memory representation of the specific sensory features is established. Moreover, it appears that a particular value also is attached to this representation. So, for example, if a novel food is ingested, not only is a representation of its sensory properties acquired, an abstract value or rating of liking (+) or disliking (–) the food is also attached to the representation. Thus, if one were asked to retrieve a representation of an orange, not only is its color, shape, texture, and taste retrieved, so is a representation of its value.

Research with both primates and rodents has identified an important role for the amygdala, specifically the basolateral amygdala, in attaching value to outcomes (Balleine and Killcross, 2006). Animals with major damage to the amygdala can learn instrumental behaviors. However, these animals are not sensitive to changes in the value of an outcome. For example, monkeys with amygdala damage have no problem learning the visual object discriminations shown in Figure 19.4. However, they are completely insensitive to devaluation of the associated rewards (Malkova et al., 1997). Moreover, monkeys with amygdala damage can learn specific motor patterns when rewarded for making the appropriate response. For example, they can learn to move a lever to the right when the signal is a red light and they can learn to move the lever to the left when the signal is a blue light (Murray and Wise, 1996). Similar results have been obtained when researchers have examined the effect of amygdala damage on instrumental learning in rats (Balleine, 2005; Balleine et al., 2003). These study results support the idea that the amygdala contributes to learning the value of the outcome and thus plays an important role in the action system.

PRELIMBIC PREFRONTAL CORTEX   The action system rapidly captures information needed to assemble an instrumental response: sensory input, responses, outcomes, and value of the outcome. The dorsomedial striatum is likely involved in the integration of this information. However, for this to occur requires input from the prelimbic prefrontal cortex. The prelimbic region of the brain is important during the initial learning of the associations that support an action. However, once these associations are learned, this region is no longer critical. The evidence for these claims is that if this region is damaged before rats learn an instrumental response, they are insensitive to reward devaluation (Killcross and Coutureau, 2003; Ostlund and Balleine, 2005). Thus, the instrumental response in this case would be called a habit. However, if the prelimbic region is damaged just after rats are allowed to learn the associations supporting the action, they remain sensitive to reward devaluation (Ostlund and Balleine, 2005). These results have two implications: (1) the prelimbic region is critical in the acquisition of the associations that support an action and (2) it is not the site in the brain where these associations are stored.

Neural Support for Habits

As noted earlier, habits are not purposeful and, once established, they are insensitive to the value of the outcome that initially motivated the behavior. Many trials are required to engrain a habitual response and they are difficult to unlearn. Two brain regions are critical to the acquisition and maintenance of habits: (1) the **dorsolateral striatum (DLS)** and (2) the **infralimbic prefrontal cortex**.

DORSOLATERAL STRIATUM   As previously illustrated in Figure 19.5, with limited training instrumental behavior is primarily supported by the action system—the behavior is sensitive to reward devaluation. However, with extensive training the behavior becomes a habit and is insensitive to reward devaluation. Thus, to determine if a particular brain region contributes to the acquisition or expression of a habit, animals receive extensive training before the reward devaluation treatment.

Henry Yin and his colleagues (Yin et al., 2004) used this strategy to reveal that the DLS is critical to habit formation. They compared rats with lesions of the DLS to control rats that experienced the surgery but not the lesion. Following extensive training to produce a lever press, they devalued the sucrose reward and then tested the rats. No reward was given during this 5-minute test. As expected, the extensively trained rats in the control condition were not influenced by reward devaluation, indicating that the behavior was a habit. In contrast, damage to the DLS influenced reward devaluation—the rats' rate of responding was dramatically reduced. This indicated that in the absence of neurons in the DLS the behavior never became a habit.

INFRALIMBIC PREFRONTAL CORTEX   Just as the prelimbic region of the prefrontal cortex is critical to the action system, so the infralimbic prefrontal cortex is critical to the habit system. Killcross and Coutureau (2003) damaged this brain region prior to rats acquiring an instrumental response (bar pressing for food reward). Even after extensive training the behavior never became a habit. The devaluation procedure reduced responding in rats with damage to the infralimbic region. In addition, Coutureau and Killcross (2003) used a pharmacological treatment to temporarily inactivate infralimbic neurons in rats that had been extensively trained to demonstrate that the instrumental response should be supported by the habit system. However, the reward devaluation treatment greatly reduced responding during the test. Coutureau and Killcross's findings were subsequently confirmed by using optogenetics (see Chapter 9) to control neurons in the infralimbic region (Smith et al., 2012). In this case, optogenetic methods were used to inhibit neurons in this region. Turning off these neurons almost instantaneously changed the control of the instrumental response from the habit system to the action system because these rats were sensitive to reward devaluation. These results have three implications.

1. The associations that support action-based behavior are still present even after the behavior becomes a habit. This implication follows because when the infralimbic function was impaired the rats became sensitive to the value of the reward.

2. With extensive training, the infralimbic region exerts inhibitory control over the action system, taking it offline so that it does not influence behavior. This implication follows because, depending upon the state of the neurons in the infralimbic region, a well-trained instrumental response can be shown to be supported by either the action or habit system.

3. When infralimbic neurons are turned off, the action system controls the response, but when these neurons are functioning, the habit system controls the response.

A comparison of the roles played by the prelimbic and infralimbic cortex is illustrated in Figure 19.10.

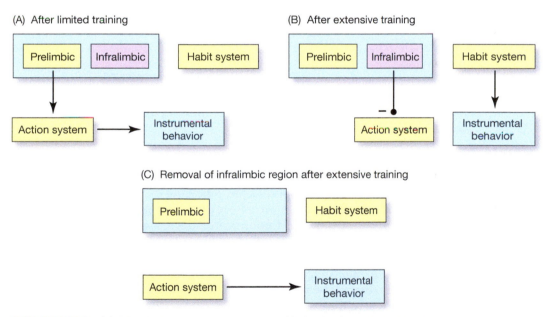

FIGURE 19.10   (A) After limited training, instrumental behavior is controlled by the action system. The prelimbic region is necessary early in training for building the action system that controls a particular instrumental behavior. Note at this stage that the habit system does not contribute to the generation of the instrumental behavior. (B) With extensive training, the prelimbic region is no longer necessary to generate an action. Moreover, the infralimbic region now suppresses the contribution of the action system (–), and instrumental behavior is produced by the habit system. (C) If the infralimbic region is removed after extensive training, the action system again assumes control over instrumental behavior. This means that after extensive training, associations that can produce instrumental behavior are present in both the action and habit systems.

The Striatum Stores Action and Habit Memories

While the DMS and DLS are part of the habit and action systems, Shiftlett and Balleine (2011) noted that it is not clear how these regions contribute to the acquisition and generation of the behavior. One possibility is that they are memory storage sites for the information that supports actions and habits. Alternatively, they may just help coordinate learning and memory storage that occurs in other brain regions.

Pauli et al. (2012) also addressed this issue. They reasoned that if the DMS and DLS actually store memories needed to support habits and actions, then it should be possible to erase this content by using the inhibitory peptide ZIP to disrupt the PKMζ function (see Chapter 7). They used the same reversal learning procedure described above to demonstrate that the action and habit systems compete. When ZIP was injected into the DMS the day before testing (theoretically erasing memory support for the action system), rats were impaired in learning to reverse their response choices. In contrast, when ZIP was injected into the DLS (theoretically erasing memory support for the habit system), rats rapidly learned to reverse their response choice. Thus, erasing information in the habit system facilitated learning to reverse the discrimination, whereas erasing task information acquired by the action system retarded learning the reversal. These results are consistent with the idea that the DMS and DLS regions of the striatum are memory storage sites for the action and habit systems. Note, however, that these regions are unlikely to be the only storage sites for instrumental responses.

The Neural Basis of Rewarding Outcomes

By definition, instrumental responses are behaviors that change the environment to produce rewards or reinforcers—rewards increase the likelihood that a behavior will be repeated and nonrewards decrease this likelihood. Two general ideas about how rewards influence behavior were also discussed earlier. One relates to Thorndike's argument that rewards strengthen associative connections. The other derives from Tolman's position that rewards provide incentive motivation for behavior. But what is the neural basis of rewards that enable them to serve these two functions?

Both of these ideas have been related to the influence rewards have on the release of the neurotransmitter **dopamine**. This source of dopamine is provided by what is called the **mesolimbic dopamine system** (Berridge and Robinson, 1998). Dopamine in this system comes from neurons located in a region of the brain called the ventral tegmental area (VTA). In particular, the VTA responds to events often used to reinforce instrumental behavior and it has outputs that project into the striatum, specifically the nucleus accumbens (Figure 19.11A).

The **dopamine reinforcement hypothesis** relates dopamine to Thorndike's idea that rewards strengthen associative connections. In this case, it is easy to

(A)

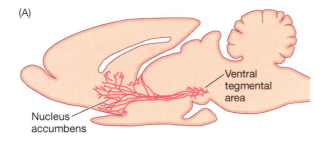

Ventral
tegmental
area

Nucleus
accumbens

(B)

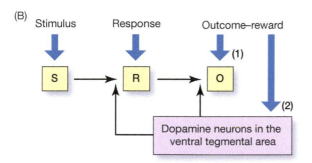

Stimulus   Response   Outcome–reward

FIGURE 19.11 (A) This sagittal section of the rat brain illustrates the mesolimbic dopamine system. The dopamine neurons are located in the ventral tegmental area (VTA) and their fibers project into the nucleus accumbens of the striatum. (B) The dopamine theory of reinforcement. An outcome–reward has two functions: (1) It generates a representation (O), and (2) it activates dopamine neurons in the VTA that release dopamine into the striatum. This acts to strengthen synaptic connections between the representations of the stimulus (S) complex and the response (R) and perhaps between the representations of the response and the outcome.

imagine that the outcome produced by behavior first turns on neurons in the VTA that then cause dopamine to be released into the striatum (the nucleus accumbens) and that this dopamine release strengthens the relevant synaptic connections supporting stimulus–response or response–outcome associative connections (Figure 19.11B).

Another hypothesis, called the **dopamine incentive salience hypothesis**, links dopamine to the motivational significance of rewarding outcomes. It assumes that activation of the mesolimbic dopamine system by a rewarding outcome attaches motivational significance to stimuli associated with the outcome (Berridge, 2007). What this means is that the presence of a stimulus associated with a strongly rewarding outcome can evoke a strong urge for the outcome. The instrumental behavior occurs because it produces the outcome that satisfies the want (Figure 19.12).

Berridge and Robinson (1998) developed the dopamine incentive salience hypothesis to provide an explanation for drug relapse (see Chapter 15). Their contention is that drug relapse occurs because addictive drugs strongly activate dopamine neurons, and neutral cues present at that time acquire the ability to produce the urge to take the drug. Thus, the sight of a cigarette or the smell of cigarette smoke might evoke an intense urge to smoke a cigarette because these stimuli were associated with the activation of the dopamine system and acquired extreme incentive properties. These urges motivate the person to engage in instrumental behaviors that produce the outcome that reduces the urge.

FIGURE 19.12 The incentive salience hypothesis assumes that the reward turns on dopamine neurons in the ventral tegmental area. In the normal sequence of events that establish instrumental behavior, the stimulus not only can associate with the response, it also can get associated with the incentive properties of the outcome. Subsequently, the stimulus complex itself can elicit strong urges or wants that lead the individual to seek out the reward. Berridge and Robinson (1998) have proposed that these urges play an important role in drug-addiction relapse. Even though an addict might go through drug withdrawal and be "clean," an encounter with stimuli associated with the drug experience can lead to relapse because they can produce irresistible urges to seek the drug. (After K. C. Berridge and T. E. Robinson. 1998. *Brain Res Rev* 28: 309–369.)

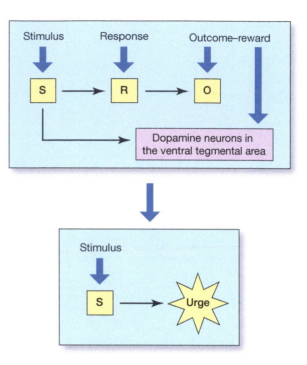

Summary

Instrumental behaviors change the environment—they produce outcomes—and their likelihood of reoccurring is modified by the nature of the outcome. Instrumental behaviors belong to two categories called actions and habits. Actions are purposeful and goal directed and supported by what are called expectancies. Actions are motivated by the expected outcomes they produce and the action system is flexible. Habits are not purposeful and thus are thought to be insensitive to the outcomes they produce. Instrumental behaviors begin as actions but with extensive repetition gradually become S–R habits. The reward devaluation strategy, which detects the animal's sensitivity to the goal, and the discrimination reversal strategy, which detects the flexibility of the two systems, can be employed to determine which system controls the instrumental response.

A cortico-striatal neural system linking a variety of cortical and midbrain regions is the system that integrates the elements of our experience—stimulus inputs, response inputs, and outcomes produced by the response—into actions and habits. The action system depends in part on three regions of the brain: the DMS, prelimbic prefrontal cortex, and the basolateral amygdala. The habit system depends on the DLS and infralimbic prefrontal cortex, which appears to suppress the action system. Both actions and habits likely depend on the mesolimbic dopamine system located in the ventral tegmental area of the brain. Neurons from this region project to the striatum and dopamine release may strengthen associative connections and serve as an incentive motivational signal.

References

Adams, C. D. (1982). Variations in the sensitivity of instrumental responding to reinforcer devaluation. *Quarterly Journal of Experimental Psychology [B], 34,* 77–98.

Balleine, B. W. (2005). Neural bases of food-seeking: affect, arousal and reward in cortico striato limbic circuits. *Physiology and Behavior, 86,* 717–730.

Balleine, B. W. and Killcross, A. S. (2006). Parallel incentive processing: an integrated view of amygdala function. *Trends in Neurosciences, 29,* 272–279.

Balleine, B. W., Killcross, A. S., and Dickinson, A. (2003). The effect of lesions of the basolateral amygdala on instrumental conditioning. *Journal of Neuroscience, 23,* 666–678.

Baxter, M. G. and Murray, E. A. (2002). The amygdala and reward. *Nature Reviews Neuroscience, 3,* 563–573.

Berridge, K. C. (2007). The debate over dopamine's role in reward: the case for incentive salience. *Psychopharmacology, 191,* 391–431.

Berridge, K. C. and Robinson, T. E. (1998). What is the role of dopamine in reward: hedonic impact, reward learning, or incentive salience? *Brain Research Review, 28,* 309–369.

Cook, D. and Kesner, R. P. (1988). Caudate nucleus and memory for egocentric localization. *Behavioral Neural Biology, 49,* 332–343.

Coutureau, E. and Killcross, S. (2003). Inactivation of the infralimbic prefrontal cortex reinstates goal-directed responding in overtrained rats. *Behavioral Brain Research, 146,* 167–174.

Dias-Ferreira, E., Sousa, J. C., Melo, I., Morgado, P., Mesquita, A. R., João, J., Cerqueira, J. J., Costa, R. M., and Sousa, N. (2009). Chronic stress causes frontostriatal reorganization and affects decision-making. *Science, 325,* 621–625.

Divac, I., Rosvold, H. E., and Szwarcbart, M. K. (1967). Behavioral effects of selective ablation of the caudate nucleus. *Journal of Comparative and Physiological Psychology, 63,* 183–190.

Gourley, S. L., Olevska, A., Gordon, J., and Taylor, J. R. (2013). Cytoskeletal determinants of stimulus-response habits. *Journal of Neuroscience, 33,* 11811–11816.

Graybiel, A. M. (2008). Habits, rituals, and the evaluative brain. *Annual Review of Neuroscience, 31,* 359–387.

Killcross, S. and Coutureau, E. (2003). Coordination of actions and habits in the medial prefrontal cortex of rats. *Cerebral Cortex, 13,* 400–408.

Malkova, L. D., Gaffan, D., and Murray, E. (1997). Excitotoxic lesions of the amygdala fail to produce impairment in visual learning for auditory secondary reinforcement but interfere with reinforcer devaluation effects in rhesus monkeys. *Journal of Neuroscience, 17*, 6011–6020.

Murray, E. A. and Wise, S. P. (1996). Role of the hippocampus plus subjacent cortex but not amygdala in visuomotor conditional learning in rhesus monkeys. *Behavioral Neuroscience, 110*, 1261–1270.

Nelson, A. and Killcross, S. (2006). Amphetamine cxposure enhances habit formation. *Journal of Neuroscience, 26*, 3805–3812.

Ostlund, S. B. and Balleine, B. W. (2005). Lesions of medial prefrontal cortex disrupt the acquisition but not the expression of goal-directed learning. *Journal of Neuroscience, 25*, 7763–7770.

Pauli, W. M., Clark, A. D., Guenther, H. J., O'Reilly, R. C., and Rudy, J. W. (2012). Inhibiting PKMζ reveals dorsal lateral and dorsal medial striatum store the different memories needed to support adaptive behavior. *Learning and Memory, 19*, 307–314.

Shiftlett, M. W. and Balleine, B. W. (2011). Molecular substrates of action control in cortico-striatal circuits. *Progress in Neurobiology, 95*, 1–13.

Smith, K. S., Virkud, A., Deisseroth, K., and Graybiel, A. M. (2012). Reversible online control of habitual behavior by optogenetic perturbation of medial prefrontal cortex. *Proceedings of the National Academy of Sciences USA, 109*, 18932–18937.

Thorndike, E. L. (1898). Animal Intelligence: an experimental study of associative processes in animals. *Psychological Monographs, 2*, Whole No. 8.

Thorndike, E. L. (1905). *The Elements of Psychology*. New York: A. G. Seiler.

Tolman, E. C. (1948). Cognitive maps in rats and men. *Psychological Review, 55*, 189–208.

Tolman, E. C. (1949). There is more than one kind of learning. *Psychological Review, 56*, 144–155.

White, N. M. and McDonald, R. J. (2002). Multiple parallel memory systems in the brain of the rat. *Neurobiology of Learning and Memory, 77*, 125–184.

Yin, H. H., Knowlton, B. J., and Balleine, B. W. (2004). Lesions of dorsolateral striatum preserve outcome expectancy but disrupt habit formation in instrumental learning. *European Journal of Neuroscience, 19*, 181–189.

Yin, H. H., Knowlton, B. J., and Balleine, B. W. (2005). Blockade of NMDA receptors in the dorsomedial striatum prevents action–outcome learning in instrumental conditioning. *European Journal of Neuroscience, 22*, 505–512.

Yin, H. H., Ostlund, S. B., Knowlton, B. J., and Balleine, B. W. (2005). The role of the dorsomedial striatum in instrumental conditioning. *European Journal of Neuroscience, 22*, 513–523.

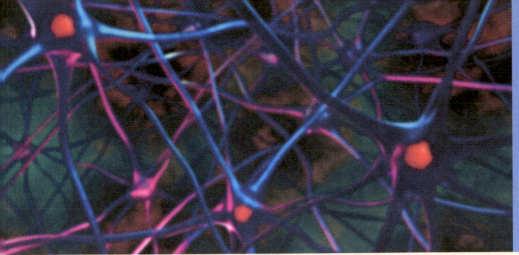

Learning about Danger: The Neurobiology of Fear Memories

All animals must solve fundamental problems associated with survival and reproduction. Thus, it should not come as a surprise that our evolutionary history has provided us with a brain that is designed to support what are called behavioral systems (Timberlake, 1994). A **behavioral system** is organized specifically to ensure that some particular need is met. There are specialized behavioral systems designed to support our reproductive and feeding-related activities and behavioral systems that allow us to avoid and escape dangerous situations.

According to the behavioral systems view, one major role of the processes that support learning and memory is to properly connect the behavioral infrastructure supported by a particular system to the ever-changing world in which we live. For example, we have the relevant behaviors for finding and ingesting food, but we have to learn the details about where the food is and what is fit to eat. We also have the relevant behaviors needed to avoid and escape from danger. But how do we know what is dangerous?

Some of this information is coded in our genes. However, in a dynamic world we have to adjust to changes in the environment. From a learning and memory perspective, the challenge is to understand how experience connects the neural systems that support our survival behaviors with the other features of our world that allow us to anticipate the occurrence of biologically significant events.

Understanding how learning and memory processes interface and tune our behavioral systems to this changing world is a large and complex endeavor because each of the several behavioral systems is specialized and has its own neural components. Rather than attempt a survey of all of these systems, this chapter focuses on just one—the so-called fear system. The importance of this system is obvious and much is known about its fundamental components. The chapter begins by describing the fear system and its neural basis, then considers how fears can be extinguished, and concludes with a discussion of the neural basis of fear elimination.

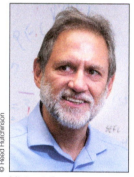

© Reed Hutchinson

Michael Fanselow

The Fear System

The fear system evolved to allow us to escape from harmful events and to avoid them in the future. Robert Bolles (1970) developed the concept of species-specific defensive behaviors to describe the class of innate behaviors that are supported by the fear system. For example, the rat, a subject of hundreds of studies on the fear system, is equipped with several easily observable defensive behaviors, including freezing, flight, and fighting. Freezing is by far the most dominant of these behaviors. As previously noted, this response (in which the animal remains essentially motionless, except for breathing) is often used as a measure of fear conditioning. Freezing provides an innate strategy to avoid danger because a motionless animal is less likely to be spotted by a predator than one that is moving. Moreover, flight is not especially effective for rodents because relative to their predators they are very slow.

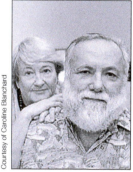

Courtesy of Caroline Blanchard

Caroline and Robert Blanchard

Michael Fanselow (1991) has argued that these defensive behaviors are organized around what he called a **predatory imminence gradient**, that is, when a potential predator is at a distance the rat will freeze, but as the predator moves within striking distance, the rat might attempt to flee the scene. If caught, it will engage in fighting in an attempt to escape. People respond to danger in much the same way. For example, Caroline and Robert Blanchard (1989), pioneers in research on defensive behaviors, have provided the following description of human defensive behavior.

> If something unexpected occurs—a loud noise or sudden movement—people tend to respond immediately…stop what they are doing…orient toward the stimulus, and try to identify its potential for actual danger. This happens very quickly, in a reflex-like sequence in which action precedes any voluntary or consciously intentioned behavior. A poorly localizable or identifiable threat source, such as sound in the night, may elicit an active immobility so profound that

the frightened person can hardly speak or even breathe, that is, freezing. However, if the danger source has been localized and an avenue for flight or concealment is plausible, the person will probably try to flee or hide… Actual contact, particularly painful contact, with the threat source is also likely to elicit thrashing, biting, scratching and other potentially damaging activities by the terrified person. (LeDoux, 1998, p. 131, excerpted from Blanchard and Blanchard, 1989, pp. 94–121.)

In addition to activating these easily observed behaviors, a danger signal will engage our autonomic nervous system, causing changes in our internal physiology, including increased heart rate and blood pressure and the shunting of blood to the peripheral muscles to prepare for flight or fight. Danger signals also produce analgesia—insensitivity to pain—and can release adrenal gland hormones that support the flight–fight response and enhance memory (see Chapter 12). Some stimuli will innately activate the fear system. However, learning and memory processes provide the primary way to link stimuli to the neural systems that support fear behavior and allow us to anticipate danger and get out of harm's way. Figure 20.1 provides a schematic of the basic ideas of a defensive behavioral system.

Experience teaches us to identify dangerous situations. This happens because an experience with an aversive event will modify our response to the otherwise insignificant features of the environment that are also present. Associative learning processes that support Pavlovian conditioning produce this outcome. The basic laboratory procedures used for creating conditioned fear are described in Chapter 9.

An aversive stimulus can establish fear to both the place–context where it occurred and the discrete phasic stimulus (a stimulus that has a distinct onset and termination) that preceded the shock. Fear as measured by defensive responses is easy to establish and increases with the intensity of the aversive event. Once established, memories for fear experience endure for a long time. Variations of this basic procedure in combination with methods for altering regions of the brain have been used to reveal much of what has been learned about the neural basis of learned fear.

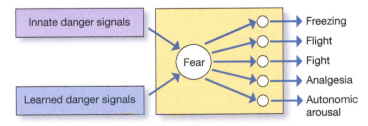

FIGURE 20.1   This figure illustrates a defensive behavioral system. This system organizes the expression of a variety of behaviors that have evolved to protect us from danger. It can be activated by innate danger signals, and experience allows this system to also be activated by learned danger signals.

The Neural Basis of Fear

When confronted with signals of danger, animals can display several responses. As noted, they freeze, they flee, and they will fight when escape is not possible. They also display autonomic arousal. In this section, some of the major components of the neural circuitry that supports these fear responses are described. The system, illustrated in Figure 20.2, is organized to receive sensory information about the environment and to decide if fear behaviors should be generated.

Midbrain subcortical nuclei are responsible for generating fear behaviors. For example, neurons located in what is called the **periaqueductal gray** produce

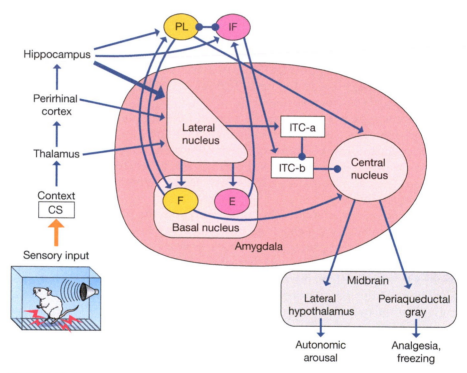

FIGURE 20.2 This figure illustrates the basic components of the fear system that can be modified by experience. The lateral nucleus receives sensory input from the sensory thalamus, perirhinal cortex, and hippocampus that provides information about the current state of the environment. The basal nucleus contains both fear and extinction neurons. Neurons in the central amygdala control midbrain structures that support the expression of fear behaviors. When neurons in the central amygdala depolarize they activate the midbrain nuclei to generate defensive behaviors. There are two clusters of inhibitory intercalated (ITC) neurons. The ITC-b cluster normally inhibits central amygdala neurons. This inhibition can be removed if the ITC-a cluster is activated. Arrows indicate excitatory connections, and round endings indicate inhibitory connections. Key: CS = conditioned stimulus; PL = prelimbic; IF = infralimbic; F = fear; E = extinction.

freezing and analgesia. Other neurons, in the lateral hypothalamus, are responsible for the changes in autonomic responses (heart rate and blood pressure) produced by the sympathetic nervous system that prepare the body for action (see Figure 20.2). Direct electrical stimulation of these brain regions can elicit fear behaviors, and damage to these regions impairs the expression of the behaviors (for reviews, see Fanselow, 1991 and Kim and Jung, 2006).

Midbrain nuclei provide the direct neural basis for specific defensive behaviors that make up the fear system. However, these regions are not directly linked to the sensory–perceptual systems by which the world is experienced. Instead, the sensory–perceptual systems interface with the midbrain nuclei by way of the amygdala (see Chapter 12). The amygdala is an almond shaped structure composed of many nuclei and subdivisions. Three components of the amygdala (see Figure 20.2) are relevant to the fear system: (1) the basolateral amygdala, composed of the lateral and basal nuclei; (2) the central amygdala; and (3) intercalated cell masses (ITC-a and ITC-b), which release inhibitory neurotransmitters (GABA) onto their targets (Box 20.1).

The lateral nucleus provides the interface that links the content of a fear conditioning experience to other components of the amygdala. Joseph LeDoux (1994) has described two pathways that bring the content of the experience to the lateral nucleus, a **subcortical pathway** and a **cortical pathway** (Romanski and LeDoux, 1992). The subcortical pathway comes directly from the sensory thalamus, which is thought to provide a somewhat impoverished representation of the sensory experience. The cortical pathway carries information from the sensory thalamus to the neocortical regions of the brain including the

BOX 20.1 Intercalated Cells Inhibit Fear

Denis Paré and his colleagues (Likhtik et al., 2008; Royer and Paré, 2002) identified clusters of intercalated cells (ITCs) located between the basolateral complex and the central amygdala. These neurons receive CS information from the basolateral amygdala and project to the central amygdala. When activated, these cells release the inhibitory neurotransmitter GABA and thus prevent their target neurons from depolarizing. In this way, they prevent neurons in the central amygdala from generating defensive behavior. Key: BL = basal nucleus; LA = lateral nucleus; AB = accessory basal nucleus.

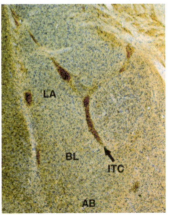

Courtesy of Denis Paré

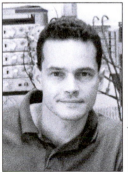

Denis Paré

Courtesy of Denis Paré

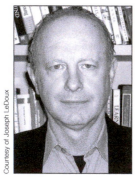

Joseph LeDoux

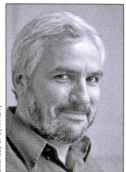

Cyril Herry

perirhinal cortex and hippocampus, which also project to the lateral nucleus and provide a richer, more detailed representation of the experience (Burwell et al., 2004). The lateral amygdala region projects to two regions—the basal nucleus and a cluster of intercalated cells (ITC-a)—that project to a second ITC cluster (ITC-b). The second cluster projects to neurons in the central amygdala and inhibits them.

Cyril Herry and his colleagues (Herry et al., 2008) discovered that the basal nucleus contains two types of neurons: (1) fear neurons that are active when fear behaviors are expressed and (2) extinction neurons that are active when fear has been extinguished (described later in this chapter). The fear neurons provide excitatory projections to the central nucleus and to neurons in the prelimbic region of the prefrontal cortex. Extinction neurons project to ITC-b cells.

The central amygdala can be thought of as the command center for initiating fear-related behaviors. It is an output region and projects to the midbrain regions that generate fear behaviors. Under normal, nonthreatening conditions, ITC-b cells inhibit central amygdala neurons. When these neurons are activated (depolarized), they activate neurons in the lateral hypothalamus and periaqueductal gray and generate fear behaviors. Thus, to generate fear behavior the neurons in the central amygdala must be depolarized.

Two regions of the prefrontal cortex—prelimbic (PL) and infralimbic (IL)—interact with the amygdala to modulate the fear response (Sotres-Bayon and Quirk, 2010). Neurons in the prelimbic region are reciprocally connected to fear neurons in the basal nucleus. These reciprocal connections are designed to *amplify* the fear signal. Support for this function comes from the observation that activation of neurons in the lateral nucleus by a cue paired with shock lasts only a few milliseconds, but prelimbic neurons show a sustained response for the duration of the CS (tens of seconds) that correlates with the duration of the fear response. In addition, inactivating PL neurons greatly reduces the expression of fear behaviors (Sotres-Bayon and Quirk, 2010). In contrast, the output from infralimbic neurons *inhibits* the fear response by activating ITC-b cells. They receive projections from the hippocampus and extinction neurons in the basal nucleus.

The fear system is complex. The main point, however, is that a conditioned fear response is produced because the fear circuit is reorganized (Figure 20.3). Synapses are strengthened that link the sensory content (context and CS) to neurons in the lateral amygdala and prelimbic cortex. Consequently, if these stimulus conditions are re-encountered the sensory input will excite neurons in the lateral nucleus and prelimbic cortex and this will result in (a) the removal of the ITC-b inhibitory block on central amygdala neurons and (b) the activation of fear neurons in the basal nucleus. Consequently, neurons in the central amygdala will be excited to generate fear behaviors (see Figure 20.3).

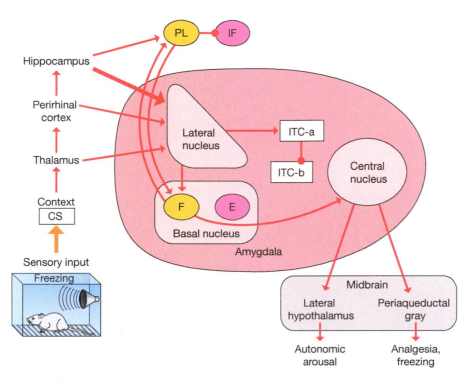

FIGURE 20.3   When an aversive event occurs, synapses are strengthened that link the sensory content (context and CS) to neurons in the lateral amygdala and prelimbic cortex. As a consequence, a re-encounter with these stimulus conditions will activate the fear circuit (in red). The inhibitory influence of ITC-b neurons on central neurons will be removed and excitatory drive provided by fear neurons and prelimbic cortex neurons will increase. Key: CS = conditioned stimulus; PL = prelimbic; IF = infralimbic; F = fear; E = extinction.

Eliminating Maladaptive Fears: Theories of Extinction

The fear system is designed to produce adaptive behaviors that keep us out of harm's way. However, the properties of this system that support rapid fear conditioning also can be maladaptive and lead to behavioral pathologies. Learned fears and anxieties such as panic attacks and post-traumatic stress disorders that result from intensive aversive experiences can be so debilitating that they greatly interfere with our ability to function normally. Consequently, the problem of how to eliminate learned fears is of great interest to basic researchers, clinical psychologists, and psychiatrists.

Researchers have focused on the Pavlovian conditioning methodology to study how to remove learned fears. Cues paired with aversive events acquire the ability to evoke a conditioned defensive response. In the language of Pavlovian

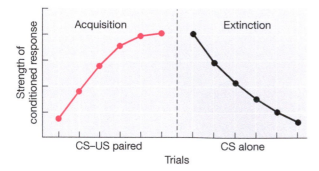

FIGURE 20.4 Paired presentations of the conditioned stimulus (CS) and unconditioned stimulus (US) produce acquisition. The CS acquires the ability to evoke the conditioned response (CR). If the CS is then presented alone, it will lose the ability to evoke the CR. This phenomenon is called extinction.

conditioning, the cue paired with shock is called the conditioned stimulus (CS) and the aversive event is called the unconditioned stimulus (US). Since Pavlov's work, it has been known that a conditioned response (CR) can be eliminated. The procedure is called the method of extinction. With this procedure, after a conditioned response is established, the subject is presented the CS but the US is not presented. When the CS is repeatedly presented alone, it loses its ability to evoke the conditioned response. This outcome, the loss of the conditioned response, is called **extinction** (Figure 20.4). Note that the term extinction is used to describe *both a method and a fact*.

Extinction is an empirical fact. Presenting the CS alone can eliminate the conditioned response. The theoretical question is, *why does this method produce extinction?* Two hypotheses have been proposed. One is called the **associative loss hypothesis**; the other is called the **competing memory hypothesis** (Figure 20.5). It is generally assumed that a CS paired with a US comes to evoke a conditioned response because it has become associated with the representation of the US. The associative loss hypothesis assumes that extinction is due to the CS-alone presentation eliminating or erasing the original CS–US association. However, the competing memory hypothesis assumes that the original CS–US association remains intact and instead a new association, called a **CS–noUS association**, is produced. If the CS activates the noUS pathway, expression of the conditioned response will be blocked or inhibited.

These two theories have different implications. The associative loss hypothesis implies that extinction should be *permanent* because the underlying association is erased. So, according to this theory, the CS must again be paired with

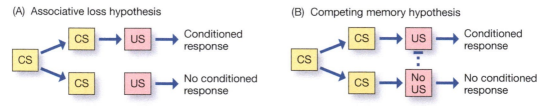

FIGURE 20.5 This figure illustrates two theories of extinction. (A) The associative loss hypothesis assumes that extinction is due to a CS-alone presentation eliminating the original CS–US association. (B) The competing memory hypothesis assumes that extinction produces a new association called a CS–noUS association. The original CS–US association that produced the CR remains intact. If the CS–noUS association occurs, it inhibits (–) the expression of the conditioned response.

the US in order to reestablish its ability to evoke a conditioned response. In contrast, the competing memory hypothesis allows that the conditioned response could recover without re-pairing the CS and US because the original association is not lost—the CS just enters into a new association, the CS–noUS association.

Mark Bouton's research program has been critical of the contemporary view of extinction (Bouton, 1994; Bouton, 2002). The evidence indicates that extinction does not eliminate the underlying associative basis of the conditioned response. Instead, *extinction produces new learning*. Three observations support this conclusion (Figure 20.6).

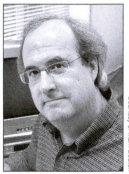

Mark Bouton

(A) Spontaneous recovery

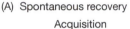
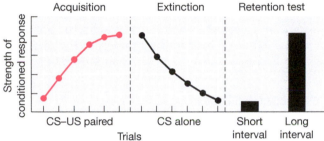

(B) Renewal effect

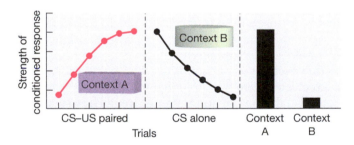

(C) Reinstatement effect

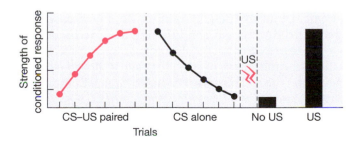

FIGURE 20.6 This figure illustrates three findings that indicate that extinction is not permanent. In each example the critical results are from the retention test where the CS is re-presented after extinction has taken place. (A) Spontaneous recovery can occur when there is a long retention interval between extinction and the test. (B) Renewal can occur when the context where extinction trials take place is different from the context in which training takes place, and the test occurs in the training context. (C) Reinstatement occurs if the US is re-presented without the CS. In all cases, recovery from extinction occurs even though the CS and US are never re-paired.

1. *Spontaneous recovery.* With the passage of time following extinction, the CS recovers its ability to evoke the conditioned response. It does not have to be paired with the US again for the conditioned response to reappear.

2. *Renewal effect.* In this case rats are given the CS–US pairings in one place or context, but extinction (CS-alone presentations) occurs in a different place. Even though extinction training eliminates the conditioned response, if the animal is returned to the original training environment, the CR recovers.

3. *Reinstatement effect.* Just re-presenting the US in the training context can reinstate the ability of the CS to evoke a conditioned response. Note again that the CS does not have to be re-paired with the US.

In these examples the CS recovers the ability to evoke the CR even though it is not re-paired with the US. If presenting the CS alone erased the underlying CS–US association, this should not happen. Thus, these results support the competing memory hypothesis—that extinction does not erase the original CS–US association, rather the CS enters into a CS–noUS association.

Neural Basis of Fear Extinction

Based on the results just discussed one would assume that at the completion of extinction, the CS is involved in two associations: the original CS–US association and the new CS–noUS association. The task for neurobiologists is to understand (a) how the neural circuitry supports a CS–noUS association and (b) what processes determine which association is expressed, the CS–US or the CS–noUS association—that is, *why does the fear response recover?*

The CS–noUS Neural Circuit

A major outcome of extinction training is to reconfigure the fear circuit so that the CS activates intercalated clusters (see Box 20.1) that inhibit neurons in the central amygdala. To accomplish this, extinction training strengthens synaptic connections that link the context and CS input to extinction neurons in the basal nucleus (a) to ITCs and (b) to neurons in the infralimbic prefrontal cortex which also projects to ITCs. Thus, when the CS is presented, ITCs are activated and neurons in the central amygdala are inhibited (Maren, 2011; Pape and Paré, 2010; Sotres-Bayon and Quirk, 2010).

It is important to remember that extinction training does not erase the synaptic connections established during fear conditioning that excite central amygdala neurons to generate fear. Extinction results because new connections are strengthened that provide the inhibition needed to prevent those neurons from depolarizing and generating fear. Thus, the CS–noUS association can be thought of as *a reconfigured fear circuit that allows the extinguished CS to suppress the central amygdala.* Figure 20.7 provides a comparison of the circuit that is established by fear conditioning that generates fear (red lines) with the circuit

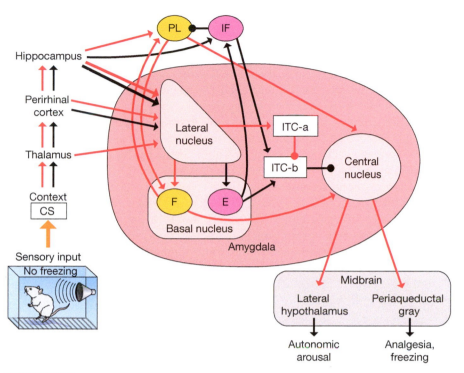

FIGURE 20.7   This figure illustrates how extinction training reconfigures the neural system to support extinction. The red arrows indicate how fear conditioning organizes the system to produce fear. The black arrows indicate how extinction training modifies the system to support no fear. The fundamental outcome produced by extinction training is to change synaptic connections that will increase inhibitory control over neurons in the central amygdala. This is accomplished by strengthening synapses linking the CS to extinction neurons in the basal region and to neurons in the infralimbic cortex. Both extinction and infralimbic cortex neurons project to ITCs that inhibit neurons in the central amygdala. The result is that the CS can now activate the new extinction circuit or the fear circuit and prevent neurons in the central amygdala from depolarizing and generating fear behaviors. Arrows indicate excitatory connections; round endings indicate inhibitory connections. Key: CS = conditioned stimulus; PL = prelimbic; IF = infralimbic; F = fear; E = extinction.

that is established when fear is extinguished (black lines). Whether or not fear is renewed will be determined by which circuit dominates.

Why Fear Renews: A Role for the Hippocampus

Fear acquisition training strengthens synapses that link the CS to fear neurons (CS–US association) and fear extinction training strengthens synapses that link the CS to extinction neurons (CS–noUS association). So how is the decision made that determines whether the CS activates extinction neurons or fear neurons? Steve Maren and his colleagues (Corcoran and Maren, 2001;

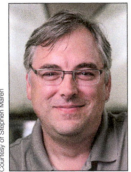

Steve Maren

Ji and Maren, 2005; Ji and Maren, 2007) have revealed that the hippocampal system makes a critical contribution to this decision. Their fundamental behavioral observation is that extinction is context specific. Thus, if extinction occurs in context B, the CS will evoke no fear if the test occurs in context B. However, the CS will elicit the fear response if it is presented in new context C. This is the previously described renewal effect. From a psychological perspective one might say that the rat has learned that the CS signals the absence of shock only in context B.

The context specificity of extinction depends on the hippocampal system (Bouton et al., 2006). When the hippocampus is damaged or inactivated following extinction, context specificity is lost and rats do not display renewed fear (Corcoran and Maren, 2001; Ji and Maren, 2005; Ji and Maren, 2007). The context regulates expression of fear or extinction because the hippocampal system also projects on to extinction neurons, and during extinction training these synapses get strengthened. Thus, if the CS is presented in the extinction context the CS–noUS circuit will dominate and the fear response will not be generated. However, if the CS is presented in another context the renewal of fear will occur.

Why Fear Spontaneously Recovers: A Role for Forgetting

As just discussed, extinguished fears can be renewed when the CS is presented outside of the context in which the CS was presented alone. The conditioned fear response also can recover spontaneously with the passage of time. One interpretation of spontaneous recovery is that it reflects a change in the temporal context that would naturally occur with the passage of time between extinction training and the test for spontaneous recovery. For example, over time the internal state of the animal changes so that it is much different at the time of testing than it was at the end of extinction training (Bouton, 2017).

An alternative explanation is that spontaneous recovery is *a case of forgetting* produced by the same endogenous processes, discussed in Chapter 13, that remove AMPA receptors from the postsynaptic density to actively degrade the memory. Migues et al. (2016) provided support for this hypothesis. Following conditioning to a tone CS paired with shock, they exposed subjects to three sessions of extinction. They then allowed 6 days for spontaneous recovery to occur. During this 6-day period they infused the peptide GluA23γ into the infralimbic cortex to prevent the removal of AMPA receptors and the synaptic basis of fear extinction. Compared to control animals, spontaneous recovery was markedly reduced (Figure 20.8). This finding supports the idea that the synaptic changes that support extinction are subject to active degradation by processes that remove AMPA receptors from the synapses potentiated by extinction.

Extinction Learning Depends on NMDA Receptors

Extinction is the result of new learning. Thus, it is reasonable to ask if NMDA receptors are involved in strengthening the synaptic connection linking the sensory–perceptual content of experience to the neurons that support extinction.

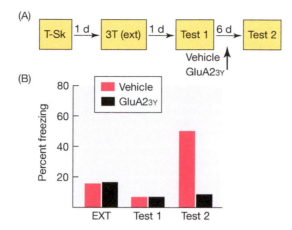

FIGURE 20.8 Spontaneous recovery may be due to active forgetting. (A) The design of the experiment. Rats received fear conditioning to a tone (T) paired with shock (Sk). They then received three sessions of extinction training, 3T (ext). (B) Freezing to the tone was extinguished (EXT). This was followed the next day by another test for freezing (Test 1), which confirmed that extinction had occurred. Over the next 6 days either the peptide GluA23Y or the vehicle was injected into the infralimbic prefrontal cortex to prevent AMPA receptor endocytosis. Test 2 revealed that rats in the vehicle condition displayed significant spontaneous recovery of the extinguished freezing response, whereas rats infused with GluA23Y did not. Thus, preventing AMPA receptor endocytosis with GluA23Y reduced spontaneous recovery. This result indicates that spontaneous recovery may be due to active forgetting processes. (After P. V. Migues et al. 2016. *J Neurosci* 36: 3481–3494.)

Several laboratories have reported that the injection of APV into the amygdala prior to CS-alone presentations significantly impairs the acquisition and retention of the learning that supports extinction (for a review, see Falls et al., 1992 and Myers and Davis, 2007). It also has been shown that the antagonist ifenprodil, which selectively blocks glutamate's access to the GluN2B subunit of the NMDA receptor, blocks the extinction of the fear response (Sotres-Bayon et al., 2007).

In addition to having glutamate binding sites, the NMDA receptor also has a glycine binding site (Figure 20.9). The glycine binding site is important because it contributes to the efficient opening of the NMDA receptor calcium channel. A number of researchers have asked if the glycine binding site contributes to extinction. They used a partial agonist called d-cycloserine (DCS) that binds to the glycine site to enhance the opening of the NMDA receptor. This work revealed that if DCS was injected either before or immediately after extinction training, the next day the rodents displayed enhanced extinction (Ledgerwood et al., 2003; Walker et al., 2002; see Davis et al., 2006 for a review). Given that NMDA receptor antagonists can prevent extinction and the partial agonist DCS can facilitate extinction, it is reasonable to assume that synaptic changes that depend on NMDA receptors play a central role in the new learning that produces extinction.

FIGURE 20.9 (A) NMDA receptors have two binding sites, one for glutamate and one for glycine. (B) APV antagonizes the glutamate binding site and interferes with extinction. (C) D-cycloserine (DCS) is an agonist for the glycine site. When it is given before or after extinction training, it facilitates the processes that produce extinction.

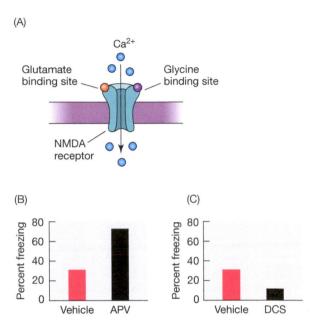

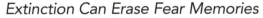

The discovery that DCS facilitates extinction in the laboratory has encouraged researchers to pursue the possibility that DCS, in combination with behavioral theory, might have therapeutic value in eliminating learned fears in people. Kerry Ressler and his colleagues (2004) have tested this hypothesis on people who suffer from acrophobia. People with acrophobia have a debilitating and irrational fear of heights. To test their hypothesis, Ressler's group used what is called **exposure therapy**. In this therapy, patients are forced to experience the stimulus situation that induces the fear response. It is used to treat a number of fear–anxiety disorders. Some participants received exposure therapy and in addition were required to take a pill containing DCS prior to exposure. Other participants received exposure therapy in combination with a placebo (a pill that contained no DCS). The patients had no knowledge of which pill they took. Several measures indicated a significant benefit to combining DCS with exposure therapy. When retested following the treatment, participants who had taken the DCS pill reported a decrease in discomfort produced by exposure. Their autonomic arousal decreased and they were more willing to expose themselves to heights. These benefits persisted for three months after the treatment.

Extinction Can Erase Fear Memories

The fear circuit of adult animals is designed to preserve the synaptic changes that produce learned fears, even when the CS no longer signals danger. However, this is not the case for the infant rodent. Rick Richardson and

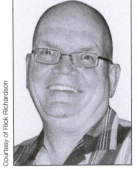

Rick Richardson

his colleagues (Kim and Richardson, 2007a, 2007b) discovered that following extinction training, infant rats (about 17 days old) do not display the major indicators that the original association (CS–US) is preserved—spontaneous recovery, renewal, and reinstatement (see also Carew and Rudy, 1991). These markers emerge when the rodents are about 21 days old, around the time they are weaned. Thus, there is a transition that takes place during the third week after birth when there is a shift from extinction erasing some aspect of the fear memory to extinction producing new learning.

This result could reflect developmental differences in components of the fear extinction circuit. For example, it is likely the hippocampal system, the prefrontal cortex, and the inhibitory circuits that suppress fear are not fully functional. However, there are molecules in the extracellular matrix complex, called **perineuronal nets**, that have been directly linked to the different outcomes produced by extinction. Perineuronal nets surround neurons (especially inhibitory neurons) and have been discovered to be key developmental regulators of plasticity (Frischknecht and Gundelfiger, 2012). Studies of the development of the visual system, for example, indicate that early in development, when these nets are absent, synapses in the visual pathway are more easily modified than later in development when they are present (Pizzorusso et al., 2002).

Nadine Gogolla and her colleagues (Gogolla et al., 2009) have linked the development of these nets to the shift from when extinction training erases the fear memory to when it produces new learning (Figure 20.10). These nets are not present during the period early in development when extinction training erases the fear memory but are present later in development when extinction produces new learning.

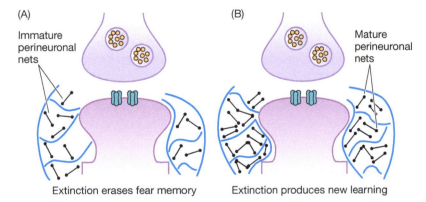

FIGURE 20.10   (A) Early in development, perineuronal nets that surround spines are immature. During this period extinction training can erase the fear memory. (B) When these nets are mature, extinction training does not erase the fear memory and extinction is due to new learning. However, by degrading these nets the infant state can be reinstated and extinction training can again erase the fear memory.

Based on these observations, Gogolla and her colleagues hypothesized that by degrading the nets the processes supporting extinction could be returned to the early infant state when extinction erases the fear memory. Consistent with their hypothesis, injecting an enzyme that degrades the perineuronal net into the BLA *prior to fear conditioning* produced this result in adult rodents— following extinction training they did not display spontaneous recovery or renewal. However, injecting the enzyme *after conditioning* did produce this result—these rodents displayed both spontaneous recovery and renewal. These results indicate that perineuronal nets support processes that protect the synapses strengthened by fear conditioning from erasure.

Defensive Circuits and the Concept of Fear

This chapter has discussed the neural circuits that support conditioned defensive behaviors such as the freezing response. The chapter is organized around the premise that there is a fear center in the amygdala that orchestrates the expression of the defensive behavioral and physiological adjustments that occur in response to threats. An implicit but not a necessary implication of this view is that this defensive circuit is also responsible for the subjective *conscious feelings of fear* that we experience in response to an imminent threat. Joseph LeDoux and Daniel Pine (LeDoux and Pine, 2016) have argued strongly *against this view*. They propose that the neural circuits for defensive behaviors, which reside in the amygdala–subcortical regions of the brain, *are not responsible for the experience of fear* as a subjective state. Instead, the subjective conscious experience of fear is the product of circuits located in higher-order associative cortical regions that may involve the prefrontal, parietal, and insular cortex. In effect they propose that a two-systems framework is needed to understand fear: a subcortical system that is responsible for defensive behaviors and a neocortical system that generates the subjective feeling of fear.

Note that this view cannot be evaluated in nonverbal animals because they cannot report on their subjective feelings. In support of their position, LeDoux and Pine note that patients with amygdala damage can still feel fearful and that subliminal threats can trigger peripheral physiological responses even when the subject is unaware of the stimulus and lacks feelings of fear.

Summary

Our evolutionary history has provided us with neural systems designed to support behaviors that are organized to meet our most fundamental survival needs. These behavioral systems are finely tuned by our experiences. This chapter focuses specifically on the fear system that supports defensive behaviors designed to allow us to anticipate danger and keep out of harm's way.

Animals continuously assess their environments for potential dangers. A set of species-specific defensive behaviors can be called out when danger lurks.

Midbrain regions (lateral hypothalamus and periaqueductal gray) provide the proximal support for defensive behaviors. However, they are under the control of neurons in the basolateral and central amygdala separated by intercalated inhibitory neurons. Inputs from the thalamus, neocortex, prelimbic prefrontal cortex, and hippocampus converge onto neurons in the BLA to provide the various levels of detailed information about the environment that is present at the time an aversive event takes place. An aversive experience modifies the strength of these synaptic connections to fear neurons in the basal nucleus and neurons in the prelimbic region so that when elements of this experience are re-encountered they will drive the central amygdala to produce defensive behaviors.

The fear system generally produces adaptive behavior, but intensely aversive experiences can lead to excessive fears that become pathological and debilitating. One way to eliminate learned fears is to use Pavlovian procedures designed to produce extinction. Exposure to just the CS can greatly weaken its capacity to evoke fear. However, in adults extinction is the product of new learning (called a CS–noUS association) that links CS input to extinction neurons and to neurons in the infralimbic cortex. Extinction neurons in the basal nucleus and infralimbic prefrontal cortex neurons project to the ITCs, which can suppress the activity of neurons in the central amygdala. This system allows animals to learn to switch between fear and no fear states and thus to adapt rapidly to changes in their environment (Sotres-Bayon and Quirk, 2010).

Extinction training does not normally erase the fear memory. However, developmental research has identified components of the extracellular matrix—perineuronal nets—that prevent extinction training from erasing fear memories. These nets are absent during infancy stage when extinction training erases fear and they emerge at the stage when extinction produces new learning. Degrading the nets returns the adult animal to the infant stage.

Historically, the subcortical neural circuit described in this chapter has been thought to be the source of our subjective feeling of fear. This view has been strongly challenged, and the idea has been proposed that two neural systems—one cortical, the other noncortical—are needed to understand fear.

References

Blanchard, D. C. and Blanchard, R. J. (1989). Experimental animal models of aggression: what do they say about human behaviour? In J. Archer and K. Browne (Eds.), *Human Aggression: Naturalistic Approaches* (pp. 94–121). New York: Routledge.

Bolles, R. C. (1970). Species specific defense reactions and avoidance learning. *Psychological Review, 79*, 32–48.

Bouton, M. E. (1994). Context, ambiguity, and classical conditioning. *Current Directions in Psychological Science, 3*, 49–53.

Bouton, M. E. (2002). Context, ambiguity, and unlearning sources of relapse after behavioral extinction. *Biological Psychiatry, 52*, 976–986.

Bouton, M. E. (2017). *Learning and Behavior: A Contemporary Synthesis, 2nd ed.* Sunderland, MA: Sinauer Associates/Oxford University Press.

Bouton, M. E., Westbrook, R. F., Corcoran, K. A., and Maren, S. (2006). Contextual and temporal modulation of extinction: behavioral and biological mechanisms. *Biological Psychiatry, 60,* 352–60.

Burwell, R. D., Bucci, D. J., Sanborn, M. R., and Jutras, M. J. (2004). Perirhinal and postrhinal contributions to remote memory for context. *Journal of Neuroscience, 24,* 11023–11028.

Carew, M. B. and Rudy, J. W. (1991). Multiple functions of context during conditioning: a developmental analysis. *Developmental Psychobiology, 21,* 191–209.

Corcoran, K. A. and Maren, S. (2001). Hippocampal inactivation disrupts contextual retrieval of fear memory after extinction. *Journal of Neuroscience, 2,* 1720–1726.

Davis, M., Ressler, K., Rothbaum, B. O., and Richardson, R. (2006). Effects of d-cycloserine on extinction: translation from preclinical to clinical work. *Biological Psychiatry, 60,* 369–375.

Falls, W. A., Miserendino, M. J. D., and Davis, M. (1992). Extinction of fear-potentiated startle: blockade by infusion of an NMDA antagonist into the amygdala. *Journal of Neuroscience, 12,* 854–863.

Fanselow, M. S. (1991). The midbrain periaqueductal gray as coordinator of action in response to fear and anxiety. In A. Depaulis and R. Bandler (Eds.), *The Midbrain Periacqueductal Gray Matter* (pp. 151–171). New York: Plenum Press.

Frischknecht, R. and Gundelfiger, E. D. (2012). The brain's extracellular matrix and its role in synaptic plasticity. *Advances in Experimental Medicine and Biology, 970,* 153–171.

Gogolla, N., Caroni, P., Luthi, A., and Herry, C. (2009). Perineuronal nets protect fear memories from erasure. *Science, 325,* 1258–1261.

Herry, C., Ciocchi, S., Senn, V., Demmou, L., Muller, C., and Luthi, A. (2008). Switching on and off fear by distinct neuronal circuits. *Nature, 454,* 600–606.

Ji, J. and Maren, S. (2005). Electrolytic lesions of the dorsal hippocampus disrupt renewal of conditional fear after extinction. *Learning and Memory, 12,* 270–276.

Ji, J. and Maren S. (2007). Hippocampal involvement in contextual modulation of fear extinction. *Hippocampus, 17,* 749–758.

Kim, J. H. and Richardson, R. (2007a). A developmental dissociation of context and GABA effects on extinguished fear in rats. *Behavioral Neuroscience, 121,* 131–139.

Kim, J. H. and Richardson, R. (2007b). A developmental dissociation in reinstatement of an extinguished fear response in rats. *Neurobiology of Learning and Memory, 88,* 48–57.

Kim, J. J. and Jung, M. W. (2006). Neural circuits and mechanisms involved in Pavlovian fear conditioning: a critical review. *Neuroscience and Biobehavioral Review, 30,* 188–202.

Ledgerwood, L., Richardson, R., and Cranney, J. (2003). D-cycloserine facilitates extinction of conditioned fear as assessed by freezing in rats. *Behavioral Neuroscience, 117,* 341–349.

LeDoux, J. E. (1994). Emotion, memory and the brain. *Scientific American, 270,* 50–57.

LeDoux, J. (1998). *The Emotional Brain: The Mysterious Underpinnings of Emotional Life* (p. 131). New York: Touchstone.

LeDoux, J. E. and Pine, D. S. (2016). Using neuroscience to help understand fear and anxiety: a two-system framework. *American Journal of Psychiatry, 173,* 1083–1093.

Likhtik, E., Popa, D., Apergis-Schoute, J., Fidacaro, G. A., and Paré, D. (2008). Amygdala intercalated neurons are required for expression of fear extinction. *Nature, 454,* 642–645.

Maren, S. (2011). Seeking a spotless mind: extinction, deconsolidation and erasure of fear memory. *Neuron, 70,* 830–845.

Migues, P. V., Liu, L. Archbold, G. E., Einarsson, E. O., Wong, J. X., Bonasia, K., Ko, S. H., Wang, Y. T., and Hardt, O. (2016). Blocking synaptic removal of GluA2-containing AMPA receptors prevents the natural forgetting of long-term memories. *Journal of Neuroscience, 36,* 3481–3494.

Myers, K. M. and Davis, M. (2007). Mechanisms of fear extinction. *Molecular Psychiatry, 12,* 120–150.

Pape, H. C. and Paré, D. (2010). Plastic synaptic networks of the amygdala for the acquisition, expression, and extinction of conditioned fear. *Physiological Review, 90,* 419–463.

Pizzorusso, T., Medini, P., Berardi, N., Chierzi, S., Fawcett, J. W., and Maffei, L. (2002). Reactivation of ocular dominance plasticity in the adult visual cortex. *Science, 298,* 1248–1251.

Ressler, K. J., Rothbaum, B. O., Tannenbaum, L., Anderson, P., Graap, K., Zimand, E., Hodges, L., and Davis, M. (2004). Cognitive enhancers as adjuncts to psychotherapy: use of d-cycloserine in phobic individuals to facilitate extinction of fear. *Archives of General Psychiatry, 61,* 1136–1144.

Romanski, L. M. and LeDoux, J. E. (1992). Equipotentiality of thalamo-amygdala and thalamo-cortico-amygdala circuits in auditory fear conditioning. *Journal of Neuroscience, 12,* 4501–4509.

Royer, S. and Paré, D. (2002). Bidirectional synaptic plasticity in intercalated amygdala neurons and the extinction of conditioned fear responses. *Neuroscience, 115,* 455–462.

Sotres-Bayon, F., Bush, D. E., and LeDoux, J. E. (2007). Acquisition of fear extinction requires activation of NR2B-containing NMDA receptors in the lateral amygdala. *Neuropsychopharmacology, 32,* 1929–1940.

Sotres-Bayon, F. and Quirk, G. J. (2010) Prefrontal control of fear: more than just extinction. *Current Opinion in Neurobiology, 20,* 231–235.

Timberlake, W. (1994). Behavioral systems, associationism, and Pavlovian conditioning. *Psychonomic Bulletin and Review, 1,* 405–420.

Walker, D. L., Ressler, K. J., Lu, K. T., and Davis, M. (2002). Facilitation of conditioned fear extinction by systemic administration or intra-amygdala infusions of d-cycloserine as assessed with fear-potentiated startle. *Journal of Neuroscience, 22,* 2343–2351.

Glossary

A

actin   A cytoskeleton protein filament that exists in two states: globular actin (G-actin) and filament actin (F-actin).

actin depolymerization factor/cofilin (ADF/cofilin)   A protein that depolymerizes F-actin. Also called cofilin.

action   A category of instrumental behavior believed to be supported by expectancies and thought to be goal directed and purposeful.

action potentials   Electrical signals conducted along axons by which information is conveyed from one neuron to another in the nervous system.

active decay theory   The idea that over time molecular processes actively degrade the synaptic basis of unused memory traces.

active trace theory   A theory that suggests that both the age of a memory trace and its state of activation at the time of a disrupting event are determinants of the vulnerability of the trace to disruption.

adjacent arm task   A version of the radial arm maze in which a rodent is released from one arm and rewarded for choosing to enter one of the two adjacent arms.

adrenal gland   An endocrine gland, located above the kidney, composed of two parts: the adrenal medulla (which secretes epinephrine) and the adrenal cortex (which secretes glucocorticoids).

adrenaline   A hormone secreted by the adrenal gland, often as a result of an arousing stimulus. Also called epinephrine (EPI).

adrenergic receptors   Receptors that bind to adrenergics.

adrenergics   Drugs that mimic the effects of epinephrine.

adrenoreceptors   Receptors that bind to epinephrine.

after images   Briefly lasting sensations; the first of three traces in William James's theory of memory.

agonist   A substance that binds to a specific receptor and triggers a response in the cell. It mimics the action of an endogenous ligand (such as a hormone or neurotransmitter) that binds to the same receptor.

AMPA receptor   An ionotropic glutamate receptor that is selective for Na^+. AMPA receptors are major contributors to whether or not the sending neuron will depolarize the receiving neuron.

AMPA receptor trafficking   The movement of AMPA receptors into and out of the plasma membrane.

ampakines   A class of drugs that may enhance cognitive function. Ampakines cross the blood–brain barrier and bind to a site on the AMPA receptor.

amygdala   A collection of midbrain nuclei, some of which are involved in supporting fear conditioning and in modulating memory storage in other regions of the brain.

annulus crossings   A measure of place learning in the Morris water-escape task based on how many times during the probe trial the animal actually crosses the exact place where the platform was located during training compared to how many times it crosses the equivalent area in the other quadrants.

antagonist   A drug that opposes or inhibits the effects of a particular neurotransmitter on the postsynaptic cell.

anterior cingulate   The frontal part of the cingulate cortex, believed to be involved in modulating memory formation.

anterograde amnesia   The loss of memory for events that occur after a brain insult or experimental treatment.

antisense methodology   A methodology that uses an injection of antisense oligodeoxynucleotides to interfere with the translation of particular proteins.

antisense oligonucleotide   A synthesized strand of nucleic acid that will bind to mRNA and prevent its translation.

Arc   An immediate early gene (activity-regulated, cytoskeleton-associated protein) that is rapidly transcribed in the hippocampus when rats explore novel environments.

associative learning   Learning based on the principle that new information can be acquired by connections between elements.

associative loss hypothesis   A hypothesis that assumes extinction is due to the CS–alone presentation eliminating the original CS–US association.

auditory cortex   A region of the brain that supports learned fear to an auditory stimulus by projecting the stimulus directly to the amygdala.

auditory cue   A type of conditioned stimulus used in fear conditioning, usually a tone.

auditory-cue fear conditioning   A conditioning procedure in which an auditory stimulus (tone) is paired with shock.

autoinhibitory–regulatory domain   A domain of a kinase protein that keeps the kinase in an inactive state.

autophosphorylation   A special property of CaMKII that enables its active subunits to phosphorylate each other.

axon   The long fiber of a neuron that extends from the soma and conducts electrical signals away from the cell body.

B

basal ganglia   A region of the brain composed of a number of subcortical nuclei including the caudate nucleus, putamen, globus pallidus, subthalamic nucleus, nucleus accumbens, and substantia nigra.

basal nucleus (BA)   A nucleus of the amygdala that is thought to be an important part of the neural basis of fear. The BA is a component of the BLA (basolateral amygdala).

basolateral amygdala (BLA)   A region of the amygdala that includes the basal and lateral nuclei. It is critically involved in memory modulation and storing fear memories and plays an important role in attaching value to outcomes.

BDNF (brain-derived neurotrophic factor)   A secreted protein that contributes to the consolidation of LTP and memory.

BDNF → CREB → C/EBPβ → BDNF   A positive autoregulatory loop that contributes to multiple waves of protein synthesis.

BDNF–TrkB receptor pathway   A signaling cascade that activates mTOR and local protein synthesis.

BDNF → TrkB → mTOR   See *BDNF → TrkB → mTOR → TOP*.

BDNF → TrkB → mTOR → TOP   A key signaling cascade that results in the local synthesis of proteins.

behavioral experience   An experience generated by a behaving organism interacting with its environment.

behavioral system   A system that is organized specifically to ensure that some particular need is met. For example, there are behavioral systems designed to support our reproductive and feeding-related activities and behavioral systems that allow us to avoid and escape dangerous situations.

bioenergetics   The flow of energy in cells.

brain-derived neurotrophic factor   See *BDNF*.

C

CA1 A subregion of the hippocampus that receives input from the CA3 region via Schaffer collateral fibers and projects to the entorhinal cortex via the subiculum. It also receives input from the entorhinal cortex.

CA3 A subregion of the hippocampus that receives input from the dentate gyrus via mossy fibers and projects to the CA1 region via Schaffer collateral fibers.

calcineurin A phosphatase activated by calcium and calmodulin.

calcium ion (Ca²⁺) A second messenger that activates other messenger proteins.

calcium-induced calcium release (CICR)
The release of calcium from the endoplasmic reticulum, thought to occur when extracellular calcium enters the dendritic spine through the NMDA receptor and binds to ryanodine receptors.

calmodulin A calcium-binding protein that can regulate a number of protein targets.

calpains Proteins that belong to a class of enzymes called proteases that can degrade proteins.

calpain–spectrin pathway A signaling pathway activated by calcium that degrades spectrin protein and results in disassembling actin networks.

CaMKII (calcium/calmodulin-dependent protein kinase II) A kinase protein that, once activated by calmodulin, is able to phosphorylate other proteins in the cell.

CaMKIINtide A noncompetitive inhibitor of CaMKII that can reverse LTP.

cAMP (cyclic adenosine monophosphate)
A second messenger activated in target cells in response to synaptic or hormonal stimulation.

cannula A small needle used to inject chemical solutions into precise regions of the brain to damage neurons.

cannula guide A hollow metal tube that is inserted permanently into the brain that allows a drug to be readily injected into an awake and moving animal.

catalytic domain A domain of a kinase that performs the phosphorylation reaction.

ceiling effect A measurement problem that occurs when the value of the performance measure approaches its highest possible level and thus cannot be further increased by some other treatment.

cell adhesion molecules Proteins located on the cell surface that can bind with other cells or with the extracellular matrix. They help cells stick together.

cell assembly Donald Hebb's idea that a population of modifiable interconnected neurons can support memory.

cell theory The accepted view that the fundamental element in the structure of living bodies is a cell.

cellular consolidation The biochemical and molecular processes that take place immediately following the behavioral experience and initially stabilize the memory trace. This type of consolidation is thought to take several hours to complete.

central nucleus (CE) A nucleus of the amygdala that is thought to be an important part of the neural basis of fear.

cerebral spinal fluid Fluid that flows in and around the hollow spaces of the brain and spinal cord; it protects the brain and spinal cord from trauma, supplies nutrients to nervous system tissue, and removes waste products.

chromosome The part of the nucleus that contains the genetic material DNA (deoxyribonucleic acid).

classical conditioning The methodology invented by Ivan Pavlov to study learning and memory.

clenbuterol An adrenergic receptor agonist.

clustered plasticity model The idea that LTP likely results from modifying synapses that are in close spatial proximity.

cofilin See *actin-depolymerization factor/cofilin*; also called ADF/cofilin.

cofilin pathway A signaling pathway that regulates actin polymerization.

cognitive expectancy theory A theory proposed by Edward C. Tolman that assumes that learning produces representations of behaviors and their resulting outcomes.

competing memory hypothesis   A hypothesis that assumes extinction produces a new association called a CS–noUS association, while the original CS–US association that produced the CR remains intact.

competitive trace theory   A theory that proposes that as memories age interactions between the hippocampus and neocortex degrade the validity of episodic memories.

complementary memory systems view
This view assumes that different learning systems evolved to serve different and sometimes incompatible functions.

conditional knockout methodology   A genetic engineering method used to knock out a particular gene in a very well specified region of the brain and to do this at different times in development.

conscious recollection   The intentional initiation of a memory with an awareness of remembering; a subjective feeling that is a product of the retrieval process.

consolidation   A stage of memory formation in which information in short-term memory is transferred to long-term memory.

constitutive trafficking   The routine movement of AMPA receptors in and out of dendritic spines.

context CS   The static features of an environment that define the place in which conditioning occurs.

context preexposure paradigm   A procedure used to study how rodents acquire a memory of an explored context.

context preexposure facilitation effect
The enhancement of contextual fear by exposure to the conditioning context prior to immediate shock.

contextual fear conditioning   Fear that is produced to the context or place in which the shock US is presented.

cortical pathway   A pathway that carries information from the sensory thalamus to the neocortical regions of the brain where a richer, more detailed representation of the experience is constructed.

cortico-striatal system   A brain system composed of the striatum and its afferent and efferent connections.

corticosterone   An adrenal hormone that can modulate memory storage, also classified as a glucocorticoid because it is involved in the metabolism of glucose.

CREB (cAMP-responsive, element-binding) protein   A transcription factor that is implicated in both synaptic plasticity and behavioral memory; a kind of molecular memory switch that in the *on* state initiates the production of memory-making messenger ribonucleic acid (mRNA).

CS–noUS association   A new association generated when the CS (conditioned stimulus) is no longer presented with the US (unconditioned stimulus). This idea forms the basis of the competing memory theory in extinction studies.

cue-dependent amnesia   Amnesia that results when a retrieved memory is followed by a disruptive event such as electroconvulsive shock.

cyclic adenosine monophosphate   See *cAMP*.

cytoskeleton protein filaments   Proteins that form the internal scaffolding that gives a cell its shape, consisting of actin, microtubules, and intermediate filaments.

cytosol   The internal fluid of the neuron.

d-cycloserine (DCS)   A drug that is a partial agonist that binds to the glycine site of the NMDA receptor to enhance its opening.

debriefing   A brief crisis intervention usually administered within days of a traumatic event in which the trauma-exposed individual is encouraged to talk about his or her feelings and reactions to the event.

declarative memory   A category of memory that includes both episodic and semantic memory.

delayed nonmatching to sample (DNMS)
A memory testing procedure used to study recognition memory in primates.

dendrites   Branched projections of a neuron that receive synaptic input from the presynaptic terminal.

dendritic spines   Small protrusions from dendrites that connect with presynaptic axons. They are important in neural transmission and can be modified in response to glutamate release.

de novo **protein synthesis (DNPS) hypothesis** The hypothesis that the consolidation of the memory trace requires that the to-be-remembered experience initiate the synthesis of new proteins.

dentate gyrus   A subregion of the hippocampus that receives input from the entorhinal cortex via the perforant path and projects via mossy fibers to the CA3 region.

depolarization   The displacement of a cell's membrane potential toward a less negative value.

destabilization function   The idea that when an existing engram or memory trace is activated, underlying synapses become unbound or weaken and this allows new information to be incorporated into the engram.

dexamethasone   A synthetic glucocorticoid.

discrimination reversal learning   A strategy used to assess the flexibility of the system supporting the instrumental response and thus to determine if it is an action or a habit.

dopamine   A neurotransmitter, related to norepinephrine and epinephrine, that belongs to a group called catecholamines.

dopamine incentive salience hypothesis The theory that the activation of the mesolimbic dopamine system by a rewarding outcome attaches motivational significance to stimuli associated with that outcome.

dopamine reinforcement hypothesis   The theory that the neurotransmitter dopamine is the primary candidate for strengthening the property of outcomes that influence instrumental behavior.

dorsolateral striatum (DLS)   A region of the striatum that is critical to the acquisition and maintenance of habits.

dorsomedial striatum (DMS)   A region of the striatum that supports goal-directed actions.

DREADD   An acronym for *d*esigner *r*eceptors *e*xclusively *a*ctivated by *d*esigner *d*rugs. A viral vector system delivers these receptors into the brain region of interest; once expressed these receptors can be activated by a synthesized drug, clozapine-N-oxide.

E

ecphory   A term introduced by Richard Semon to represent how retrieval cues interact with the engram to produce the experience of a memory.

electroconvulsive shock (ECS)   A treatment for psychiatric disorders in which seizures are induced with electricity for therapeutic effect, also known as electroconvulsive therapy (ECT).

electrode   A fine wire used to deliver electric current to the brain.

encoding specificity principle   The idea that memories are best retrieved when environmental stimulation (internal state as well as the external environment) at the time of retrieval matches the conditions present at the time the memory was established.

endocytosis   An active process by which substances (such as cell surface AMPA receptors) are internalized by being engulfed by the cell membrane.

endocytotic zone   A region that contains complex molecules designed to capture proteins such as AMPA receptors leaving the PSD and to repackage them in endosomes for recycling to the membrane.

endoplasmic reticulum (ER)   An organelle that is part of the endomembrane system and one of the elements of translation machinery. The ER extends continuously throughout the neuron and works together with the plasma membrane to regulate many neural processes. It is also a calcium store and can release calcium when ligands bind to receptors located on its surface.

endosomes   Membrane systems involved in transport within the cell, they receive endocytosed cell membrane molecules and sort them for either degradation or recycling back into the cell membrane.

engram   A sustained neural representation of a behavioral experience; another name for the memory trace.

engram cells   Neurons belonging to the collection of cells that were active at the time the memory was established and can be reactivated when the memory is retrieved.

entorhinal cortex   An area of the brain located in the medial temporal lobe that is a major interface between the hippocampus and other regions of the neocortex.

enzyme   A protein that accelerates the rate of chemical reactions.

epinephrine   A hormone produced by the adrenal gland that modulates memory storage, also called adrenaline.

episodic memory system   The memory system that extracts and stores the content of personal experiences.

EPSP   See *excitatory postsynaptic potential (EPSP)*.

ERK (extracellular-regulated kinase)   A kinase that participates in many aspects of synaptic plasticity. See *ERK–MAPK*.

ERK–MAPK   One of several possible signaling pathways or cascades, initiated by neurotrophic factors, that can converge to phosphorylate CREB protein and induce the transcription of plasticity-related mRNAs.

escape latency   The time between when a training trial starts and when the subject completes the trial.

excitatory postsynaptic potential (EPSP)   Depolarization of the postsynaptic membrane potential by the action of a synaptically released neurotransmitter.

excitatory synapses   Synapses that typically contain receptors that respond to glutamate and contribute to the depolarization of the neuron by allowing sodium ions to enter the neuron.

exocytosis   The process by which AMPA receptors are inserted into the plasma membrane.

expectancy   A three-term association (S1–R–S2) that includes a representation of the stimulus situation (S1) that preceded the response, a representation of the response (R), and a representation of the outcome (S2) produced by the response.

exposure therapy   A therapy in which patients are forced to experience the stimulus situation that induces their fear response, used to treat a number of fear–anxiety disorders.

extinction   In a Pavlovian experiment, the elimination of a conditioned response (CR), achieved by presenting the conditioned stimulus (CS) without the unconditioned stimulus (US).

extracellular matrix (ECM)   A matrix, composed of molecules synthesized and secreted by neurons and glial cells, that forms a bridge between the pre and postsyanaptic neurons. The molecules it contains interact with the neurons to influence their function.

extrahippocampal system   A collection of cortical areas that can support fear conditioning independent of the hippocampus.

F

F-actin (filament actin)   A two-stranded helical polymer composed of globular actin.

false memory   When what is remembered is different from what actually happened or when what is remembered never happened.

familiarity   A process that can support recognition memory without recollection of the time or place of the experience.

fear conditioning   A form of learning in which fear comes to be associated with a previously neutral stimulus.

fEPSP   See *field potential*.

fiber volley   A measure of action potentials arriving at dendrites in the region of the recording site of an LTP (long-term potentiation) experiment.

field potential   A measurement of the change in the ion composition of extracellular fluid as positive ions flow away from the extracellular recording and into the surrounding neurons. Also called fEPSP or field EPSP, it is the dependent variable in a long-term potentiation (LTP) experiment.

first messenger   A molecule that carries information from one neuron to another neuron.

floor effect   A measurement problem that occurs when the value of the performance measure is so low that it cannot be further reduced by some other treatment.

freezing   An innate defensive response of rodents in which they become immobile or still, a behavior that has survival advantages because a moving animal is more likely to be detected by a predator than a still one.

functional end points   End points of the biochemical processes initiated by the second messenger Ca^{2+} that can strengthen synaptic connections.

G

G proteins (guanine nucleotide binding proteins)   Second messenger proteins in the plasma membrane that are activated by glutamate binding to metabotropic glutamate receptors.

G-actin (globular actin)   Subunits of actin that serve as monomer building blocks that assemble into F-actin.

genetic engineering   A collection of methods used by scientists to alter the DNA of living organisms and thereby alter specific genes.

genomic signaling   Processes initiated by synaptic activity that lead to the production of new proteins through transcription and translation.

glucocorticoids   A class of hormones involved in the metabolism of glucose. In contrast to adrenaline, glucocorticoids can directly enter the brain.

glutamate   An excitatory amino acid neurotransmitter that is the primary neurotransmitter in the induction of long-term potentiation.

green fluorescent protein (GFP)   A protein derived from jellyfish that exhibits green fluorescence when exposed to light.

GTPases   Small proteins that regulate other biochemical processes. Most prominent among the regulatory GTPases are the G proteins (Guanosine-5′-triphosphate).

H

habit   A category of instrumental behavior believed to be the product of strengthening S–R connections and believed not to be goal directed or purposeful.

habituation   The idea that the magnitude of the response to an eliciting stimulus decreases with repeated stimulation.

high-frequency stimulus (HFS)   Another name for the inducing stimulus in an LTP experiment.

hippocampal formation   A region of the brain composed of the dentate gyrus (a subregion of the hippocampus), the hippocampus proper (CA1 and CA3 fields), and the subiculum.

hippocampus   A region of the brain composed of the hippocampus proper (CA1 and CA3 fields) and the dentate gyrus subregion. The hippocampus is believed to make a critical contribution to episodic memory.

hyperpolarization   The displacement of a cell's membrane potential toward a more negative value.

I

immediate early gene (IEG)   A gene that is rapidly activated at the transcription level before any new proteins are synthesized.

immediate shock effect   The display of no fear to a context after rodents have been shocked without being allowed to first explore that context.

indexing theory   A theory that assumes that the hippocampus stores an index to cortical patterns of neural activity that were generated by an episode.

inducing stimulus   The low-intensity, high-frequency stimulus used to induce long-term potentiation (LTP).

infralimbic prefrontal cortex   A cortical region that is believed to suppress the action system and thus to play an important role in selecting which system—the action or habit system—controls instrumental behavior.

inhibitory avoidance conditioning   A behavioral methodology used to train rodents to avoid where they previously experienced an aversive event.

inhibitory domain   A domain of a kinase protein that keeps the kinase in an inactive state.

instrumental behavior   Behavior that can change or modify the environment. Instrumental behaviors/responses can be modified by the consequences they produce.

instrumental learning   Learning that a reward or reinforcer is contingent on the occurrence of a particular behavior.

integration theory   The idea that when an engram is activated the information it contains can be integrated with new information contained in the present environment.

integrative function   The incorporation of new information into a retrieved memory trace.

integrins (integrin receptors)   Receptors that respond to molecules in the extracellular space or matrix and to intercellular signals such as calcium. They are classified as cell adhesion molecules.

intercalated cells   Clusters of cells in the amygdala that produce inhibitory output that, when fed forward to the central nucleus of the amygdala, can reduce the output of the neurons that generate defensive behavior.

interference theory of forgetting   A theory that attributes forgetting to additional experiences overwriting or producing new memories that interfere with the retrieval of a preexisting memory.

intertrial interval   The time between conditioning trials.

inverse tag   An outcome that occurs when Arc and CaMKIIβ interact in dendritic spines to reduce their potentiation and prevent depotentiation in nearby spines.

in vitro preparation   A method of performing an experiment in a controlled environment outside of a living organism. For example, a slice of hippocampus tissue is often used to conduct long-term potentiation (LTP) experiments.

ion   An atom or a group of atoms that has acquired a net electric charge by gaining or losing one or more electrons.

ion-gated channel   A specific ion channel that opens and closes to allow the cell to alter its membrane potential.

ionotropic receptors   Receptors comprised of several subunits that come together in the cell membrane to form a potential channel or pore which, when open, allows ions such as Na^+ or Ca^{2+} to enter. Also called ion-gated channels or ligand-gated ion channels.

IP3 (inositol 1,4,5-triphosphate)   A second messenger that is synthesized when glutamate binds to the metabotropic glutamate receptor 1 (mGluR1).

IP3R (inositol 1,4,5-triphosphate receptor)   A receptor that binds to the second messenger IP3, located on the endoplasmic reticulum in the dendritic compartment near the spines.

K

kinase   An enzyme that, once activated, catalyzes the transfer of a phosphate group from a donor to an acceptor.

L

lateral hypothalamus   A region of the brain responsible for changes in the autonomic responses (heart rate and blood pressure, for example) produced by the sympathetic nervous system that prepare an animal for action.

lateral nucleus (LA)   A nucleus of the amygdala that is thought to be an important part of the neural basis of fear. The LA is a component of the BLA (basolateral nucleus of the amygdala).

learning–performance distinction   A principle that recognizes that performance is influenced by a number of processes in addition to learning and memory processes.

ligand   Any chemical compound that binds to a specific site on a receptor.

LIMK   A kinase that phosphorylates the actin-depolymerization factor/cofilin site.

local protein synthesis   The translation of existing mRNA into protein that occurs in the dendrites.

locus coeruleus (LC)   A small region of the brain that contains only about 3,000 neurons, yet projects broadly and provides nearly all the norepinephrine to the cortex, limbic system, thalamus, and hypothalamus.

long-lasting LTP (L-LTP)   An enduring form of long-term potentiation thought to require the synthesis of new proteins.

long-term depression (LTD)   A reduction in LTP produced by long-lasting, low-frequency stimulation.

long-term habituation   A long-lasting form of habituation that is produced by many sessions of repeated stimulation.

long-term memory (LTM) trace   A relatively enduring memory trace that is resistant to disruption.

long-term potentiation (LTP)   A persistent strengthening of synapses produced by low-frequency, intense electrical stimulation.

M

MAPK (mitogen-activated protein kinase)
A kinase that participates in many aspects of synaptic plasticity. See *ERK–MAPK*.

medial temporal hippocampal (MTH) system
The region of the brain composed of the perirhinal, parahippocampal, and entorhinal cortices and the hippocampal formation, which is composed of the hippocampus proper (CA1 and CA3 regions), subiculum, and dentate gyrus.

membrane potential   The difference in the electrical charge inside the neuron's cell body compared to the charge outside the cell body.

memory consolidation   A process that stabilizes the memory and renders it resistant to disruption.

memory modulation framework   A theory that assumes that experience activates both the neurons that store the memory and other modulating neural–hormonal events that can influence the neurons that store the memory.

memory modulators   The hormonal and other neural systems that are not part of the storage system but can nonetheless influence the synapses that store the memory.

memory proper   See *secondary memory*.

memory trace   A sustained neural representation of a behavioral experience, also called an engram.

mesolimbic dopamine system   A small number of neurons located in a region of the brain called the ventral tegmental area (VTA) that provide dopamine to other regions of the brain.

messenger   A molecule that conveys information from a sending neuron to a receiving neuron.

messenger ribonucleic acid (mRNA)   A molecule of RNA that carries a chemical blueprint for a protein product.

metabotropic receptor   A G-protein receptor that stimulates or inhibits intracellular biochemical reactions. In contrast to ionotropic receptors, metabotropic receptors do not form an ion channel pore; rather, they are indirectly linked with ion channels on the plasma membrane of the cell through signal transduction mechanisms.

mGluR1 (metabotropic glutamate receptor 1)
A subtype of metabotropic receptor located in the plasma membrane near dendritic spines.

midbrain subcortical nuclei   Nuclei in the midbrain region that provide the direct neural basis for specific defensive behaviors that make up the fear system.

modular view   The theory that only episodic memory depends on the entire medial temporal hippocampal system and that semantic memory does not require the hippocampus to contribute.

mossy fibers   Axons that connect the dentate gyrus to the CA3 region of the hippocampus.

mRNA   See *messenger ribonucleic acid*.

MTH system   See *medial temporal hippocampal (MTH) system*.

mTOR (mammalian target of rapamycin complex)   This protein complex regulates many intracellular processes including local protein synthesis.

mTOR–TOP pathway   A signaling pathway activated by BDNF that results in the local translation of proteins.

multiple memory systems   A theory that different kinds of information are acquired and stored in different parts of the brain.

multiple trace theory   A theory of systems consolidation that assumes that the medial temporal hippocampal system is always required to retrieve episodic memories but that semantic memories can become independent of this system.

myosin IIb   A motor protein that can shear filament actin into segments.

N

neural cadherins (N-cadherins)   Calcium-dependent cell adhesion molecules; strands of proteins held together by Ca^{2+} ions. Cadherins can exist as either monomers or *cis*-stranded dimers.

neurobiology of learning and memory
An important scientific field that seeks to

understand how the brain stores and retrieves information about our experiences.

neuron doctrine The idea that the brain is made up of discrete cells, called neurons or nerve cells, that are the elemental signal units of the brain.

neurotransmitter A substance released by synaptic terminals for the purpose of transmitting information from one neuron to another.

neurotrophic factors Molecules that promote survival of neural tissues and play a critical role in neural development and differentiation. These factors bind to Trk receptors.

NMDA receptor An ionotropic glutamate receptor selective for the agonist NMDA that plays a critical role in the induction of long-term potentiation (LTP).

nonreward A term used to represent an outcome produced by an instrumental behavior that decreases the strength of that behavior.

nonsense syllables Meaningless non-words created by placing a vowel between two consonants, for example, *nuh, vag,* or *boc.*

norepinephrine An adrenergic neurotransmitter.

NSF An abbreviation for N-thylmaleimide-sensitive factor, NSF is a trafficking protein that regulates the release of GluA2 AMPA receptors for insertion into the synapse.

NTS See *solitary tract nucleus.*

nucleus accumbens A collection of neurons within the striatum that contribute to learning instrumental behaviors and may also modulate memory formation.

O

object-in-context task A task used to determine if an animal remembers where it experienced a particular object.

object-place-location task A task used to determine if an animal remembers where an object was located.

object-recognition task A task used to determine if an animal remembers a particular object.

opsins Genes that code for proteins that in response to light can regulate the flow of ions across the membrane.

optogenetics A methodology that combines genetic engineering with optics, the branch of physics that studies the properties of light, to provide a way to control the activity of individual neurons.

P

path length A measure of place learning in the Morris water-escape task; the distance the rodent swims before finding the hidden platform.

pattern completion A process assumed to be supported by the hippocampus by which a subset or portion of an experience that originally established the memory trace can activate or replay the entire experience.

pattern separation A process assumed to be supported by the hippocampus that enables very similar experiences to be segregated in memory.

perforant path Fibers that connect the entorhinal cortex to the dentate gyrus.

periaqueductal gray A midbrain region responsible for producing freezing and analgesia (loss of sensation of pain) responses to fear in rodents.

perineuronal nets Molecules in the extracellular matrix complex that surround neurons. These molecules prevent the erasure of fear memories by extinction.

perirhinal cortex A cortical region adjacent to the hippocampus that is critically involved in object-recognition memory.

phosphatases A class of enzymes whose function is to dephosphorylate proteins.

phosphorylation The chemical addition of a phosphate group (phosphate and oxygen) to a protein or another compound that causes it to become active.

PKA (protein kinase A) A kinase that is activated by the second messenger, cyclic adenosine monophosphate protein (cAMP), that participates in the process of exocytosis.

PKC (protein kinase C) A kinase activated by calcium that participates in the process of exocytosis.

PKMζ (protein kinase Mζ)   A kinase that lacks an inhibitory domain and is thought to play a critical role in the maintenance of LTP and memory.

place-learning task   A version of the Morris water-escape task in which the rat is required to find a platform hidden below the surface of the water, also called the hidden-platform task.

plasticity   The property of the brain that allows it to be modified by experience.

plasticity products (PPs)   Another name for mRNAs and proteins that are thought to be critical to the production of long-lasting changes in synaptic strength.

polymer   A chemical compound that is made of small molecules that are arranged in a simple repeating structure to form a larger molecule.

polymerization   The process of combining many smaller molecules (monomers) into a large organic module called a polymer.

polyubiquitin chain   A chain of ubiquitin molecules that tag a protein for degradation.

postsynaptic dendrite   The component of the neuron specialized for transmitter reception.

postsynaptic density (PSD)   A region at the tip of the dendritic spine that is the site of neurotransmitter receptors.

postsynaptic depolarization   The flow of positive ions into the postsynaptic neuron.

postsynaptic potential   A brief electrical event that is generated in the postsynaptic neuron when the synapse is activated.

post-translation processes   Processes that chemically modify proteins after their translation.

post-traumatic stress disorder (PTSD)   A syndrome in which individuals with this diagnosis have unusually vivid recall of the traumatic events they experienced, accompanied by severe emotional responses.

predatory imminence gradient   A measure of fear response in rodents that is dependent on the distance of a predator, that is, when a potential predator is at a distance the rat will freeze, but when the predator moves within striking distance, the rat might attempt to flee.

prediction error hypothesis   The idea that synapses become destabilized when the retrieved information does not match the actual outcome.

prelimbic prefrontal cortex   A region of the medial prefrontal cortex believed to be needed to acquire an action. However, once the associations that support an action are learned, this region is believed to no longer be critical.

presynaptic terminal   The component of the neuron that is specialized to release the transmitter.

primary memory   The persisting representation of an experience that forms part of a stream of consciousness; the second of three traces in William James's theory of memory.

probe trial   The stage in the Morris water-escape task in which the platform is removed to assess the rodent's memory of the platform location.

procedural memory   A category of memory that supports the performance of actions and skills.

proteases   A class of enzymes that can degrade proteins.

proteasome   A protein complex that contains proteases and degrades proteins tagged with ubiquitin.

protein synthesis   The assembly of protein molecules from messenger ribonucleic acid (mRNA), also called translation.

Q

quadrant search time   A measure of place learning in the Morris water-escape task. A rodent that has stored a memory of the location of the platform will spend more of its search time in the training quadrant than it will in the other quadrants.

R

Rac1   A small GTPase that contributes to actin regulation.

Rac-PAK cascade   A signaling cascade that contributes to the reorganization and crosslinking of actin filaments.

radial arm maze   An apparatus with eight arms radiating from a central platform designed to study spatial memory and working memory in animals.

reactivation treatment   Similar to the idea of a retrieval test in which cues are presented for the purpose of retrieving or activating an existing engram or memory trace.

receptor   A protein located on the surface of or within cells that is responsible for binding to an active ligand.

recognition memory   Memory that supports the ability to identify previously experienced objects.

recognition memory tasks   A category of tasks that are used to access recognition memory, including object recognition, object place location, and object in context.

recollection   A retrieval process that produces information about the time and place of an experience.

reconsolidation theory   A theory that assumes that the retrieval of a memory itself can disrupt an established memory trace but that the retrieval also initiates another round of protein synthesis so that the trace is "reconsolidated."

reference memory   Memory for the arms of the radial maze that either consistently contained the reward or never contained the reward.

reinforcer or reward   Terms used interchangeably to represent an outcome produced by an instrumental behavior that increases the strength of that behavior.

reinstatement   One of several ways to recover an extinguished conditioned response (CR), in which simply re-presenting the unconditioned stimulus (US) in the training context can reinstate the ability of the conditioned stimulus (CS) to evoke the CR.

renewal effect   One of several ways to recover an extinguished conditioned response (CR), achieved by changing the context for extinction but later returning the animal to the training context to recover the CR.

resting membrane potential   The membrane potential or membrane voltage (about −70 mV) maintained by a neuron when it is not generating action potentials.

retention interval   The time between the training experience that establishes the memory and the test used to retrieve the memory.

reticulum theory   A theory popularized by Camillo Golgi that the brain is one continuous network.

retrieval failure   Amnesia that is the result of an inability to retrieve an existing memory.

retrograde amnesia   The loss of memory for events that occurred prior to a brain insult or experimental treatment.

reward   Also called a reinforcer. Terms used interchangeably to represent an outcome produced by an instrumental behavior that increases the strength of that behavior.

reward devaluation   A method used to determine if an instrumental behavior is an action or a habit.

Rho–ROCK cascade   A signaling cascade that leads to the phosphorylation of cofilin and actin polymerization.

ribosomes   Dense globular structures that take raw material in the form of amino acids and manufacture proteins using the blueprint provided by the mRNA.

rictor (rapamycin-insensitive companion of TOR)   A component of the mTOR complex.

RNA-binding protein (RNA-BP)   A protein that binds to double or single-stranded RNA.

RU 28362   A drug that is a glucocorticoid receptor agonist.

ryanodine receptor (RyR)   A calcium-binding receptor located on the endoplasmic reticulum that extends into dendritc spines.

S

Schaffer collateral fibers   Fibers that connect CA3 to CA1 pyramidal cells in the hippocampus.

second messenger   A molecule that relays the signal received by receptors located in the plasma membrane (such as NMDA and AMPA receptors) to target molecules in the cells.

secondary memory   The record of experiences that have receded from the stream of consciousness but can be later retrieved or recollected; the third of three traces in William James's theory of memory, also called memory proper.

secondary treatment   A method used to decrease the likelihood that the person who experienced a trauma will develop post-traumatic stress disorder.

semantic memory   A category of memory that is believed to support memory for facts and the ability to extract generalizations across experiences.

sensitization   An enhanced reflex response to a reflex-producing stimulus.

separatist view   The theory that only episodic memory depends on the entire medial temporal hippocampal system and that semantic memory does not require a contribution of the hippocampus.

short-lasting LTP (S-LTP)   Long-term potentiation with a limited duration, supported by post-translation processes.

short-term habituation   A form of habituation that does not endure.

short-term memory (STM) trace   A relatively short-lasting trace that is vulnerable to disruption.

signaling cascade   A series of biochemical reactions initiated by a first messenger and transduced into the cell through second messengers and kinases.

silent synapse   A synapse with no AMPA receptors.

simple system approach   A strategy used to reduce the complexity of studying the neural basis of memory by studying an animal with the simplest nervous system that can support a modifiable behavior.

slingshot   A phosphatase that reverses phosphorylated cofilin.

social-recognition memory   Memory for a previously encountered individual.

social transmission of a food preference   A method for studying how rodents acquire food preferences from other rodents.

solitary tract nucleus (NTS)   A brain stem region that receives information from the vagal nerve, also referred to as the NTS (derived from the latin *nucleus tractus solitarius*).

soma-to-nucleus signaling   A genomic signaling process that occurs when Ca^{2+} enters the soma through voltage-dependent calcium channels opening as a result of action potentials.

spatial learning   Learning that requires the animal to use the spatial position of cues to locate a goal object.

spectrin   An actin-binding protein that crosslinks and stabilizes actin filaments.

spontaneous recovery   The recovery of an habituated response that occurs "spontaneously" with the passage of time.

standard model of systems consolidation   A theory that assumes that as episodic and semantic memories age they no longer require the medial temporal hippocampal (MTH) system for retrieval.

stargazin   A transmembrane AMPA receptor regulatory protein that participates in the anchoring of the receptor in the post synaptic density.

state-dependent learning   The idea that internal cues present at the time of learning become associated with the target memory and can contribute to memory retrieval.

stereotaxic surgery   A surgery that uses a coordinate system to locate specific targets inside the brain to enable some procedure to be carried out on them (for example, a lesion, injection, or cannula implantation).

storage failure   Amnesia that is the result of a failure to store the memory.

striatum   A subregion of the basal ganglia, composed of the caudate nucleus, putamen, and nucleus accumbens; the basic input segment of the basal ganglia.

subcortical pathway   A pathway that carries information from the sensory thalamus to the lateral nucleus of the amygdala (LA). It is thought to carry a somewhat impoverished representation of the sensory experience.

subiculum   The output component of the hippocampal formation.

synapse   The point of contact between the presynaptic sending neuron and the post-synaptic receiving neuron.

synapse-to-nucleus signaling   A genomic signaling process that begins at the synapse and results in transcription.

synaptic-activity-regulated trafficking   Movement of AMPA receptors in and out of the dendritic spines that is regulated by synaptic activity generated when glutamate binds to postsynaptic receptors.

synaptic cleft   The space that separates the presynaptic terminal and the postsynaptic dendrite.

synaptic plasticity hypothesis   The hypothesis that the strength of synaptic connections—the ease with which an action potential in one cell excites (or inhibits) its target cell—is not fixed but is plastic and modifiable.

synaptic strength   A concept used to represent the ease with which a presynaptic neuron can excite the postsynaptic neuron.

synaptic tag   A property of a postsynaptic spine that allows it to capture synaptic proteins or mRNA.

synaptic tag and capture hypothesis   A theory that assumes that an LTP-inducing stimulus changes a dendritic spine so that it can capture plasticity products generated by strongly stimulated synapses. It does this through biologically marking (tagging) a synapse in the spine.

synaptic vesicles   Spherical membrane-bound organelles in presynaptic terminals that store neurotransmitters.

systems consolidation   A theory that assumes that a change in the strength of the memory trace is brought about by interactions between brain regions (the medial temporal hippocampal system and neocortex). Systems consolidation is assumed to take place over a long period of time, after the memory is initially established.

T

tag   A biological marking of a synapse in the dendritic spine that has been stimulated so that it will have the capacity to capture new plasticity products.

TARPs   Transmembrane AMPA regulatory proteins that co-assemble with AMPA receptors and contribute to trapping them in the postsynaptic density.

temporally graded retrograde amnesia   Amnesia that is more pronounced for recently experienced events than for more remotely experienced events.

test stimulus   The stimulus used to establish a baseline in an LTP experiment. It is also the stimulus used to determine that LTP has been established.

TetTag mouse   A transgenic mouse that allows the inducible–stable labeling of active neurons.

theta-burst stimulation (TBS)   A different stimulus protocol for inducing long-term potentiation and the forms of LTP it induces, modeled after an increased rate of pyramidal neuronal firing that occurs when a rodent is exploring a novel environment.

Thr286   A phosphorylation site on the regulatory domain of CaMKII.

TOP (terminal oligopyrimidine tract)   A class of mRNAs located in the dendritic spine that encode for proteins such as ribosomal proteins and elongation factors that are part of the translation machinery.

trace updating   The incorporation of new information into existing memory ensembles.

transcription   The process of converting genetic material from DNA to messenger RNA (mRNA). The resulting mRNA is called a transcript.

transcription factors   Proteins that interact with DNA to produce mRNA.

transcription repressor proteins   Proteins that inhibit transcription.

translation   The process by which mRNA is converted to protein, also called protein synthesis.

translation machinery   The molecules that participate in translating mRNA into protein.

trisynaptic circuit   A neural circuit in the hippocampus consisting of three groups of neurons: (a) *granular cells* in the dentate gyrus, (b) connected by mossy fibers to *CA3 pyramidal cells*, (c) connected by Shaffer collaterals to *CA1 pyramidal cells*.

Trk receptors   A class of plasma membrane receptors in the tyrosine kinase family that bind to neurotrophic factors.

TrkB receptors   A subset of tyrosine kinase receptors that have catalytic properties when activated.

U

ubiquitin   A component of the ubiquitin–proteasome system that targets proteins for degradation. Ubiquitin tags proteins for degradation by proteasome.

ubiquitin proteasome system (UPS)   A system composed of ubiquitin and proteasome molecules that cooperate to degrade proteins.

ubiquitination   A process that creates a ubiquitin chain.

unitary view   The theory that both semantic and episodic memory depend on the entire medial temporal hippocampal (MTH) system.

V

vagus or vagal nerve   Cranial nerve X, arising from the medulla and innervating the viscera of the thoracic and abdominal cavities, that carries information about the body into the brain.

viral vector   A new technique for delivering a gene to a particular region of the brain that involves genetically modifying a virus to carry the gene of interest.

visible-platform task   A version of the Morris water-escape task in which the rat is required to find a platform that is visible above the surface of the water.

voltage-dependent calcium channel (vdCC)   A membrane protein forming a pore that is permeable to calcium gated by depolarization of the membrane.

W

working memory   The memory system that maintains and manipulates information to solve a particular problem or achieve a particular goal.

Z

ZIP (ζ inhibitory peptide)   A peptide that can serve as an inhibitory unit for PKMζ.

Index

Page numbers in *italic* denote entries that are included in a figure.

About The Book

Editor: Jess Fiorillo

Project Editor: Linnea Duley

Copy Editor: Julia Rudy

Production Manager: Joan Gemme

Book and Cover Design: Rick Neilsen

Book Production: Rick Neilsen

Illustration Program: Troutt Visual Services, LLC

Indexer: Grant Hackett

Book and Cover Manufacture: LSC Communications